HUMAN BIRTH
An Evolutionary Perspective

FOUNDATIONS OF HUMAN BEHAVIOR

An Aldine de Gruyter Series of Texts and Monographs

Edited by
Sarah Blaffer Hrdy, *University of California, Davis*
Melvin Konner, *Emory University*
Richard W. Wrangham, *University of Michigan*

HUMAN BIRTH
An Evolutionary Perspective

Wenda R. Trevathan

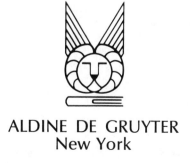

ALDINE DE GRUYTER
New York

ABOUT THE AUTHOR

Wenda R. Trevathan is Assistant Professor of Anthropology, New Mexico
State University. She has been a major contributor to professional journals
and is the coauthor (with A. J. Kelso) of *Physical Anthropology.*

ALDINE DE GRUYTER (Formerly Aldine Publishing Company)
A Division of Walter de Gruyter, Inc.
200 Saw Mill River Road
Hawthorne, New York 10532

Library of Congress Cataloging-in-Publication Data

Trevathan, Wenda.
  Human birth.

  (Foundations of human behavior)
  Bibliography: p.
  Includes index.
  1. Childbirth.   2. Mother and child.   3. Human
behavior.   4. Human evolution.   I. Title.   II. Series.
[DNLM: 1. Ethology.   2. Evolution.   3. Infant, Newborn
4. Labor.   5. Mother-Child Relations.   WQ 300 T812h]
RG652.T73   1987   155.6'463   86-22169
ISBN 0-202-02029-0

Printed in the United States of America
10 9 8 7 6 5 4 3 2 1

CONTENTS

1 EVOLUTIONARY PERSPECTIVES ON HUMAN BIRTH AND BONDING: THE BACKGROUND

2 ISSUES RELATING TO THE CURRENT STUDY: THE BIRTH CENTER, MIDWIVES, MOTHERS, AND METHODS

3 THE PROCESS OF PARTURITION

4 THE NEWBORN INFANT

5 MOTHER–INFANT INTERACTION IMMEDIATELY AFTER BIRTH

6 MOTHER–INFANT BONDING AT BIRTH

7 AN EVOLUTIONARY PERSPECTIVE ON HUMAN BIRTH AND BONDING: CONCLUSIONS

ACKNOWLEDGMENTS

On a Sunday morning, at the American Anthropological Association meetings in San Francisco, I attended a symposium on childbirth, a topic that was only mildly interesting to me at the time. Among the participants were John Kennell, Marshall Klaus, and Lucile Newman, and the ideas that they presented that morning had a dramatic effect on my academic interests from that time on. I mark that morning, in 1976, as the date of conception for this book. There are many I want to thank for providing prenatal care and for serving as midwives during this 10-year gestation.

A number of people were of great help to me during the year I gathered data at The Birth Center in El Paso. I especially thank Shari Daniels, John Major, Kathy Berry, Michele Gerin-Lajoie, and Linda Holland. Thanks to all the midwives: Cheryl, Natalie, Valerie, Abigail, Loretta, Carolyn, Jody, Medra, Ronda, Wendy, Anne, Dev Kirn Kaur, Sharon, Millie, Mary, Liz, Ruth, Janet, Roslyn, Martha, Susan, Dimka, Shelly, Karen, Barbara, and Vickie.

And thank you for sharing your births with me: Maria, Mayra, Alice, Rosa, Leticia, Elsa, Ophelia, Martha, Luz, Soledad, Margarita, Elena, Patricia, Lisa, Estela, Irene, Rufina, Enriquetta, Candelaria, Melody, Gloria, Charlotte, Lolly, Joaquina, Linda, Shareen, Denise, Rosaria, Marta, Elva, Hortensia, Delia, Rita, Christina, Elizabeth, Lola, Yvonne, Yolanda, Alicia, Mary, Dolores, Ramona, Donna, Julie, Claudia, Lydia, Victoria, Guadalupe, Olivia, Carmen, Lourdes, Kathy, Cynthia, Estella, Berta, Ana, Naomi, Virginia, Susan, Socorro, Lorenza, Thomasa, Ellen, Hermelia, Michele, Catalina, Sylvia, Madeline, Graciela, Idalia, Micaela, and Lynn.

Correspondence and conversations with various people during the past year have been especially helpful to me in developing the ideas in this book. Among these are Brigitte Jordan, Jane Lancaster, Jim Chisholm, Jim McKenna, Jack Kelso, Wendy Lawrence, W. John Smith, Gordon Dean, Lynn Johnson-Dean, Scott Rushforth, Steadman Upham, Richard Wrangham, Fred Plog, and many mothers, fathers, and midwives.

Financial support for research was provided by the Department of Anthropology and the Graduate School at the University of Colorado, The University of North Carolina at Charlotte Foundation, and the Arts and Sciences Research

Center at New Mexico State University. Patricia Rosas-Lopatequi helped with the transcriptions of the Spanish tapes. Many thanks go to Holly Reynolds and her Interlibrary Loan staff at the NMSU library. The cover design was modified from a rock art drawing by John Davis.

A number of people have read and commented on parts or all of the manuscript. For that and much more, I thank Arch McCallum, Janet Levy, Dawne Bost, Helen Fisher, Earl Trevathan, and Viviane Renard. As anyone who has ever experienced childbirth knows, more important than all the vitamins, good food, and exercise, is love and emotional support. For that I thank Clint Burleson.

INTRODUCTION

The story of human evolution has been told hundreds of times, each time with a focus that seems most informative to the teller. The "hunting hypothesis" is attractive to some, the "sex contract" to others. And on it goes as various writers and thinkers develop themes that, to them, make sense as organizing principles for bringing our species through five million years of time to the present. This story is no different.

The primary characters are mothers and infants, and the theme I have chosen as my organizing principle is birth. Alan Walker is credited with describing our attempts to unravel the mystery of human evolution as similar to working "a 3-D jigsaw puzzle with no picture on the box and half the pieces missing" (Weaver, 1985, p. 610). By focusing on birth, I hope to add to the story of human evolution a new dimension and a crucial, but still small, piece of the puzzle.

Darwin argued survival, but today we know that reproduction is what evolution is all about. But indeed, reproduction cannot occur unless survival has preceded it. So, what better place to examine the two than at the point at which survival has been most challenging for human beings throughout evolutionary history: the moment of birth. Individual and inclusive fitness and the survival of the species are directly dependent on the outcome of birth, an event which is itself affected by the phylogenetic and ontogenetic history of the individuals giving birth and being born.

To begin this discourse, I will examine phylogenetic factors that are part of the heritage of every parturient woman about to begin labor. She is, first of all, a sexually reproducing mammal with the characteristic features of viviparity and mammary glands. She has also inherited an endocrine repertoire from ancestors as remote as reptiles, a placenta from the earliest viviparous mammals, and a birth canal from her earliest hominid ancestors.

The newborn infant enters the world with its own set of hormones, a large brain inherited from remote hominid ancestors, and a state of helplessness unusual in the primate order. Both mother and infant begin labor with a nutritional, health, and genetic heritage that is unique to them and, for the mother, a whole array of sociocultural factors that affect her attitudes toward and experience with childbirth. Even their behaviors when they meet each other for the first time are influenced by past adaptations and immediate sociocultural factors.

Each of these factors, and others, will be considered in detail in this book as I demonstrate that a focus on the single event of birth is crucial for understanding not only human development but also human evolution.

The first chapter consists of a review of the many compromises that have been made during the evolution of life on earth that must be understood if one is to appreciate fully the physiological, physical, and behavioral processes that characterize human parturition. These compromises include sexual (contra asexual) reproduction, viviparity (contra oviparity), a hemochorial (contra epitheliochorial) placenta, a long gestation period, and a reproductive strategy that includes high parental investment in very few offspring. All higher, or haplorhine, primates have these compromises as part of their evolutionary heritage. Human parturition has been affected by three additional factors: morphological adaptation for habitual bipedalism, increased brain size and elaboration, and secondary altriciality of the newborn infant. The third is to some extent a result of the first two factors, but all three interact in a way that increases interdependency of mothers and neonates and leads to a dependency on others during parturition.

With the evolutionary history presented as a baseline on which to build the specifics of human birth and mother–infant bonding, I discuss in the remaining chapters the process of labor and delivery in human and nonhuman mammals, the state of the newborn infant, behavioral interactions during the immediate postpartum period, and mother–infant bonding. In writing these chapters I drew upon sources in clinical obstetrics, primate and nonprimate ethology, developmental psychology, and biocultural anthropology. In addition, the bulk of Chapter 5 and parts of the other chapters consist of my own research on birth and mother–neonate interaction. Recognizing the dearth of information on naturalistic human behavior during birth, I undertook a 1-year study of 110 women who delivered with midwives in a nonhospital setting. A description of this study, the women who participated in it, the methodology, and the setting is provided in Chapter 2.

In Chapter 3, I describe the process of parturition and related behaviors in a number of mammalian species. The criteria used in selecting the species include the existence of a substantial body of literature (e.g., the rat) or the need to illustrate a specific point. I have also tried to include as many descriptions of nonhuman primate births as I could find. An ethological description of parturition behavior in the human female is introduced with an attempt to be as objective as possible, that is, to report behaviors just as one would for a member of another species. The final part of this chapter presents a comparison of birth in human and nonhuman primates, emphasizing both similarities and differences. Among the factors evaluated are the use of the hands in delivery, the position of the fetus during emergence, time of delivery, position assumed during delivery, and consumption or disposal of the placenta. I also emphasize the somewhat unusual human practice of having assistance at birth and offer explanations for the evolution of this behavior. Finally, the role of adult males at birth is reviewed, for primates in general, and as it varies among human populations.

Chapter 4 focuses almost exclusively on the human newborn infant. It begins with the immediate physical and physiological adaptations the neonate must make in transition to the extrauterine environment. I then examine the relative immaturity of the human brain at birth, and review studies of neurological assessment of the neonate and characteristic state changes exhibited in the postpartum period. The adaptive and evolutionary significance of five infant behaviors is discussed. These include clinging, crying, smiling, following, and sucking, behaviors that John Bowlby (1958) and others have described as species-specific for human infants. In addition to discussing universal behaviors, I also review studies that have described ethnic and gender differences in human neonates. Finally, I present the argument that the human neonate is actually an "exterogestate fetus" (Montagu, 1961; Gould, 1977) and that its needs, and the compensating caretaking responses of the mother, are thus significantly different from those of any other primate species.

These caretaking responses of the mother are elaborated upon in Chapter 5. I describe species characteristic behavior patterns for human females in the first hour postpartum which occur in tactile, visual, and vocal interaction. As mentioned above, the bulk of this chapter is based on my own study of women giving birth with midwives in nonmedical settings. In the last part of the chapter I propose an ethogram of maternal behavior immediately after birth, suggesting the evolutionary significance of the behaviors which make up the pattern.

In Chapter 6, I cover the somewhat controversial topic of human mother–infant bonding and the significance of the immediate postpartum period for the development of that bond. As in Chapter 3, numerous animal species have been selected to illustrate specific points. I discuss the strength and specificity of the mother–infant bond in mammals as it relates to behavioral ecology of the species in question. Proximate factors affecting the bond are reviewed, as is the concept of a critical or sensitive period for its development. Most of the experimentation on mother–infant bonding has been conducted on animals other than humans, but I attempt to relate the findings to the development of the human mother–infant bond, although the analogies are far from perfect.

In Chapter 7, the last chapter, I propose a set of scenarios that describe birth-related behavior and mother–infant interaction at five stages in human evolution: the pongid–hominid divergence, encephalization in the genus *Homo*, obligate midwifery with further encephalization, the transition to agriculture and village life, and the industrial and technological revolution of the twentieth century. I also bring together much of the diverse material presented in the earlier chapters into an overall evolutionary perspective on human birth and bonding. A great deal of this perspective is, unfortunately, still dependent on speculation and what have been called "evolutionary 'just-so stories.'" I propose ways in which a number of these "just-so stories" can be turned into testable hypotheses and models. I hope that among the readers are some who will be stimulated to design tests for a few of the models and that they find support or refutation for my proposals, either in their own work or in past research I have overlooked. The role of birth in human evolution has for too long been ignored; this book is an attempt to remedy that oversight.

1

EVOLUTIONARY PERSPECTIVES ON HUMAN BIRTH AND BONDING: THE BACKGROUND

All characteristics and behaviors of a species ultimately can be evaluated in terms of their reproductive consequences. Natural selection has favored and will continue to favor genetically based characters and behaviors that enhance reproductive success. The fact that fitness is measured in terms of reproductive success, however, does not necessarily mean that ''more is better.'' Just as in economics, there is always an upper limit, a point at which the costs of producing or acquiring more far outweigh the benefits of each unit of increase. Competing selection pressures operate on all organisms, and rarely are responses made without compromise. Compromise can be made at various levels. At the individual level a trait can be favored up to the point at which it becomes detrimental to the individual or extracts energy from development of another trait. Within a group, an individual's fitness can be favored to the point at which each unit increase has a negative effect on other members of the group carrying that individual's genes. The reason that selection has favored compromise solutions throughout the history of life is that fitness is measured in generational, not in individual, terms. In other words, how many offspring one individual produces is not so important as the number of that individual's genes represented many generations later. In the long run, the amount of energy expended by an individual in the reproductive effort is far less important than the benefit to future fitness.

Although most of this book is concerned with human birth and mother–infant interaction immediately after birth, these two areas of concern are only a small part of the overall human reproductive strategy. In order to appreciate what goes on during birth and why mothers and infants behave the way they do after birth, it is important to have some understanding of the long series of steps that have been taken in the evolution of this reproductive strategy from the earliest sexually reproducing organisms to technologically managed births of today. The phylogenetic background of human birth and bonding is the subject of this chapter.

SEX

One of the first compromises reached in the evolution of the human reproductive strategy, beginning with very simple forms of life, was the

1

compromise of sex. Explaining the origin of sexual reproduction is one of the greatest problems confronting evolutionary theory (Fisher, 1930; Maynard Smith, 1971; Williams, 1975). If the goal is to produce more, then the optimal strategy for an individual, it would seem, would be to reproduce asexually so that all of its genes are included in each offspring. Sexual reproduction entails the cost of meiosis (only one-half of an individual's genes are passed on) and the cost of recombination (the risk of breaking up a good combination of alleles for the production of a potentially lethal combination). And yet, vertebrates are overwhelmingly committed to sexual reproduction.

The usual explanation offered is that sexual reproduction facilitates the production of new variability in organisms confronting frequent environmental challenges. For example, if a pathogen arises that is capable of destroying an entire population or species, only a mutation in an asexual species can afford possible immunity to the pathogen. In sexually reproducing forms, some individuals may have inherited a genetic combination that, by chance, confers resistance to the new pathogen. Most of the population may be wiped out, but individuals that can "utilize genetic variance generated by past natural selection" (Maynard Smith, 1971:166) will survive. In general, transgenerational changes afforded by recombination can proceed far faster in species reproducing sexually than they can in asexual organisms that are dependent on mutation for change. In other words, evolution can proceed faster in sexually reproducing organisms that it can in asexual organisms. In addition, as Muller (1964; cited in Daly and Wilson, 1983) pointed out, recombination allows the elimination of unfavorable mutations whereas all descendents of an asexual species are "stuck with" a deleterious mutation in a parental form. In this way, recombination allows avoidance of change which confers decrease in fitness.

In a similar vein, Bernstein and his colleagues (1985) propose that the origin of sexual reproduction can be found in the advantages gained in the repair of genetic damage (see Maynard Smith, 1971). DNA damage and mutation are constant challenges that can be met successfully if two alleles or chromosomes are inherited from both parents, at least one of which has a "normal" variant capable of masking the effects of the deleterious mutation. In other words, repair and masking are short-term benefits accruing to the individual who reproduces sexually, whereas variation is a long-term benefit accruing to future offspring. Since natural selection operates on the individual, immediate benefits better explain the origin of sex than variation, which is more appropriately seen as a consequence. In the long run, it is better for an organism to have 10 offspring, sharing one-half its genes, that in turn have 10 on down the line in perpetuity, than 1000 clones that become extinct through inability to survive an environmental perturbation.

The dimorphism associated with sex is so taken for granted by human beings that its significance can be easily overlooked. It is, in fact, important to the adaptive strategy of each species. Not only are the apparatus and mechanisms of reproduction different for the two sexes, but the roads to reproductive success are divergent, if not in outright conflict. Inasmuch as reproductive success, or the differential transmission of an individual's genes to the next generation, is considered by evolutionists to guide an individual's approach to its environment (through the effect of natural selection), these differences are indeed important.

Thus, another consequence of sexual reproduction is that, as Wilson (1975:314) notes, it is an antisocial force in evolution. This antisocial force is apparent not only between the sexes but also between parent and offspring. If parents and offspring are genetically identical, it is clear that any act on the part of the parent that enhances the survival of offspring would be favored by selection. In sexual reproduction an offspring and parent share only one-half their genes so that an act enhancing the survival of offspring increases, in subsequent generations, not only the parental genes but those of competitors, as well. With parents and offspring acting selfishly, conflict is inevitable. In some species, for example, it may be to the parents' advantage to breed again as soon as possible and terminate care provided the most recent batch of young. The young, however, will inevitably do all that they can to retain parental attention (Trivers, 1974).

The antisocial force is evoked even more strongly in the relations between the sexes. The basis of sexual difference is dimorphism of and investment in the gametes. Females produce large, energetically expensive, immobile gametes, whereas males produce small, energetically inexpensive, mobile gametes. This disparity is exacerbated in mammals by the demands of pregnancy in females. Given these differences, it is adaptive for females to optimize each attempt at reproduction, whereas males are better served by maximizing fertilization (Williams, 1975). This has profound significance for our understanding of a species' interaction with its environment, for the overall adaptive complex must represent a compromise between the optima for the two sexes.

In higher vertebrates, the female's strategy of maximizing each attempt at reproduction may include expending time and energy in the protection and feeding of offspring. The more assistance she can obtain in this process, the greater the likelihood that more of her young will survive. This, of course, pits the sexes against each other at the outset; she improves survival of her genes if she convinces the male to remain following insemination. He, on the other hand, improves his chances by leaving as soon as impregnation of the female takes place. Obviously, some sort of compromise has been worked out between the sexes, and between the generations, or sexual reproduction would not be so common and pervasive today.

To some extent, the "choice" of mating and parenting strategies for the male (stay or leave; monogamy or polygamy) has something to do with the amount of postconception effort he *can* contribute to the production of offspring. In birds, both parents generally feed and care for the young. In most species, neither sex has an advantage over the other in caretaking abilities. Given equal ability in parenting, it is not surprising that approximately 90% of bird species mate monogamously, for a season or for life. Most of these species are also territorial, a behavior that further favors monogamy. In this case, a male has two options: He can provide care for the young, thus increasing the survival chances of his brood, or he can abandon the female after courtship and seek new mates. This latter choice often involves finding new territories, defending them against other males, and attracting females for breeding purposes, all of which are time- and energy-consuming activities. Thus, in many cases the benefits of remaining monogamous and providing care for the young outweigh the advantages of promiscuous mating, especially if, as seems likely, offspring survival rate is increased. In mammals, the male can do little beyond providing protection for the young, so it is more often the case that he abandons a female as soon as courtship and mating have been completed. Not surprisingly, monogamy is rare in mammals. The issue of paternal care of young will be pursued further in Chapter 3.

VIVIPARITY

After sexual reproduction, the next adaptations of concern in the evolution of the human reproductive strategy are the steps of internal fertilization and internal gestation, or the evolution of viviparity from the primitive oviparous baseline. Each step resulted in a further reduction in numbers of offspring that can be reproduced with each generation. Species that release sperm and eggs for external fertilization can produce millions of gametes at a time with the only limitation being the production capacity of their ovaries and testes. In addition, there is little or no subsequent responsibility, once gamete release has occurred. If the female retains the eggs for internal fertilization, the numbers produced are limited not only by the capacity of her ovaries but also by the capacity of her body to hold the eggs until fertilization has occurred. The cost to both sexes is greater, but the zygotes receive an extra bit of protection during a critical period, so it is likely that a greater percentage of them survive than is the case with external fertilization. Thus, we have a second step in the trade-off of quantity for quality and a step in the direction of greater parental investment.

With internal gestation, the cost to the female becomes even higher and the resulting numbers of offspring produced even lower. Again, however, by affording greater protection to the young until they are fairly well developed, a female further increases the percentage of young that survive. Internal gestation also enables embryonic development to proceed in a homogeneous environment, relatively independent of temperature and humidity fluctuations in the external environment. Viviparity has apprently evolved independently in many animal lines, which suggests that it is a successful strategy. One estimate has it that viviparity evolved 75 times in reptiles, 22 times in fish (10 in Chondrichthyes, 12 in Osteoichthyes), 4 times in amphibians, and 1 time in mammals (Blackburn, 1981).

The steps involved in the evolution of viviparity are complex and will only be mentioned briefly here. In oviparous species, the *corpus luteum* is the only source of progesterone, the hormone responsible for inhibiting uterine contractions. When the *corpus luteum* dies, progesterone is withdrawn and uterine contractions begin, leading to oviposition. One key to viviparity is that the embryo must be retained in the uterus for a longer time, and progesterone production must continue so that contractions are inhibited until the fetus can survive outside of the mother's body. In order to retain the embryo, temporary endocrine glands are required which serve to maintain gestation through successive stages of embryonic development. In some mammalian species, the *corpus luteum* persists throughout pregnancy. In others, including our own, its function as a secretor of progesterone is assumed by the placenta soon after implantation or in mid- to late pregnancy. In this case the *corpus luteum* usually disappears at the time the placenta becomes the primary endocrine organ maintaining pregnancy.

A developing embryo, whether retained or not, must be able to obtain nutrients and oxygen and must be able to excrete wastes and carbon dioxide. Nutrient provision can be assumed by the yolk (present, at least at certain stages, in both oviparous and viviparous animals), so the biggest challenge to evolving viviparity was gas exchange. Thus, the placenta likely evolved primarily as an organ for gas exchange, and only later, with large mammals, did it become an important agent of nutrient transfer.

THE HEMOCHORIAL PLACENTA

We usually think of the placenta as one of the characteristics that distinguishes the eutherian mammals from other mammals. Indeed, the subclass is sometimes referred to as comprising the "placental mammals," implying that others could be called "nonplacental." Actually the placenta is an organ that probably evolved in conjunction with viviparity and thus evolved independently in several animal lineages. For this chapter, however, a review of its development in mammals will be sufficient.

When the fertilized mammalian egg, or zygote, reaches the blastocyst stage, two separate clusters of cells are distinguishable (Figure 1.1). One is the inner cell mass, which will develop into the embryo, amnion, and allantois. The second cluster, called the trophoblast, is the layer of cells lining the blastocyst, which will form the chorion and, ultimately, the placenta. The amnion, allantois, and chorion are often referred to as "extraembryonic membranes," indicating that, although they arose from the same fertilized egg as the embryo, they are not part of the embryo and are shed at birth (Figure 1.2). The amnion serves to maintain the embryo in an aqueous environment, which is important for animals that lay their eggs or bear their young outside of the water. The allantois functions in the elimination of waste and the transmission of gases, fusing with the inner surface of the chorion to form the placenta. Part of the allantois forms the umbilical cord. The chorion encloses the amnion, embryo, yolk sac, and allantois and serves as an intermediary between the embryonic material and the

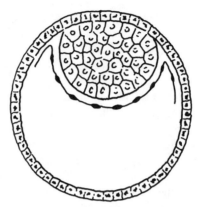

FIGURE 1.1. Diagram of the mammalian blastocyst showing the trophoblast (outer rim) and the inner cell mass (at north pole). Reproduced from ''Phylogeny of the Primates'' by W. P. Luckett and F. S. Szalay. By permission of Plenum Publishing Company, New York. Copyright, 1975.

surrounding environment. In eutherian mammals, the chorion is the membrane that is in direct contact with the inner lining of the uterus, or endometrium, and part of it, with the allantois and uterine tissues, forms the placenta.

The most common placenta found in marsupials is the choriovitelline, a yolk sac-type of placenta in which the vascularized yolk sac fuses with the chorion. Marsupial embryos are surrounded by a shell membrane for most of the period of intrauterine development. When that membrane disappears near the end of pregnancy, placentation occurs, but for only a brief period before parturition takes place. Luckett (1975) proposes that the choriovitelline placenta is the ancestral placenta for the marsupials and eutherians, noting that a transitory form of this type is found early in pregnancy in a number of eutherians. The choriovitelline placenta is, for example, present in a transitory stage in primates such as lemurs and lorises, but it is absent in higher primates (for information on primate taxonomy, see Table 1.1). It should be noted that the chorioallantoic placenta characteristic of eutherian mammals is found in some marsupials, including bandicoots, of the family Peramelidae. Luckett (1975) suggests that this is an example of convergence in that chorioallantoic placentas occur in several lineages that have no immediate common ancestor.

The eutherian chorioallantoic placenta is one in which the chorion becomes vascularized by allantoic blood vessels. These placentas can be divided into several types, classified very generally according to their shape and structure, including the number of membranes between the maternal and fetal circulatory systems and, as mentioned previously, the degree of contact between the chorion and the uterine lining (Table 1.2). Two of concern in a survey of the Primate order are the epitheliochorial and hemochorial placentas. The former is found in swine, horses, donkeys, lemurs, and lorises, among others. The chorion is simply in close apposition to the uterine lining and the villi are widely diffused.

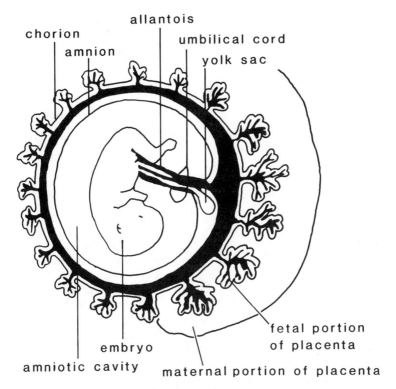

chorion
allantois
amnion
umbilical cord
yolk sac

fetal portion
of placenta

embryo

amniotic cavity

maternal portion of placenta

FIGURE 1.2. Diagram of the human embryo, fetal membranes, and placenta. Reproduced from "Elements of Biological Science," Second Edition by W. T. Keeton. By permission of W. W. Norton and Company, Inc., New York. Illustrations by Paula di Santo Bensadoun. Copyright 1973, 1972, 1969, 1967 by W. W. Norton and Company, Inc.

There are six membranes between the maternal and fetal systems, three composed of maternal tissue and three of fetal tissue.

In the hemochorial placenta, characteristic of haplorhine primates, rodents, bats, and insectivores, the trophoblast penetrates the epithelium, connective tissue, blood vessel walls, and maternal veins; the villi come into direct contact with and are surrounded by maternal blood (Beer and Billingham, 1976). Rather than being diffused as in the epitheliochorial placenta, or forming bands at the equator as in endotheliochorial placentas (characteristic of carnivores), the villi form a single disk. Early in pregnancy, in species with hemochorial placentas, there appear to be several maternal membranes that gradually erode until the trophoblast is directly against the maternal blood, resulting in almost no barrier between the two systems. Three membranes remain, all of fetal origin.

It is difficult to determine which is the ancestral placenta. Some viviparous reptiles have yolk sac placentas, in which there is no invasion of the maternal tissue by fetal tissue, and capillaries of the two systems are separated by several

TABLE **1.1.** Taxonomy of the Primate Order[a]

Scientific names	Common names
Suborder:	
Strepsirhini	
Family	
Lemuridae	Lemur, lepilemur, mouse lemur
Indriidae	Sifaka, indri
Daubentoniidae	Aye-aye
Lorisidae	Loris, potto, galago, bushbaby
Suborder:	
Haplorhini	
Family	
Tarsiidae	Tarsier
Callitrichidae	Marmoset, tamarin
Cebidae	Cebus, capuchin, night monkey, titi, squirrel monkey, saki, uakari, howler, spider monkey, wooly monkey
Cercopithecidae	Macaque, baboon, mangebey, mandrill, gelada, guenon, patas, langur, colobus
Hylobatidae	Gibbon, siamang
Pongidae	Orangutan, gorilla, chimpanzee
Hominidae	Human being

[a]Modified with permission of Macmillan Publishing Company from *Evolution of Primate Behavior* by Alison Jolly. Copyright 1985 by Alison Jolly.

TABLE **1.2.** Mammalian Placenta Types[a]

Classification	No. maternal layers	No. fetal layers	Example species
Epitheliochorial	3	3	Horse, pig
Syndesmochorial	2	3	Sheep, bison, cow
Endotheliochorial	1	3	Cat, dog
Hemochorial	0	3	Humans, rodents, rabbits

[a]Diagram taken from *Advances in Reproductive Physiology*, Vol. 3, edited by Anne McLaren. Copyright 1968 by Grafton Books, a division of Collins Publishing Group.

layers. Others, however, have chorioallantoic placentas that afford a degree of maternal–fetal intimacy equivalent to that found in mammals with epitheliochorial placentas. This similarity to reptilian placentas suggests that the epitheliochorial is the most primitive and thus ancestral to other eutherian placentas.

Luckett (1975) argues, on the basis of ontogenetic evidence, that the epitheli-ochorial placenta is the ancestral type, and that the hemochorial placenta evolved directly from that. Others (see Martin, 1969; Mossman, 1937, cited in Martin, 1969) have argued that an ancestral endotheliochorial placenta gave rise to both the hemochorial and endotheliochorial forms. Finally, since the hemochorial placenta is found in the most ancient and primitive mammals, insectivores, and rodents, it has been argued that this is the ancestral form.

Continuing his analysis of placental types and fetal membranes in primates, Luckett (1974) has used cladistic analysis to justify a taxonomy that divides the order into two suborders, Strepsirhini and Haplorhini. According to him, tarsiers share 6 of 10 derived characteristics of anthropoids, including a hemochorial placenta and lack of a choriovitelline placenta early in pregnancy. Luckett thus places them in the suborder Haplorhini, separate from the Strepsirhini, which are characterized by epitheliochorial placentas and presence of a choriovitelline placenta early in pregnancy. (Analysis of similar factors exclude the tupaids from the order Primates, according to Luckett.)

Among the functions of the placenta is transfer of oxygen, nutrients, and gamma globulin from mother to fetus, and transfer of carbon dioxide and wastes from fetus to mother. Transfer is primarily by diffusion across the membranes of the maternal and fetal blood vessels. (Gamma globulin crosses the placenta via a specific carrier mechanism.) Beaconsfield *et al.* (1980:99) note that the interdigitation of these blood vessels is such that a surface area "equal to that of more than half a tennis court" is provided for diffusion. Additional functions of the placenta include storage of glycogen and production of hormones important for the maintenance of pregnancy, initiation of labor, and development of lactation. This last function will be explored in more detail.

Human chorionic gonadotrophin (HCG), an analog to the hypothalamic gonadotrophins, follicle-stimulating hormone (FSH), and luteinizing hormone (LH), is produced by the trophoblast soon after implantation and it may, in fact, facilitate implantation of the blastocyst. The "pregnancy test" is based on this hormone, which can be detected in the urine as early as 4 weeks after the last menstruation. It is produced at low levels immediately after implantation, rises to a peak at 2 months, and drops to low levels for the remainder of the gestation period (Hickman, 1985). This peak and subsequent drop are associated with the assumption of steroid production by the placenta. For the first 2 or 3 months, chorionic gonadotrophin stimulates the *corpus luteum* to produce progesterone and estrogen; later in pregnancy, these hormones are produced by the placenta. These have a number of functions. Progesterone inhibits uterine contractions and maintains the uterus in a pregnant state. It also stimulates growth of the breasts and mammary glands, inhibits secretion of prolactin, and regulates growth of the fetus (Young, 1975). Human placental lactogen (also known as human chorionic somatomammotrophin) is also produced by the placenta, as its name implies. It resembles human growth hormone and, thus, may function in regulating fetal growth (Hickman, 1985).

The placenta also serves a protective function, acting as a barrier to the transfer of certain agents, including bacteria and most macromolecules. Unfortunately, it does not block the transfer of most drugs, chemicals, vitamins, and other agents of potentially negative consequence to the fetus. In addition, antibodies that would typically be evoked by a maternal system encountering a graft or transplant do not often pass into the fetal system. At least it appears that the placenta blocks them, although it is actually far more complicated than that.

In general, the success of a skin or organ transplant is low, and after a few hours or days, rejection usually takes place. The fetal "graft" is less than 50% similar to its mother (since it inherits some of her recessive alleles), and yet, rejection does not often occur. Later that same offspring can provide skin for grafting to its mother, although the graft usually fails to take. And today, with recent developments in reproductive technology, a fetus with no genetic identity with its surrogate mother can be carried to term. Noting the very brief gestation time of bandicoots (which have chorioallantoic placentas, as already noted), Luckett (1975) suggests that marsupials have not evolved a mechanism for preventing rejection of the fetus, and that one of the most critical factors in the evolution of eutherian chorioallantoic placentation was the development of such a mechanism.

What is it about the process of eutherian gestation that prevents rejection of the fetal "graft"? A number of explanations have been offered, none of which is fully satisfactory. Does the fetus itself lack antigenicity? This suggestion is refuted by the evidence that transplacental antigens are present early in embryonic development (Van Tienhoven, 1983). Is the uterus a "privileged site" and thus not susceptible to normal immunological processes? True immunologically privileged sites lack lymph vessels in which the uterus is abundant. Also, ectopic pregnancies are not rejected, suggesting that the presence or absence of a uterus has little effect on immunological tolerance. Or is the maternal system altered so that the immune response is not triggered during pregnancy? This suggestion gets closer to the likely mechanism, although it does not explain everything. For example, grafts of skin are usually ultimately rejected during pregnancy but are retained for longer periods of time than usual, especially if the donor is a close relative of the mother.

A number of factors are secreted during pregnancy that are known to interfere with the functioning of lymphocytes, at least in the laboratory. These include HCG, human chorionic somatomammotrophin, prolactin, and adrenal corticosteroids. Further evidence that the maternal immune response system may be depressed during pregnancy is seen in the fact that portions of the fetal membranes often break away from the placenta and enter the maternal bloodstream. Most are destroyed, but some reach the lungs with no evidence of maternal reaction (Anderson, 1971). (It was formerly believed that this was associated with eclampsia, but now it is known to be a normal occurrence.)

Anderson (1971:1078) studied the effects of what he has termed the "immunological inertia of viviparity" on armadillos, rats, dogs, and sheep. A depression of immunological reactions was observed in pregnant females of all species. The depression was most marked in the armadillo and the rat and least marked in the dog and sheep. It should be noted, as Anderson did, that armadillos and rats have hemochorial placentas like those of human beings, while dogs and sheep have endotheliochorial and epitheliochorial placentas, respectively. It is presumed that the greater number of placental layers between the maternal and fetal circulatory systems of dogs and sheep reduces the necessity of a depressed maternal immune response for inhibiting fetal rejection.

Certainly it is evident that a number of these factors are interacting during pregnancy to prevent rejection of the fetus. However, it is not a foolproof system—rejection does occasionally occur, and there is evidence that it is quite common in the first few days after fertilization in human beings. Abnormal embryos are commonly aborted, so the maternal immune response is not entirely suppressed, although the degree of sensitivity may vary throughout pregnancy.

A familiar example of problems that arise when mother and fetus have different antigens is seen when they carry incompatible genes for the ABO, Rh, and perhaps other hemoglobin polymorphisms. If the mother is Rh negative and the fetus Rh positive, the production of antibodies is triggered in the mother, usually at the time of delivery, for the first incompatible pregnancy. Unless they are neutralized within a few hours, the antibodies will remain in her system, resulting in immunological problems in subsequent incompatible pregnancies. The abortion and stillbirth rate is higher in these pregnancies, as is the incidence of hemolytic disease of the newborn.

Perhaps a more common situation, although the evidence for it is more controversial, is isoimmunization resulting from ABO incompatibility. In an ABO incompatible pregnancy, the fetus has antigens that the mother lacks: for example, fetus type A or B, mother type O. Naturally occurring antibodies against antigens A and B are circulating in the bloodstream at all times in mothers with type O. Thus, it is theoretically possible for those antibodies to cross the placenta and destroy erythrocytes of a fetus of type A or B, resulting in intrauterine anemia or problems at birth that would kill the fetus. Although this is theoretically possible, is there any evidence that this occurs?

Waterhouse and Hogben (1947), in a survey of family data from 12 previous studies, demonstrated that there are intrauterine incompatibilities between mother and fetus involving the ABO system. Involved in the studies, which were conducted between 1927 and 1944, were 1239 families with 4139 children. The researchers found a significant shortage of families in which the father was A and the mother O, as compared with ones in which the father was O and the mother A. They also found a highly significant shortage of group A children for the father A–mother O matings. There was also a decrease in the ratio of A to O children with increasing birth rank in those matings. The results of the survey revealed a net deficiency of 25% of A children in father A–mother O matings, which meant a fetal death rate of 8% of all A children or 3% of all conceptions for that population. These figures were much higher than the contemporary Rh incompatibility death rate of 0.5%. It is suggested that the relatively low incidence of ABO hemolytic disease of the newborn is due to the fact that potential problem pregnancies terminate in abortion or miscarriage before the disease can be manifested.

Matsunaga (1959) collected similar data on 1429 Japanese families, 812 of which were compatible matings and 617 of which were incompatible. There was a significant increase in the number of abortions and in the number of childless couples among the incompatibly mated group. Compatibly mated couples averaged significantly more children than those who were incompatible at the ABO system. In addition, Matsunaga calculated that the mortality rate in the incompatible matings was 21%.

In another study, Chung and Morton (1961) found that maternal–fetal incompatibility in their sample of Caucasian families significantly reduced fertility by 6.3% and caused elimination of 9.4% of incompatible zygotes. Boorman (1950) examined 2000 consecutive admissions to a British maternity hospital and observed a deficiency of A births from O mothers.

In any event, although the evidence is occasionally contradictory, it appears that the placenta is not a perfect barrier against fetal antigens that might cause immunological reaction in the mother nor is her immune system totally suppressed during pregnancy. Intrauterine selection at the ABO locus, causing stillbirth, abortion, or death from hemolytic disease, represents a powerful pressure on the ABO polymorphism. If there were not counterselective forces operating to maintain the A or B alleles which are selected against at this level, these two alleles would be reduced to extremely low levels within a few generations. This does not appear to be happening, and the likely counterselective agent is infectious disease during infancy and early childhood, which may differentially affect the blood types.

Another question that can be pursued in the context of immunological response during pregnancy is whether or not the different numbers of layers between the maternal and fetal circulatory systems provide different degrees of protection from immunological reaction. Does the epitheliochorial placenta with its six layers afford greater protection to the fetus than the hemochorial placenta with fewer layers, as implied in Anderson's study previously described?

Luckett (1974) notes that thalidomide causes several fetal deformities when administered to humans, rhesus macaques, and baboons, all species with hemochorial placentas. Galagos, however, who have epitheliochorial placentas, are apparently not affected by the drug, suggesting that the greater number of layers prevents its passage into the fetal system.

The fact that animals with epitheliochorial placentas can carry to term a pregnancy resulting from a heterospecific mating suggests that greater genetic differences are tolerated, or not detected, because of the thicker placental barrier. Matings between horses and donkeys, horses and zebras, leopards and tigers, cattle and bison, cattle and yak, yak and bison, and, possibly, sheep and goats, are all known to have occurred, resulting in live, albeit usually sterile, offspring. All of the above species have epitheliochorial or endotheliochorial placentas.

Conceptions occur, but viable offspring are rare or unknown in heterospecific matings among rats, mice, hamsters, rabbits, guinea pigs, and haplorhine primates, all species with hemochorial placentas.

At the beginning of this chapter it was suggested that sexual reproduction conveys advantages on practitioners in that greater variation in offspring, resulting from meiotic division and recombination, provides greater flexibility in responding to environmental change. But the evolution of viviparity brought another challenge: There is a decided limit to the amount of variation tolerated between generations because of the degree of intimacy between maternal and fetal systems.

In an evolutionary sense, the advantage of the epitheliochorial placenta is that greater genetic variability is possible, allowing occupation of different habitats or greater chance of responding to an environmental change. Associated with this is more rapid divergence of lines. The dramatic diversification of mammalian lineages at the beginning of the Cenozoic era is referred to as an adaptive radiation, a phenomenon made possible by the likely ancestral mammalian epitheliochorial placenta. (Mammals with hemochorial placentas and very short gestation times could also experience rapid diversification of lines because birth occurs before immunological rejection can occur.) Even more recently, an adaptive radiation of species occurred when the lemurs arrived on Madagascar. Within a short time there were dozens of descendent species occupying a wide range of ecological niches. Lemurs have epitheliochorial placentas; it is unlikely that the same degree of divergence would have occurred had the first primate on Madagascar been one with a hemochorial placenta.

Adaptive radiation is a special form of cladogenesis, a process characterized by diversification of species resulting from an increase in variation in a gene pool, coupled with reproductive isolating mechanisms. Anagenesis is a form of progressive evolution characterized by increasing complexity of the species and a decrease in genetic variability. Speciation per se does not occur. It is occasionally referred to as "phyletic evolution" indicating that the lineage itself is evolving even though reproductive isolation of populations within it does not occur. Human evolution, at least in the past two million years, is one of anagenesis. In general, species with phylogenies reflecting cladogenetic processes are those with epitheliochorial placentas. Species with phylogenies reflecting anagenesis are those with hemochorial placentas and long gestation times. As already implied, rapid speciation is possible in animals with hemochorial placentas and short gestations.

Because the methodologies of biological classification used by taxonomists vary from one order of mammals to another, it is difficult to make generalizations about rates of evolution and numbers of species evolving per unit time. Until a synthesis of opposing methodologies (Mayr, 1981) is achieved, it will be hard to demonstrate that speciation has been more common in the last five million years in, for example, the horse line, than in the hominid line. As a preliminary inquiry, I examined hypothetical family trees in *Equus, Bison,*

Homo, and *Panthera.* Members of the genus *Equus* have epitheliochorial placentas with six layers between mother and fetus. Willoughby (1974) proposes that more than 25 separate species have evolved from a late Pliocene ancestor. Like sheep, goats, and cows, bison have syndesmochorial placentas with five layers between mother and fetus. McDonald (1981) suggests that four separate *Bison* lines have diverged from a late Pliocene ancestor. Cats have endotheliochorial placentas with four layers between maternal and fetal systems. In a molecular analysis of phylogeny of the *Panthera* lineage, Collier and O'Brien (1985) list eight separate species that have evolved from a common ancestor five million years ago. During the equivalent time period, only two lineages of hominids have existed, although three separate consecutive "phyletic" species have been proposed for each lineage.

Undoubtedly, the criteria used for proposing lineage splitting in these four mammalian groups are not the same, and factors other than placenta types affect speciation (e.g., life span, migration patterns). Nevertheless, a cursory inspection of these family trees argues for greater divergence in lines with more barriers between the maternal and fetal circulatory systems. I hope that this hypothesis will be tested more rigidly when more mammalian groups have been subjected to cladistic analysis.

In any event, the capacity of the mother to respond immunologically to the fetal antigens has become a major selective agent for all viviparous animals. It is, as Goodman (1960) suggests, the explanation for the great similarities in embryological development seen in vertebrates. Mutations or incompatible recombinations would likely be eliminated, limiting the genetic variability in the species—eliminated, that is, if their effects are manifested during gestation. Any protein that is not expressed until after birth would not be detected as foreign by the maternal system and would thus not likely be eliminated. Goodman (1961) suggests that this was the key compromise between the conflicting "goals" of viviparous reproduction and the potential advantage of genetic variability, in the event of an opportunity to move into a new environmental zone. The delayed epigenesis of certain proteins allowed for more variability between generations, but it also resulted in a period of infant dependency characteristic of all mammals.

If this is true, we would expect greater homogeneity of proteins expressed prenatally in mammalian orders and within a species. Those appearing postnatally would be expected to show more variation. Indeed, this appears to be the case. Albumin, as an example, shows remarkable similarity across the entire mammalian class. Gamma globulins, on the other hand, do not develop until after birth and exhibit great variability even within a species, such as our own (Goodman, 1960). Albumin is a conservative protein that has changed very little; the gamma globulins appear to have evolved rapidly. Presumably, polymorphisms for albumin have been selected against by the maternal immune response, because this protein appears early in embryonic development. A consequence of the delayed development of gamma globulins is that the newborn infant has few resources for fighting infection. Instead, it is dependent on antibodies acquired from the mother during the late stage of pregnancy and from the colostrum.

How does all of this relate to primate and human evolution? The earliest primates, along with all mammalian orders, were evolving into a broad environmental zone. The "exogenous environment" (Goodman, 1961:139) favored variability, but the "endogenous environment" of viviparity favored homogeneity. The likely compromise was delay in maturation of a number of proteins and the resulting long period of infant dependency. Most of these mammals probably had placentas that afforded more barriers between the maternal and fetal systems, so not so many systems were undeveloped at birth. In addition, gestation times were short, so birth occurred before the maternal system had time to recognize foreign antigens and develop antibodies against them. Due to these factors, genetic variability between generations was great, and as this variability was ordered by natural selection and genetic drift, speciation occurred.

Subsequently, brain advancement became a critical component of the adaptive strategy of primates. Although the epitheliochorial placenta is extremely efficient at transporting nutrients to the developing young (witness the fact that the species that give birth to the most precocial young have epitheliochorial placentas), it is not so efficient at oxygen transport as the hemochorial placenta (Harned, 1970). Thus, for a line emphasizing brain development, it would have been advantageous to have fewer layers between the maternal and fetal systems. Perhaps one of the causes of the haplorhine divergence was selection for a hemochorial placenta.

Approximately five million years ago, our hominoid ancestors encountered further challenges in attempting to respond to environmental changes. The climate of Africa was changing, and seasonality and biotic variation were increasing. At the same time, the niche to which our ancestors had been adapted for several million years was decreasing its carrying capacity; some populations had to find other niches to exploit. This necessitated changes not only in behavior but also, ultimately, in anatomy and physiology.

The hemochorial placenta which had been so important for primate brain development became a disadvantage when, again, variability was necessary for adjusting to the changes. Another compromise was worked out whereby development of proteins critical for responding to the exogenous environment was delayed until after birth (Goodman, 1962). A delay even greater than that seen in most mammals meant an even more undeveloped infant at birth. As we shall see later, this increased infant helplessness was an important factor in determining the hominid reproductive and parenting strategies.

GESTATION LENGTH

Gestation length is highly variable in eutherian mammals and seems to defy organization according to taxonomy. Various factors have been proposed as determinants of gestation time, including fetal size, maternal size, fetal growth rate, brain weight, brain growth rate, litter size, and type of placenta. In general, mammals that give birth to precocial offspring have longer gestation times than those that give birth to altricial young. This, in turn, is related to brain size, brain growth rate, and behavioral ecology of the species. Carnivores, for example, exhibit the altricial pattern with brief gestations, several offspring at a time, and undeveloped young that remain immobile for several days or weeks following birth. Most ungulates, on the other hand, have longer gestations, fewer offspring per birth, and well-developed young that can follow their mothers soon after birth. Lions, which have altricial young, have a gestation period of about 105 days, while seals, whose infants must withstand cold water and swim soon after birth, have a 350-day gestation period. These species, with very different reproductive patterns, are closely related, and both have endotheliochorial placentas. Likewise, animals with hemochorial placentas give birth to both precocial (e.g., most haplorhine primates) and altricial (e.g., squirrels and mice) young. In other words, the placenta type does not appear to play a role in gestation schedule or rate of fetal growth.

According to Sacher and Staffeldt (1974), brain weight at birth is the primary factor determining gestation length, coupled with degree of advancement of brain growth at birth. The latter explains the observed longer gestation times of precocial taxa relative to altricial taxa of about equal brain weight. This also explains the discrepencies noted when fetal growth rate was believed to be the primary determinant of gestation: Great apes (*Pan, Pongo,* and *Gorilla*) give birth to very small infants, although they have long gestation times. Brain weight and development are high, however, putting these animals in line with others when these variables are plotted against gestation time. Sacher and Staffeldt also propose that life spans in mammals are related directly to brain weight, speculating that species with large brains must have longer reproductive lives to compensate in fitness for the decreased reproductive rate necessary for the maintenance *in utero* of these large brains. Thus, species with long lives, such as most haplorhine primates, elephants, and whales, have long gestation periods, larger and more developed brains at birth, and relatively precocial young. Those with short gestation periods, smaller and less developed brains, and several altricial young per litter, would, if the proposal is correct, be expected to have shorter reproductive lives.

Human beings fit the precocial pattern in most respects: Few young at a time, fairly long gestation periods, and an extensive period of infant dependency. Human young are extremely undeveloped at birth, however, especially when compared with infants of other primate species. Only at 6–9 months of age does the human infant acquire the motor development, chemical development, or brain development displayed by other haplorhine primate infants shortly after birth (see Gould, 1977).

Examination of the developmental stages of primates after birth reveals that, for most stages, the human duration is about one-third or one-half longer than for any other primates. For example, the period of infancy is about 6 years in humans and 4 years in chimpanzees. A female chimpanzee reaches puberty at about age 10, a gorilla at 7, and human beings in foraging societies, between 16 and 17. Growth is completed in chimpanzees and gorillas at age 11 but not until 20 in humans. Life span is approximately 35 years for these two great apes, and close to 70 for humans. One would assume from this pattern that the gestation period would also be one-third to twice as long in humans as in the great apes; but this is not so. Gestation averages 228 days in chimpanzees, 256 days in gorillas, and 267 days in humans. (Most of the above figures are from Harvey and Clutton-Brock, 1985.) Montagu (1961), Gould (1977), and others have suggested that the human gestation period actually may be about 18 months, but that the fetus must be delivered half way through that period in order to be born at all because of the restriction placed on neonatal cranial size by the narrow bipedal pelvis. Extending the gestation period for human beings by 6–9 months would bring it more in line with the other developmental stages. Montagu has suggested the term *exterogestation* for the period following birth when human neonates are functioning in many ways more like a fetus than an infant. Alternatively, the human neonate can be referred to as "secondarily altricial."

BIPEDALISM AND PARTURITION

Gould (1977:369) cites Portmann's essays on secondary altriciality in the human neonate but notes that the German scholar "ridicules the argument that something so coarsely mechanical as difficulty in parturition might have anything to do with [it]." I would argue, however, that the phylogenetic constraint that birth takes place through the pelvic canal imposes upper limits on neonatal brain and body size for all mammals. This canal is somewhat inflexible in its capacity of supporting the body above the limbs associated with terrestrial adaptations in vertebrates. Locomotor habit determines rigidity and arrangement of the bones of the pelvis, affects the size of the birth canal, and thus determines maximum fetal size at birth.

Three locomotor categories in primates can be used to demonstrate how mechanical requirements of locomotion place limits on the size of the birth canal. These are the categories of quadrupedalism (most monkeys), brachiation (apes), and bipedalism (humans). In general, the size, shape, and rigidity or flexibility of the pelvic girdle relates directly to the mode of locomotion of the animal. Three bones fuse to form the adult mammalian pelvis: the ilium, ischium, and pubis (Figure 1.3). These, in turn, articulate posteriorly with the fused sacral vertebrae to create a fairly rigid basin for abdominal support, muscle attachment, and obstetrical outlet. The pubic bones articulate with each other anteriorly at a symphysis, separated by cartilage. Both of these joints (sacroiliac and pubic

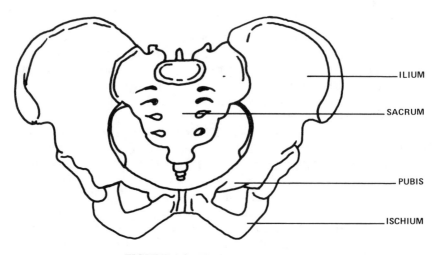

FIGURE 1.3. The human bony pelvis.

symphysis) are relatively immobile in primates but can be loosened temporarily in females by hormonal action at the time of delivery.

According to Leutenegger (1974), efficient, habitual quadrupedalism favors a short distance between the sacroiliac and the hip joints, a relationship that results in a narrow pelvic opening. This, in turn, limits the size of the fetal head at birth for quadrupedal primates. For brachiators, a decreased distance between the two joints is not necessarily disadvantageous, so that selection for larger cranial size at birth can proceed without sacrificing locomotor efficiency. In other words, with the evolution of brachiation in primates, the constraint on fetal cranial size at birth has relaxed, with the expected result of larger neonatal brains in brachiators, including apes, gibbons, and New World spider monkeys.

Almost all primates can assume a bipedal stance and walk bipedally for short distances. For nonhumans to do so they must bend forward at the hip with a compensating bend at the knees. This is energetically expensive, however, and is used only under special circumstances, such as while carrying objects or when standing and searching. Major morphological changes were necessary in the evolution of habitual bipedalism. These included elongation of the hindlimbs relative to the forelimbs, reorientation of the pelvic girdle, including a further shortening of the distance between the sacroiliac and hip joint (acetabulum), and reorientation of most of the musculature involved in locomotion. Theoretically, then, this should mean further constraints on fetal cranial size than those found in quadrupedal primates.

In quadrupedal monkeys, the body weight is distributed fairly evenly between the fore- and hindlimbs. The ilium is an elongated blade that lies parallel to the vertebral column and lateral to it. The ischium is also elongated, toward the tail. Three sacral vertebrae are fused and lie high above the pubic symphysis, so that the fetal head passes the sacrum before entering the main pelvic inlet (Schultz,

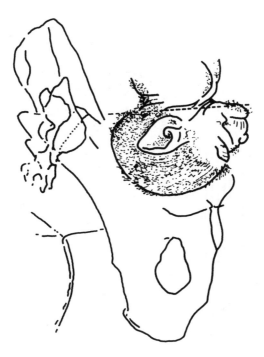

FIGURE 1.4. Passage of the monkey fetal head through the pelvis, lateral view.

1949) (Figure 1.4). In apes, the lumbosacral border is above the pubis, but the five fused sacra extend into the birth canal so that the fetal head passes sacrum and pubic symphysis at about the same time.

The pelvis of a bipedal animal must support more than one-half its body weight, so a less flexible arrangement of the bones is called for. The pelvic girdle in humans is very different from that of other primates: the ilium is shorter, broader, and expanded front-to-back; the ischium is also shorter and broader. The point at which the ilium articulates with the sacrum is larger, providing greater stability and support in this region.

Several other changes contribute to efficient upright posture. As mentioned above, these include the shortening of the distance between the sacroiliac joint and the acetabulum, resulting in a narrow sagittal dimension of the pelvis. Enlargement in the transverse dimensions enables a wider stance in erect posture and places the ischia and related musculature in a better position for functioning bipedally. The entire pelvic brim is inclined toward the sacrum, resulting in improved transmission of weight from the spine to the legs. In humans, the sacrum is directly opposite the pubic symphysis, contributing further to a smaller pelvic inlet. The fetus must thus pass the sacrum and pubic symphysis at the same time (Figure 1.5). Emergence is toward the front of the ischia, while in nonhuman primates, the fetus emerges in a more posterior direction.

In nonhuman primates, the sagittal dimension of the pelvic opening is

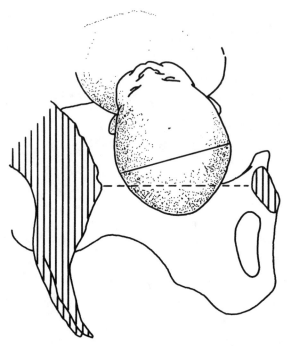

FIGURE 1.5. Passage of the human fetal head through the pelvis, lateral view.

significantly greater than the transverse dimension (Figure 1.6). The infant skull
is also larger in the sagittal dimensions, and the fetus enters the birth canal with
its head oriented in the sagittal plane. Because of the realignment necessary to
accommodate bipedal locomotion in hominids, the pelvic inlet is widest in the
transverse dimension, but the pelvic outlet is widest in the sagittal dimension.
Thus, the human fetal head must enter the birth canal with its head in the oblique
or transverse plane of its mother, but must rotate 45–90° to exit. Although this
feat is usually accomplished with no assistance, it places further challenges on
the process of parturition for our species, in which cephalopelvic disproportion
is not uncommon.

In general, smaller primates have larger neonates and thus have more
difficulties during delivery than do larger primates. For example, neonatal
weights in squirrel monkeys, marmosets, and tamarins are about 14–21% of
maternal weights whereas in Old World monkeys, they range from 4–9%.
Gorillas give birth to infants weighing only 2% of their weight, while human
neonates are less than 6% their mothers' weights (Lynch *et al.*, 1983). Of more
obstetrical importance is the size of the neonatal head. In marmosets and squirrel
monkeys, the cranial length of neonates is approximately one-third larger than
the sagittal dimension of the maternal pelvis. However, these infants are often
born with a face presentation, that is, the face enters the pelvic basin first,
presenting a smaller diameter, although the cephalopelvic fit is still very close

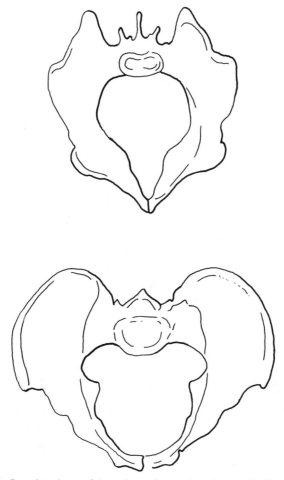

FIGURE 1.6. Superior views of the pelves of a monkey (top) and a human (bottom).

and neonatal mortality is rather high. Leutenegger (1974) notes that abortions, stillbirths, and miscarriages account for approximately one-half of all recorded births for squirrel monkeys and marmosets. They are obviously close to or at the upper limit of brain size at birth.

The course of human evolution has been dominated by two trends: increasing brain size and increasing efficiency of bipedal locomotion. Each of these contributed significantly to the survival and success of our species. With greater dependency on intelligence, coupled with the need for only two limbs in locomotion, hominids have been able to manipulate, modify, and eventually control, to a great extent, the environments they have inhabited.

Unfortunately, these two characteristics of our species are in direct conflict with each other when it comes to childbirth. Encephalization, as argued above, requires an expanded birth canal, whereas efficient habitual bipedalism requires a narrow pelvis. The result of these conflicting requirements is a species with obstetrical problems and mortality related to birth that is rare among undomesticated animal species.

It is clear that bipedalism places upper limits on the size of the neonatal skull that can be passed at birth. Lower limits on degree of brain development for all mammals at birth are imposed by the minimum stage of development that allows survival without placental support. The lower limit is also maintained by the ability of the mother to provide care for an immature infant. All mammals provide some degree of care for infants, thus allowing for a stage of infancy in which brain maturation and learning take place. In general, the longer the stage of infancy, the more learning that takes place; optimally, more learning occurs while the brain is developing than after adult brain size has been reached. For mammalian species in which learning is important for survival, selection has favored birth while the brain is at a relatively immature stage.

If selection is to favor encephalization in a lineage, it must escape the constraints on brain size at birth imposed by the size of the pelvic canal, or fetal brain size development must be decreased even further so that more than the usual amount of growth takes place postnatally. As noted before, this requires modification not only of brain growth patterns but also of maternal caretaking behavior. As we shall see, the only way encephalization could proceed in the hominid lineage was for birth to occur when brain size was less than that of our quadrupedal or brachiating ancestors. Again, as with the placenta type we have inherited, the result of these contrasting selective forces is a more helpless and vulnerable infant than that seen in any other primate species.

It can be argued then, that difficulties during parturition are part of the evolutionary history of all higher primates. These are due primarily to the requisite pelvic size for efficient locomotion, the large size of the neonate relative to maternal body size, and particularly, the relatively large size of the fetal cranium. In other words, as selection favored large brains in most primate lineages, difficulties in parturition resulted. At the hominid–pongid divergence, two different adaptive strategies developed that had an effect on parturition. The pongids embarked on a strategy that emphasized increased adult body size, although the selective pressures operating on that did not simultaneously favor increases in neonatal size. The result was a large pelvis in a large body, a neonate that was thus relatively small, and easy parturition. There are still sex differences in the pelves that, as Leutenegger (1974) suggests, reflect past adaptations when body size in the pongids was smaller than that of modern forms. As body size increased, pelvic dimorphism was maintained allometrically.

Increased body size is a relatively recent phenomenon in great apes, suggesting that, although the constraint on fetal cranial size at birth has been lifted, the expected increase in neonatal brain size has not occurred. One possible explanation for this is Martin's suggestion that a large brain needs high-energy foods, both prenatally and postnatally (cited in Lewin, 1982). Perhaps, then, chimpanzees, gorillas, and orangutans do not have brains so large as ours because they eat relatively low-energy foods. A slightly more simplistic-sounding, but ultimately more complicated, explanation, is that their brains are not so large as ours because they do not need such large brains. Removing phylogenetic constraints is one thing; selection *for* encephalization is an entirely different matter.

At the pongid–hominid divergence, the hominid strategy may or may not have resulted in an increase in adult body size, but selective pressures operating to rearrange the pelvis for bipedalism resulted in a smaller birth canal, still-large neonates, and even greater difficulties during parturition. How these challenges were met will be developed more fully later, but we now turn our attention to the fossil evidence for difficult parturition in the early hominids.

In a typical human birth, the fetus enters the birth canal obliquely, with the occiput against the left pubis (Figure 1.7). This is referred to as "left occiput anterior" (LOA) indicating that the left side of the occiput is at the pubic symphysis in the sagittal plane. Once the head has passed the pelvic inlet, it must then rotate ("internal rotation") to alignment in the sagittal plane so that the longest dimension of the fetal head is now aligned with the widest dimension of the midpelvis. As the head rotates upon entering the midpelvis, the shoulders remain in the oblique or transverse position: Each fetal dimension is aligned with the matching maternal pelvic dimension. This results in a twisting of the neck, but once the head is free of the pelvis, it is able to return to a normal position ("restitution"). The shoulders, however, must follow a similar path in order to emerge: they must also undergo internal rotation, a movement that results in external rotation of the head. The anterior shoulder moves forward under the symphysis, after which the posterior shoulder emerges through flexion.

It should be apparent that a dimension that has not been considered but that may be relevant to the ease or difficulty of parturition is the size of the shoulders. Although the incidence of shoulder dystocia (hindrance of labor progress due to shoulder size) is less than 1% of U.S. births today, it becomes increasingly problematic with larger infants. Oxorn and Foote (1975) note that incidence in infants weighing over 4000 g is 1.6%. If the shoulders are not freed soon after emergence of the head, brain damage and death are likely outcomes. Less dire complications include fracture of the humerus or clavicle or damage to the brachial plexus, resulting in paralysis of the limbs. The mother attempting to deliver impacted shoulders suffers extensive lacerations and, in the absence of anesthesia, extreme pain.

Leutenegger (1972, 1973) has argued that birth was "quick and easy" for australopithecines, as it is in contemporary pongids. He estimates that the range of cranial capacity in infant *Australopithecus africanus* was 110–173 cm^3 meaning that the head dimensions would have been smaller than the estimated dimensions of the pelvis of adults of the same species. STS-14, for example, has a pelvis with a transverse diameter of 99 mm and a sagittal diameter of 85 mm. A newborn chimpanzee with cranial capacity ranging from 139 to 171 cm^3 typically has a head length of 83 mm and head breadth of 71 mm. Thus, even if

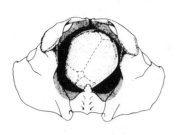
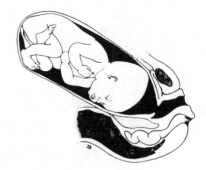

A. Onset of labor.

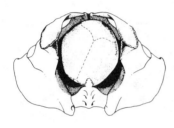
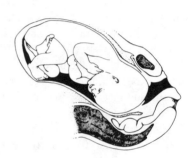

B. Descent and flexion.

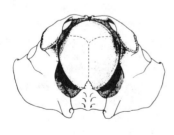
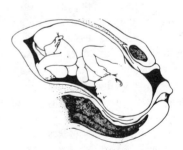

C. Internal rotation: LOA to OA.

FIGURE 1.7. Normal labor and delivery of a human fetus, left occiput anterior (LOA). Reproduced from "Human Labor and Birth," Third Edition by H. Oxorn and W. R. Foote. By permission of Appleton-Century-Crofts, New York. Copyright, 1975.

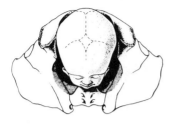

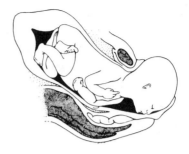

D. Extension.

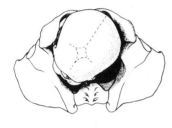

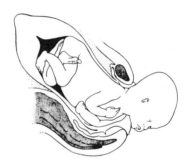

E. Restitution: OA to LOA.

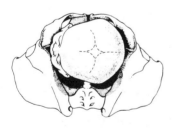

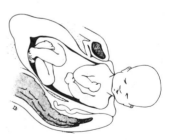

F. External rotation: LOA to LOT.

FIGURE 1.7 *Continued.*

the maximum estimate for cranial dimensions of newborn australopithecines were taken, the head would be smaller than the principal diameters of the STS-14 pelvic inlet. This, of course, assumes that the hominid pattern of prenatal and postnatal brain growth has always been as it is today. Martin suggests that the primate pattern of doubling brain size postnatally would have worked in

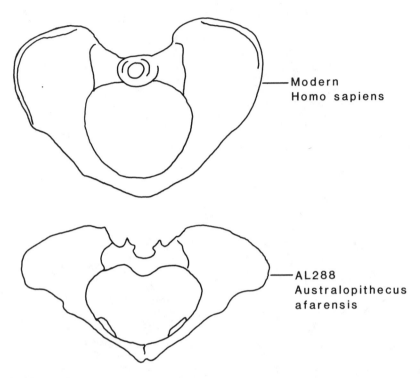

FIGURE 1.8. Comparison of superior views of the pelves of modern *Homo sapiens* (top) and *Australopithecus afarensis* (bottom).

australopithecines, and that their neonates would have been born with brains larger, relative to adult size, than neonates of *Homo* (cited in Lewin, 1982).

Several scholars disagree that birth was easy in australopithecines. In comparing australopithecine pelves represented by the probable female STS-14 (Robinson, 1972) and the certain female AL-288, or "Lucy" (Lovejoy, 1981), and those of modern human females, Berge *et al.* (1984) have found a number of similarities and differences. For example, the australopithecine biacetabular diameter is much larger relative to pelvis size than that of any other primate, including modern humans (Figure 1.8). The result is a large ischio-pubic index: 140 in the australopithecines versus a maximum of 120 in modern females. When the innominate is viewed laterally, the pubis is seen as a continuous straight extension of the ilium while in modern humans the pubis is oriented more perpendicular to the ilium. Overall, the pelvic brim is broader transversely than most modern pelves, resembling what obstetric texts term a platypelloid or flat pelvis (Myles, 1975).

The inclination of the pelvis in australopithecines and modern humans is similar, indicating that emergence of the fetus was/is in a ventral direction and the fetus entered the pelvis in an oblique or transverse position. Berge *et al.*

(1984) have noted that this orientation of the fetus is perhaps a derived characteristic of all hominids, relating directly to the derived characteristic of bipedalism. They further argue that parturition was more difficult for australopithecines although not, perhaps, so much so as for members of the genus *Homo*. Most have argued that the only difficulty of relevance for survival is the ratio between fetal head diameter and maternal pelvic dimensions. Berge and her colleagues add two further difficulties that threaten successful parturition: (1) the flexion of the fetal spine and extension of the head necessary to emerge from the birth canal in a ventral orientation and (2) the series of rotations (internal rotation, restitution, external rotation) that are necessary so that at all times the widest part of the infant is in the relevant widest part of the mother. I would add that, although getting through the bony pelvis is the hardest part for the neonate, the passage through the vagina and other soft tissues poses the greatest hazards to the mother. Third degree lacerations (tearing from the vagina to the anus) are not uncommon in the absence of episiotomies, and unless they are properly repaired and treated, disability and serious infection can result.

Tague and Lovejoy (1985) agree that birth was not an easy process for australopithecines, but they disagree with Berge and her colleagues about the emergence pattern of the fetus. Pointing to the "hyperplatypelloid" shape of the pelvis of AL-288, they agree that the australopithecine fetus would have entered the pelvis in a transverse dimension but would have remained in that position for the entire delivery rather than rotate to an anteroposterior dimension for emergence. The process of asynclitism, whereby the head is tilted during delivery so that the parietal eminences pass the symphysis separately, is the usual way that birth is accommodated in platypelloid pelves of contemporary women (Hickman, 1985). I will argue later that it appears that the typical emergence pattern for nonhuman primates is occiput posterior, whereas for humans, the typical pattern is occiput anterior. According to Tague and Lovejoy, australopithecines are unique among primates in having the fetus emerge entirely in a transverse dimension. This, they suggest, is due to the platypelloid shape which is, itself, a result of selection for improved visceral support in a bipedal animal.

One thing that Tague and Lovejoy have not considered, however, is that this platypelloid shape places even more restrictions on the emergence of the shoulders. Broad, rigid shoulders are apparently homologous for hominids and brachiating apes, but for the latter, whose birth canals are large relative to fetal size, passage of the shoulders is no particular problem. For hominids, as mentioned previously, the shoulders are a relevant dimension that may have required, even in australopithecines, a series of rotations as the fetus emerged from the birth canal. For the broad shoulder to pass through the platypelloid pelvis of "Lucy," the head would have had to turn in an anteroposterior dimension at, or shortly after it passed, the pelvic outlet. Alternatively, if the head remained in a transverse position, the neck would have had to twist sharply, placing the lower body in a position perpendicular to the head. Which of these two patterns was followed would depend, somewhat, on the length of the necks of australopithecine neonates.

In any event, most of the evidence leads to the suggestion that birth was not particularly easy for australopithecines, just as it is not particularly easy for most primates today. However, the constraints put upon parturition as the pelvis was being reoriented for bipedalism were likely enough of a challenge to survival for early hominids. It is not likely that encephalization and bipedalism were under strong selective pressures at the same time. In other words, these opposing forces already mentioned did not act in strong contention with each other until efficient bipedalism had been well established. Thus, the initial challenges that the hominids faced in adapting to bipedalism would have been met through strong selective pressures operating to reconstruct the pelvis with minimal or no pressure to enlarge the pelvic canal for parturition until the reconstruction process had been more or less completed. Later, when encephalization increased its pace in our lineage, it did so in a species that had not only adapted sufficiently to a new mode of locomotion and a new niche but also that had begun to use and depend on tools and live in and depend on social groups.

If parturition was difficult before encephalization, how could it be accomplished in the genus *Homo* without sacrificing efficiency in bipedal locomotion? What options are available to a lineage that is producing infants too large for successful delivery? Leutenegger (1973) suggests that one option is that taken by Callitrichidae, that is, producing twins whose combined size is great relative to the mother's body but who individually can be delivered with little difficulty. Another way to meet the problem of producing young too large to deliver successfully is to deliver them "prematurely" when the fetus has not reached the normal neonatal size. This may well have been the path followed by the earliest hominids. Twinning simply was not an option for animals living in an unpredictable environment with an adaptive strategy characterized by high mobility. To avoid sacrificing efficiency in locomotion, encephalization could increase only with a decrease in the degree of brain growth *in utero* and a resulting more helpless neonate. The birth process became more complicated, but there were others nearby to assist and protect the vulnerable mother and infant. It is therefore likely that living in an extended family group was the key to the development of this strategy. Only in this way could encephalization proceed in our lineage. Social, technological, and behavioral characteristics eventually allowed the hominid lineage to escape the constraints to encephalization imposed upon all primates by the arrangement of the pelvic bones for efficient locomotion.

But pelvic remodeling did not stop with early *Homo*. It has continued even into the present as the contrasting forces of selection for efficiency in bipedal locomotion and parturition continue. As noted, the pelvis of *Homo* is rounded, or gynecoid, whereas the australopithecine pelvis is flat or platypelloid. The pelvic outlet is also wider, relative to body size, than is the outlet of australopithecines (Lovejoy, 1975). This remodeling likely reflected further modifications for efficiency in bipedal locomotion and pressure to alter the birth canal for delivering neonates that had larger brains than those of their predecessors. I will argue later that it was at this point that assistance at childbirth made a critical difference in mortality and morbidity for *Homo* mothers and infants. Not only was parturition more difficult, but the genus became encumbered with a unique need of obligate midwifery. This need was further intensified with encephalization in *Homo erectus* and *Homo sapiens.*

LACTATION

The demands of internal gestation on the female's energy budget depend, to some extent, on the amount of growth that takes place *in utero* and the efficiency of the nutrient delivery system. Weight of the fetus in viviparous animals, relative to maternal weight, ranges from less than 1% for grizzly bears and some marsupials to as high as 64% for the Florida pine snake (Pond, 1977). In general, internal gestation appears to have a more noticeable effect on reptilian behavior than on that of most mammalian females. Pond notes that in later pregnancy, some reptilian females have difficulty moving and eating, while mammals exhibit fewer alterations of behavior, suggesting greater efficiency of the mammalian placenta. For reptilian mothers, however, the demands are over at birth, whereas for mammals, the energy expenditure for the female is generally greater after birth than before birth.

Lactation is a distinguishing characteristic of mammals, and it is closely associated with, and even may have preceded, the evolution of viviparity in that class. As Short (1976) has argued, however, lactation is the weak link in the mammalian reproductive process in that it is far less efficient than the placenta at supplying nutrients to the young. The mammalian mother is confronted at birth with a dependent "parasite" that will grow rapidly and thus need more nutrients, while her ability to provide those nutrients decreases in efficiency. Pond (1977) points out, that, despite the relative inefficiency of lactation, it is still far superior to the alternative: the infant having to forage on its own immediately after birth as do newly hatched reptiles. Again, the cost of lactation is great for the female, as is most of what she does to reproduce, but the survival rate of her offspring is far higher than would be expected if self-sufficiency in feeding were demanded of infants at birth.

Pond also adds that, if the options were to lengthen gestation or lactation, it would be ultimately advantageous to the mother to lengthen the latter in that occasional relief and independence from the young are possible while lactating, but not during pregnancy. The amount and degree of independence from infants depends, however, on the quantity and quality of milk produced in each species. Devorah Miller Ben Shaul (1962), in analyzing the composition of milk of a large sample of mammals, notes that there is no clear pattern according to taxonomic relationships among species (grizzly bears and kangaroos have almost

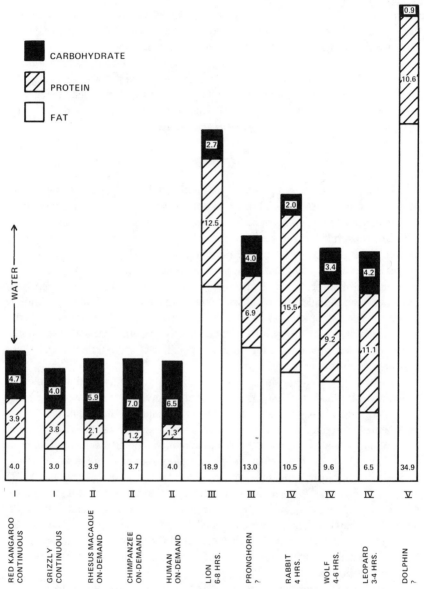

FIGURE 1.9. Carbodydrate, protein, and fat composition of milk of selected mammals. Roman numbers, group number. (From Ben Shaul, 1962.)

identical milk, for example), but that there is a good correlation among nursing behavior, ecology, and milk composition. She delineates five patterns, referring to them as Groups I–V (Figure 1.9). Group I consists of animals that are in continuous contact with their young, including marsupials and species that bear their young during hibernation and, thus, remain with them constantly. Since contact is continuous and nursing takes place at any time, milk is not highly concentrated with nutrients. Group I animals have milk that is low in fat (about 4%) and low in protein (3–8%).

Group II includes mammals that remain in constant contact with their infants, and although nursing is not continuous, it can occur at any time, a pattern known as "on-demand feeding." Most primates are in this group and have milk that is low in fat and protein and relatively high in carbohydrates, especially lactose. Species in which precocial young are delivered, capable of following their mothers and gaining access to the teat almost any time, are also in this category. Milk low in fat and protein is adequate for animals that nurse frequently, grow slowly, and do not need the high fat content for warmth.

Perhaps the most interesting aspect of the milk of Group II mammals is that the carbohydrate content exceeds that of almost every other mammal for whom data are available. The key nutrient for rapid brain growth is lactose, and few other groups of mammals have brains as undeveloped at birth as those of higher primates, especially hominids. Milk with relatively large amounts of carbohydrates has apparently been selected in species that experience fairly rapid brain growth after birth, although not necessarily rapid body growth. By contrast, species in which the brain is almost completely developed at birth do not have milk high in carbohydrates. Seals, for example, experience very little brain growth after birth, and their milk has only a trace of carbohydrates and no lactose at all. Dolphins have less than 1% carbohydrate in their milk, and their infants are well developed at birth.

Group III mammals include those that leave their young in nests or burrows and return at fairly widely spaced intervals to nurse. Their milk is high in fat and protein, allowing the young to be satiated for long periods of time. Predator species such as lions, who must spend several hours in hunting effort, nurse their young at 6–8-hour intervals. Several deer species leave their young in secluded spots and return every 8–12 hours to nurse them. By staying away for long periods of time, a deer mother reduces the chances that her odorless young will be found by a predator.

The giraffe has an unusual feeding pattern reflected in the composition of her milk. For the first 10 days, her infant remains in a secluded spot for 12–15 hours while she forages for food. During that time, her milk is high in fat and protein, reflecting a Group III pattern. By age 10 days, however, the infant can follow the mother and can thus gain access to her teat at almost any time. By this time, her milk is low in fat and protein, and the 10-day-old giraffe is an on-demand feeder, thus belonging in Group II.

Group IV mammals, including rabbits, most rodents, and carnivores, are those whose young are altricial at birth and must be left alone for periods of time while their mothers hunt or forage for food. The intervals between nursing bouts are not so long as those for Group III mammals, so milk is not so high in fat as it is for the lioness who stays away from her young for longer periods.

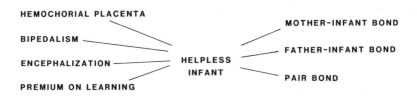

FIGURE 1.10. Factors in human evolutionary history that have contributed to increasing altriciality of the infant.

Finally, Group V includes animals who live in cold, wet environments and require large quantities of fat in the milk to maintain body warmth. In some species, such as the dolphins and whales, nursing takes place under water and must be brief, requiring milk that is highly concentrated. The blue whale, for example, lives in arctic seas and gives birth to a well-developed infant measuring about 7 m in length. Fat content in the milk of this species is as high as 50%.

It is apparent from this brief survey that milk composition fits the feeding styles of mothers and the nutritional needs of infants, and that these characteristics probably evolved together. Although only the major constituents (fats, protein, carbohydrates) have been discussed here, milk is far more finely tuned, with each species having a unique combination of amino acids, vitamins, minerals, and other nutrients. Also, milk composition of all mammals changes as the infants grow older, again reflecting changing needs of the infants themselves. Improper growth or more severe consequences result when infants of one species are fed on the milk of almost any other species.

As a primate, with Group II milk composition, the hominid female has inherited a parenting strategy that, until recent milk substitutes became widely available, required that she be in more or less constant contact with her infant (see Lozoff *et al.,* 1977; Blurton Jones, 1972). For early hominids, leaving a young infant in the care of other group members was rarely an option because of the relatively unlikely event that another lactating woman was available to babysit and serve as a wet nurse. The need to carry an infant while foraging placed limitations on foraging ability, birth rate, and female independence. The social and demographic characteristics of our species thus have been shaped largely by this pattern of delivering relatively helpless infants, requiring frequent feedings and greatly intensified parental care.

INTENSIFICATION OF PARENTAL CARE

Sections of this chapter have described factors in human evolutionary history that have contributed to increasing altriciality of the hominid infant (Figure 1.10). The first was the hemochorial placenta which, because of the close intimacy between the maternal and fetal circulatory systems, resulted in selection for delayed maturation of certain proteins and delayed development of the central nervous system. Accompanying bipedalism was selection for a narrow pelvis that placed upper limits on the size of the fetal cranium that could pass through it at birth. For a typical pelvis of contemporary human females, that limit is 350 cm^3 (Martin cited in Lewin, 1982). As selection favored adult brain size greater than 700 cm^3 (the adult size resulting from doubling of a fetal 350 cm^3 limit), more than one-half of the growth had to take place after birth. Thus, human neonatal brain size, motoric maturation, and other related systems are far less developed at birth than any other closely related primate neonate. Only with intensified parental care in response to greater helplessness of the infant could selection favor the evolution of a large brain in a bipedal animal.

Regulating access to food and other critical resources is certainly as important a part of a species' reproductive strategy as reproduction itself. To be an efficient exploiter of food resources, it is important that a young animal spend as much time as possible learning about the habitat and the optimal ways of locating, processing, and consuming suitable foods. Most primates are efficient exploiters of food resources because of delayed maturation and its accompanying longer period of dependency and learning and a large brain that makes learning even more effective. An important adaptation for social primates is having a long period of time in which to learn physical aspects of the habitat (food, water, places of safety) and behavioral aspects of the social group (mating strategies, dominance hierarchies, predator deterrence, mothering skills).

In subsequent chapters, I shall argue that maternal behaviors in response to neonates at birth and those that lead to the development of a strong mother–infant (and, more recently, father–infant) bond are just as much a part of the human adaptation as our placenta, mode of locomotion, large brain, and helpless infant. Without appropriate responses at birth, none of these last four characteristics would have been successful adaptations. This proposal suggests that there may have been a period of incomplete adaptation in maternal ability to provide care and infant state at birth. There may have been a period when maternal attention was not sufficient to care for more helpless infants with resulting high infant mortality. For a while, a major cause of variation in reproductive success among hominid females may have been differential abilities in bearing, nursing, and parenting helpless infants.

SUMMARY

Before continuing the evolutionary history of birth in hominids, I shall review the heritage of the human female as presented in this chapter. She is a sexually reproducing organism, and each time she reproduces she incurs the costs of finding a mate and the costs of meiosis and recombination. This means that she is able to pass on to the next generation only one-half as many genes as she could if she were an asexually reproducing organism. Presumably this compromise enhances the likelihood that at least some of her genes will survive an environmental change.

The human female also reproduces viviparously. Retaining the embryo in her body entails greater costs, both in a decrease in numbers she can reproduce and in the energy required to maintain the developing embryo internally. The mechanism for supporting the human embryo and fetus is the hemochorial placenta, one which affords a low degree of immunological tolerance between mother and fetus. Thus, the human female cannot carry to term a fetus phenotypically greatly different from herself, and she must be more selective in choosing her mate. Females characteristically deliver a single young in whom is invested much time and energy. Furthermore, this singleton young is born in a state of helplessness that requires intensive caretaking by the mother immediately after birth. This helplessness is a product of two factors: (1) delayed maturation of several systems because of the hemochorial placenta; and (2) decreased relative gestation length because of the narrowed birth canal required by a bipedal animal. This helpless infant, its birth, and the mother's response to it at birth are the subjects of the following chapters. Chapter 2, is an overview of my research on maternal behavior at birth on which subsequent arguments are based.

2

ISSUES RELATING TO THE CURRENT STUDY: THE BIRTH CENTER, MIDWIVES, MOTHERS, AND METHODS

ANTHROPOLOGICAL INTEREST IN BIRTH AND BONDING

John Bowlby introduced attachment theory to the study of mother–infant interaction in a 1958 paper in which he attempted to place certain patterns of the mother-infant behavioral repertoire in an evolutionary perspective. Prior to that time, most studies of this first human relationship had taken a psychoanalytic or a social learning focus and had paid little attention to origins or adaptive significance of any of the behaviors examined. Bowlby, in subsequent works (1969, 1973), argued that the drive to form attachments (which he defined as relationships between two individuals that endure through time) is instinctive in humans, as it is in many other animals. He also offered explanations for ways in which attachment could have been favorably selected in the course of human evolution by placing it in the context of the "environment of evolutionary adaptedness." Only by doing this, he argued, can we understand the adaptive significance of parent–infant attachment. In other words, if we examine the mother–infant bond only as it exists in contemporary settings, we will ask the wrong questions and get the wrong answers about its origin and function. If we examine it in the context in which it was shaped during hominid evolution, we will better see the functions it serves.

An analogy of determining the function of a car submerged in water may be useful. If we try to figure out the purpose of the car in the wrong context, we will determine that the car makes no sense. When we look at the car on the road, where it was designed to function, its purpose and usefulness become clear. It will be argued later that one of the best ways of evaluating the adaptiveness of behaviors seen during the first hour after birth is to ask what function or purpose they served early in hominid evolution. Previous observers of the same behaviors have asked what function they have now, looking for answers in the formation of the mother–infant bond. Sometimes the answers have been wrong, because of the inappropriateness of looking at behaviors only in the context of modern birth and childcare.

In the past two decades, attachment theory and mother–infant bonding have continued to occupy an important place in social psychology and primatology (see Brofenbrenner, 1968; Ainsworth, 1973; DeVore, 1963; Dunn and Richards, 1977). Students of primate behavior quickly became interested in the concept of attachment or bonding with the recognition that the mother–infant bond, rather than male–male dominance, forms the basic axis of social organization in primates (Lancaster, 1975), and that it sets the tone for all other relationships formed during the infant's lifetime (Lancaster, 1975; Hinde, 1974; Harlow and Harlow, 1965). Only recently have anthropologists recognized the importance of the early mother–infant relationship for the development of language, for learning, and for formation of subsequent bonds that form the basis of human social organization. Thus, a shift of focus which has already occurred in the fields of pediatrics, ethology, developmental and social psychology, and primatology is beginning to affect anthropological thinking. Newman (1972:51), for example, has posed the question for social anthropologists: "How does a particular people take a newborn infant and make him a member of their group? What do they do to him and for him to assure that he will survive and that the group identity is firmly imbedded in his consciousness?" Schreiber (1977:379) observes, in her review of *Maternal–Infant Bonding* (Klaus and Kennell, 1976), that "there is a paucity of systematic data on pregnancy, birth, mother–infant and family interaction in nonindustrial, nonurban, nonhospital environments, data that are needed to better understand the role of early social interaction in the development of the infant."

Observations of birth and mother–infant interaction immediately postpartum have been extended to a few other cultures, but this, the traditional domain of anthropologists, has been done in most cases by psychologists (see Ainsworth, 1967; Goldberg, 1977) or physicians (see Brazelton, 1977). In a survey of 296 cultures in the Human Relations Area Files (HRAF) and other reports that contain information on childbirth, I found only 22 sources (19 cultures) that show any evidence of the writer having actually witnessed a delivery. There are several reasons for this, but the primary one is that strangers, especially men, are rarely welcomed at such a ritually important and immodest event as birth. Until recently, most field anthropologists have been men and have had extremely poor luck pursuing this subject. Raphael (1973), for example, relates that one male anthropologist was killed in the Philippines when he tried secretly to observe a birth. At best, anthropologists have relied on informants, and, as a consequence, the information on birth contained in ethnographic accounts is nonexistent, or irrelevant to our present interests, or inadequate, and when present, often inaccurate.

Examples of conflicting information are frequent. Trezenem (1936) reports that among the Fang of West Africa a woman must never see her placenta or she will become sterile. More than 20 years later, Alexandre and Binet (1958) record that the woman who has given birth always buries her own placenta. They further note that, "It is difficult for a man to obtain more precise information on this point since the subject is restricted to women." Another conflicting placenta disposal report is found in Gayton's (1948) description of childbirth among the Yokuts and that of Kroeber (1953). The former states that the afterbirth is buried or placed deep in a stream; the latter states that it is never put in water.

Children or women who have not given birth are not allowed to be present at a Guajiro birth according to Gutierrez de Pineda (1950). Bolinder (1957), however, records that Guajiro children are encouraged to witness the birth and often stay home from school to do so because it was desirable for the family to be together at this time. Titiev (1951) also records a prohibition against children at Araucanian births while Hilger (1957) says children are welcomed.

Certainly variations in birth practices exist in all cultures. Within the same culture, one woman may choose to kneel during delivery, another may squat; different observers reporting on two different women would produce what seem to be conflicting accounts. Thus, more than one birth must be observed in order to describe normal practices and behaviors. All anthropologists are also aware of the great differences between what a member of a group will describe as the cultural norm and what actually happens, and events surrounding childbirth are no exception.

An example of what must be erroneous information, likely based on unfamiliarity with parturition, is the report of Raum (1940) that Chagga women begin to bear down as soon as uterine contractions begin. For a primipara this could mean 12 hours of hard pushing, resulting in a torn cervix, prolapsed uterus, dead baby, and, possibly, maternal death as well.

Margaret Mead's accounts of childbirth provide support for the proposition that only by directly observing a delivery can one obtain adequate information. When she first went to Manus in 1928, a woman who had not given birth could not witness a delivery, so Mead had to rely on informants for her information: "I believed then as I do now, that in fieldwork it is essential not to deceive those from whom one wants to learn the truth. I had never had a child so I saw no births. None of the accounts which I was given told me anything of importance about the way in which a child's introduction to the world foreshadowed its future course of development (Mead, 1956:343)." Indeed, there are only a few paragraphs in her 1928 book devoted to childbirth, and these are rather unremarkable in their content. By contrast, her 1956 account of her return to Manus (after which time not only had she given birth herself, but the restriction against women who had not done so had been removed) contains one of the richest, most complete accounts of childbirth in the anthropological literature, not otherwise devoted entirely to birth.

In five pages, Mead not only notes the activities of the mother, the midwives, and the other attendants but describes in detail the rhythmic sounds of the first few minutes of the infant's life, a rhythm that she then follows and develops for the individual's entire life. This type of information was completely lacking in the accounts of informants, and yet the interpretation she gives it, based on her own observations, provides a key for understanding that culture.

> So from the moment that a Manus baby is born, it is caught into a system which emphasizes the active rhythmic reciprocity with the world about it, deemphasizes differences in size and strength and sex, and stresses its existence as an independent organism. Before the cord is cut, the old woman who takes care of the newborn starts to lull it in time to its own crying so that the sound it makes and the sound it hears are as nearly one as it is possible to make them (Mead, 1956:346).

Witnessing a birth does not guarantee, of course, producing a complete or even accurate description. Only a few of the accounts I reviewed can be considered adequate. These include Hanks (1963) writing about the Central Thai, Granqvist (1947) writing about the Jordanians, Dubois (1944) on the Alorese, Adriani and Kruyt (1951) on the Toradja, Blackwood (1935) on the Buka, Holmberg (1950) on the Siriono, Mead as above, and Hart, Rajadhon, and Coughlin (1965) writing on birth customs in the Philippines, Thailand, and Vietnam, respectively. Recently, anthropologists (primarily women) have devoted much of their research to childbirth, resulting in vast improvements in the information gathered (see, for example, Jordan, 1978; Cosminsky, 1977, 1978; Kay, 1982).

Other than these few exceptions, much of the emphasis in ethnographic accounts of birth is placed on the disposal of the placenta and the handling of the umbilical cord. It is easy to ask about these, and informants usually have a ready answer, even if they themselves have not attended a birth. It is far more difficult to ask and receive answers to more technical questions that are much more meaningful if we are to understand variations in the management of childbirth and the immediate postpartum period. Furthermore, it is impossible to discuss biologically based behaviors without more detailed observations.

In 1978, I undertook a study of birth and immediate postpartum mother–infant interaction in a maternity center in El Paso, Texas (Trevathan, 1980). Although the culture studied was not actually non-Western, the methodology used in the study and the management and environment of the births were typical of those in many less-developed countries. Most of the 110 women who participated in the study were Hispanic. Births were attended by lay midwives in a homelike atmosphere, and no medication was used during labor and delivery. Typically, I arrived when the woman was in active labor, and I was able to observe each mother–infant pair for 1 full hour after birth.

Among other concerns, I was particularly interested in examining maternal behaviors that had been termed "species-specific" by other researchers. These included an orderly progression of tactile contact on first interaction with the infant, holding the infant on the left side of the body regardless of maternal handedness, maintaining eye-to-eye contact with the infant, speaking to the infant in a high-pitched voice, and initiating breastfeeding within an hour after birth. Each of these behaviors will be discussed extensively in Chapter 5.

These five behaviors that have been described as species-specific for human mothers have been interpreted as contributing to formation of a strong mother–infant bond or attachment. Much of the theoretical basis for deriving conclusions about early human attachment has been based on research on nonhuman animals. In human beings, however, there is increased complexity of attachment because of the wide variation in the human experience. Thus, Ainsworth (1977), in reviewing her work with Ganda mothers and infants, suggests that attachment theory be further refined so that when discussing human behavior we talk in terms of "patterns of attachment behaviors." The next step is to determine which patterns or which parts of patterns are specific to all human beings (thus a "human pattern" as distinct from other mammalian patterns) and which are culturally mediated.

In some sense, this is similar to the distinctions made by Kummer (1971) between "phylogenetic adaptations" and "adaptive modifications." By his definition, the former refers to characteristics of the evolving genotype that will be manifested regardless of the environment in which the organism lives. An "adaptive modification," according to Kummer, is a behavior that reflects, to a greater extent, the environment in which the organism develops. A behavior that is culturally mediated is thus an adaptive modification.

Students of animal behavior have suggested that maternal behaviors directed toward offspring immediately after birth are often found universally throughout a species and represent biological mechanisms that trigger maternal–infant bonding, thus ensuring care of the young. The adaptive significance of these behaviors is obvious in that they increase survival of offspring. If there is, as has also been suggested, a characteristic behavior pattern on the part of the human mother when presented with her newborn infant within 1 hour after birth, such a pattern should be observed in natural births throughout the world. The pattern, if it is species-specific, should emerge, regardless of cultural variation. In Kummer's terminology, such behaviors would be phylogenetic adaptations.

On the other hand, most of human behavior is a result of learning, and, at least in the later stages of infancy, maternal attitudes toward offspring vary extensively from one culture to another. Thus, one may postulate that since maternal expectations are largely dependent on cultural patterning, immediate reactions to the neonate may also reflect this cultural patterning. Finally, human behavior is almost infinitely variable, and even identical twins growing up in the same environment have individual and unique experiences. Thus, a mother's reaction to her neonate may be a result of the sum of the influences of her culture, her genotype, and her individual experiences. If this is true, maternal behavior should vary from one mother to another, and patterns will not be discernible. These last two examples would be adaptive modifications.

In essence, then, there are three competing hypotheses about human maternal behavior in the immediate postpartum period: (1) maternal behaviors are more or less universally patterned across the species; (2) behavior varies systematically by such factors as cultural background of the mother, gender of the infant, maternal parity, obstetrical medication or complications, and setting; (3) maternal behaviors vary randomly or with no discernible pattern.

THE SETTING: EL PASO AND THE BIRTH CENTER

El Paso is located in western Texas, on the Rio Grande which forms the border between the United States and Mexico at that point. The state of New Mexico is just west of El Paso and also borders Mexico. Across the river from El Paso is Juaréz, Mexico, a city of 567,365 people in 1980, which is the largest Mexican border city. The entire Juaréz–El Paso metropolitan area has a population of close to one million. The Birth Center (TBC), where this study was conducted, is located in downtown El Paso in "Segundo Barrio," an area of predominantly lower socioeconomic Hispanic residents. It is less than a mile from the bridge that leads into Mexico. The services of TBC are offered to anyone, regardless of legal residence status, as long as they express a willingness to breastfeed. Because of its location and the extremely low cost of maternity care with TBC, most of the clients are Hispanic and most speak little or no English.

For a number of the TBC clients, this was the first pregnancy for which they had received any prenatal care at all. Reasoning that these women were unlikely to seek care elsewhere, the midwives accepted many clients who would be considered high risk and unacceptable at alternative birth centers elsewhere in the United States. Very few items in a medical and previous pregnancy history were grounds for automatic refusal of service, and almost every woman was given a chance to attempt her delivery at home or at TBC. Women with uncontrolled diabetes, pre-eclampsia, active syphilis, and severe pelvic abnormalities were referred to physicians for hospital delivery. Previous cesarean section, abnormal presentation, multiple pregnancy, Rh negative blood factor, grand multiparity, and age were not reasons to exclude a woman from care at TBC, although these women were monitored more closely during pregnancy and labor for signs that hospitalization was necessary. Women as young as 13 and as old as 51 have delivered at TBC. There have been 62 breech presentations, 23 sets of twins, 24 previous cesarean sections, and women with as many as 13 children. The only grounds for automatic refusal of care at the initial application was unwillingness to breastfeed. More recently, however, the midwives in El Paso have experienced more restrictions on their practice. Thus, many of the women who were acceptable as clients at the time this study took place would no longer be allowed to be attended by midwives.

TBC occupies an old, two-storey house with examination rooms, birth rooms, a large living room for classes, and a kitchen and living quarters for students and for mothers and infants who need extended care. During this study period, the midwives were handling about 30 births a month and teaching childbirth education classes 5 nights a week. The clinic was open for prenatal and postpartum care 6 days a week. When TBC first opened, most of the clients sought care in their seventh month of pregnancy. As the popularity of out-of-hospital birth and the reputation of the TBC midwives increased, more and more women began to seek care earlier in their pregnancies.

Typically, after the initial examination, each client returned for prenatal care every 4 weeks until the twenty-eighth week of pregnancy, then every 2 weeks until the thirty-sixth week, and every week thereafter until delivery. Approximately 8 weeks before her due date, a woman and her husband or other family member or friend were assigned to childbirth preparation classes with seven other couples. These included seven class meetings covering such topics as exercises for well-being, relaxation, and concentration; anatomy and physiology of labor and delivery; breathing techniques; contraception and family planning; nutrition; breastfeeding; techniques for labor and second stage; hospital procedures should transport be necessary; complications that can occur; care of the newborn; and films of home and TBC births.

Unless a woman requested otherwise, there were usually four midwives, including trainees, present for the actual delivery. Most women gave birth sitting on the bed, supported by several pillows. If complications were suspected or she had trouble delivering in that position, she was moved to a semi-sitting or supine position on the padded table that was available. If the father or another relative was present, he was encouraged to "catch" the baby once the head had delivered in a normal vertex presentation. Occasionally the mother herself would complete the task of bringing her infant into the world after the shoulders were born.

Every infant was placed on the mother's abdomen immediately after birth, and the umbilical cord was cut when it stopped pulsating. If resuscitation was necessary, it was performed while the baby was held by its mother. After the placenta had been delivered and the woman checked for bleeding and wiped clean, she and the father and their infant were left alone as much as possible for the remainder of their stay. The only routine interruption was an inspection for bleeding every 5 minutes during the first hour after birth. If the delivery and postpartum period were uneventful, the mother and infant could leave the center 3–5 hours after birth.

Postpartum care included a home visit by a midwife on the day following birth and return visits to TBC by the mother and infant on the fifth day and at 2 weeks. At 6 weeks they returned for a final examination, at which time advice was given on contraception, immunization, and future pediatric care.

A sliding scale based on income was used to determine what each client should contribute for TBC services. The minimum was $150 based on an income of less than $3000 per year. The maximum requested was $400 from those who earned, based on their own estimate, more than $11,000 per year. This fee covered all prenatal examinations, all vitamins, childbirth preparation classes, the delivery, and postpartum care. Most of the clients paid the minimum or nothing at all. This low cost was possible because most of the midwives associated with TBC exchanged their services for experience. TBC is a nonprofit organization and depends, to some extent, on private donations of materials and money.

A summary of deliveries that took place at TBC from the time it opened in August 1976 until April 1982, appears in Table 2.1. During that time period, 2695 women registered for and received prenatal care at TBC; 2537 subsequently

TABLE **2.1.** Summary of TBC Births, August, 1976 to April, 1982

Total number of births	2695	
Born with TBC midwives	2537	94%
Vertex	2475	
Breech	62	
Sets of Twins	23	
Born in hospital	158	6%
Cesarean section	61	2.3%
Forceps	18	
Maternal characteristics		
Hispanic	2299	87%
Anglo	344	13%
Age (years)		
Under 18	347	13%
19–25	1411	53%
26–30	582	22%
31–40	280	11%
Over 40	19	
Marital status		
Single	606	23%
Married	1987	75%
Widowed or divorced	53	
Primiparas	908	36%
More than 4 children	366	14%
Fewer than 2 prenatal exams	222	9%
More than 6 prenatal exams	2007	79%
No preparation classes	239	9%
Complete series of classes	1391	55%
Hb less than 11 g/dl	471	19%
Hb greater than 13 g/dl	556	22%
Rh negative mothers	161	6%
Weight gain less than 15 lb	341	13%
Weight gain more than 40 lb	203	8%
Prepregnant weight less than 100 lb	170	7%
Prepregnant weight greater than 160	156	6%
VBAC[a]	24	
Infant characteristics		
1-minute Apgar greater than 8	1044	41%
5-minute Apgar greater than 8	2024	80%
Weight less than 6 lb	269	11%
Weight between 6 and 9 lb	2115	83%
Boys	1325	52%
Girls	1212	48%
Delivery data		
Second stage less than 10 minutes	986	39%
Second stage longer than 45 minutes	334	13%
Blood loss less than 2 cups	1623	64%
Blood loss greater than 4 cups	357	14%
Minor lacerations requiring sutures	823	32%
Episiotomies	88	3%

Continued

TABLE **2.1.** Continued

Complications		
Postpartum hemorrhage	328	13%
Fetal distress	26	
Arrested labor	12	
High blood pressure	13	
Cord problems	16	
Persistent posterior	21	
Abruptio	13	
Problems in third stage	16	
Other	143	
Transport		
Before birth	104	4%
Placenta previa	3	
Cephalopelvic disproportion	25	
Breech	2	
Bad meconium	3	
Abruptio placenta	5	
Failure to progress	33	
Fear, mother's choice	16	
Pre-eclampsia	2	
Bleeding varicosities	1	
Aborting twin	1	
Cervical laceration	1	
Cord prolapse	2	
Prematurity	9	
Premature rupture of membranes	3	
Malpresentation	2	
Postpartum transport of mother		
Postpartum hemmorhage	1	
Placenta accreta	3	
Retained placenta	10	
Other	5	
Neonatal hospitalization		
RDS (respiratory distress syndrome)	8	
Prematurity	8	
Meconium aspiration	2	
Congenital defects	4	
Pneumothorax	1	
Shock	2	
Deaths		
Maternal	0	
Stillborn	11	
Neonatal	10	

[a]Vaginal delivery following cesarean section.

delivered there, while 158 were referred to hospital care before or during labor. Maternal mortality was zero, 11 infants were stillborn, and 10 died during the neonatal period (the first 28 days). Most complications during labor and delivery were handled by the midwives, although women were transported to the hospital for a number of reasons, including placenta previa, cephalopelvic disproportion, abruptio placenta, failure to progress, cord prolapse, malpresentation, and premature rupture of the membranes. Twenty-five infants were hospitalized after birth for reasons including respiratory distress syndrome (RDS), prematurity, meconium aspiration, congenital defects, pneumothorax, and shock. Delivery outcome was usually much more positive: 80% of the infants had Apgar scores at 5 minutes greater than 8. Postpartum hemorrhage was somewhat common (14% of the women who delivered at TBC lost more than 4 cups measured blood). Other complications that were resolved without transport included fetal distress, arrested labor, elevated blood pressure, and cord problems. For most of the women, however, labor and delivery were normal, and pregnancy outcome was positive.

Soon after TBC opened in 1976, the director began accepting students for midwifery training. The basic program consisted of 6 months of intensive classwork, lectures, reading, examinations, observations, and actual experience in labor and delivery under the supervision of a more experienced midwife. Those who successfully completed the first 6 months continued in a 6-month internship either at TBC, at one of the two satellite centers, or with another experienced midwife elsewhere in the country. To complete the internship, a student had to have had primary responsibility for a minimum of 50 deliveries.

I enrolled in the midwifery training program that began in September 1978. One of my primary reasons for doing so was to gain as much insight into the birth process as possible, but it was also a way of gaining access to the women whose deliveries I wanted to observe. I had been trained in the anthropological method of "participant observation" and felt that the only way to understand fully what was going on during labor, delivery, and the postpartum period was to immerse myself as thoroughly as possible in the process by training to become a midwife.

As part of my training, I took part in prenatal examinations and was able to interview prospective mothers about their willingness to participate in the study. To participate fully, a woman had to complete a personal history questionnaire and to agree to my presence during labor, delivery, and 1 full hour after birth. It was also important that she and the infant were available for follow-up at 5 days, 2 weeks, and 4 months postpartum. During the 8-month period over which the study was conducted, one-half of all those who delivered agreed to participate. I have little doubt that had I not been a midwife trainee, becoming a more familiar figure at TBC in the process, I would have had far fewer women agree to participate.

The ability to make accurate observations at the time of delivery and to complete follow-up information depended very heavily on the other midwives with whom I worked. I entered the program with 10 other women, and over the course of the training period, most became supportive of my research. We endured many hardships including infant deaths, the stress of the daily work schedule, hostility from the medical establishment and other midwives, lack of money, and the intense emotional aspects, both positive and negative, of every delivery. In most respects, we worked together as a team, and had I been completely outside that team, working only as a researcher but not as a student midwife, I am sure that I would not have received the cooperation I did.

Most important, perhaps, the training enabled me more accurately to perceive and interpret events surrounding each delivery. Only by knowing what a woman was experiencing physically, could I determine what was a normal reaction to labor and the range of variation acceptable within that definition. I had also been trained to understand emotional aspects of labor and delivery and could see that facial grimaces and writhings did not always mean unbearable pain but were part of the normal hard work necessary for delivering a child.

Being trained as a midwife also enabled me to witness the birth event not only as a "participant observer" but also as a "contributing observer" (Hazell, 1974). If it became necessary, I could, in most instances, offer assistance to the laboring woman or to the midwives attending her. On several occasions, I had to abandon my observations when help was needed. Ultimately, my skills may prove beneficial as I continue observations of birth in other settings. As Hazell (1974) points out, however, becoming a contributing observer carries with it a much higher level of responsibility. Ethical questions which have plagued generations of anthropologists become even more complex when the researcher is a direct contributor to a cultural happening.

MIDWIVES

In the United States and Europe, the status of midwives has fluctuated. They were regarded as witches during the sixteenth and seventeenth centuries, although at other times their position was respected (Forbes, 1966). In the United States, the decline of midwifery during the early twentieth century is associated with the rise of obstetrics and the transference of childbirth to the realm of medicine and the hospital (Devitt, 1977).

"Granny" midwives have been the guardians of childbirth in the United States for decades in the rural South (Mongeau *et al.,* 1960), in Appalachia (Osgood *et al.,* 1966), and in the Hispanic communities in the Southwest (Clark, 1970; Van der Erden, 1959; Schreiber and Philpott, 1978). Traditionally, these women served poor people, usually blacks and other minorities, and women in areas with few or no medical services. Thus, they were little threat to medical professionals, and laws protecting their right to practice in states with sizable minority groups were not challenged until recently. Most of these women were empirical midwives, having learned from other midwives, often their mothers or grandmothers. They had little or no formal education; many could neither read nor write.

Today in this country, we have three more or less distinct groups of midwives. The "grannies" of the South and the *parteras* of the Southwest are still practicing, although their numbers have declined in many areas. A new, fairly well-respected group of professionals, the Certified Nurse Midwives (CNM), has also begun to increase in numbers in recent years. These practitioners are registered nurses with a year or more of specialized training in obstetrics, and usually work within the medical framework. Today there are more than 2000 who are certified by the American College of Nurse Midwives (ACNM), although not all of these are actually in clinical practice. To be certified by ACNM, a midwife must have a current RN license, must have completed a program offered by one of the 24 accredited schools of nurse midwifery in the United States, and have passed the certification examination given by the ACNM. Foreign-trained nurse midwives must take a refresher course before taking the examination.

The third distinct group is a rather amorphous number who refer to themselves variously as "lay," "empirical," "uncertified," or "independent" midwives. Although their practice is legal in only a few states (as of this writing, they include Alaska, Arizona, Connecticut, Florida, Minnesota, Mississippi, New Jersey, New Mexico, Rhode Island, Tennessee, Texas, and Washington) there are well over 2500 of them practicing all over the United States, according to a recent estimate (Vorys, 1977). The midwives associated with TBC are in this third category. For the first 6 months of the study, there were 16 women involved in births at the center: 11 students in their first 6 months of training, 3 interns in their second 6 months, and 2 associate midwives who had completed their training. Of these 16, only 2 had had formal medical training (1 was an RN, 1 an LPN). All were white (non-Hispanic), and none spoke Spanish as her primary language, although 4 spoke it fluently as a second language. The remainder had adequate or minimal facility with the language. All had completed high school, 6 had completed college, and 1 had a masters degree. Their experience was variable and ranged from students who had never seen a birth before enrolling in the program to the director who had had primary responsibility for more than 600 births. Typical of most lay midwives in the country today and unlike midwives of the past and other cultures, they were relatively young, most being in their late twenties. Also, many had never had children.

THE MOTHERS

Every woman who registered for prenatal care at TBC and whose delivery was expected between October 1978 and May 1979 was informed of the "bonding study," as it was called by the midwives, and invited to participate. Since their initial prenatal examination took up to 2 hours, the information sheet on my study and the questionnaire requesting background information were given at a subsequent examination. Volunteers were also recruited during the childbirth education classes. In the 8-month period, 152 women agreed to be in the study, approximately 50% of all those who delivered during that time period. For various reasons, only 110 women were actually observed for behavior relating to birth and mother–infant interaction.

Of the 110 women, 82% were of Hispanic background; 75.5% spoke only Spanish. It was not determined how many were Mexican citizens, naturalized United States citizens, or registered aliens. Many of the addresses on the birth certificates were in Juaréz, and a number of letters sent to El Paso addresses were returned by the Post Office, suggesting that some of those may have been false.

Most of the Hispanic women had annual incomes of less than $3000 and had fewer than 6 years of formal education. The Anglo women were typically of a higher socioeconomic class, and most had at least a high school education. The demographic and cultural characteristics of the women who participated in the study are presented in Table 2.2. Also included in that table is a summary of other variables related to childbirth and mothering behavior, including basis for selecting TBC for care, attitude toward childbirth, and attendance at childbirth preparation classes. The mean age for all women in the study was 23.1 (SD = 4.7) with a range from 16 to 39, a median of 22.4, and a mode of 21. Mean maternal parity was 2, with a range from 1 to 9. Fifty (45.5%) of the women were pregnant for the first time.

As noted previously, there were major differences between the Hispanic and Anglo women other than those attributable to culture. The Hispanic people living along the border have been influenced not only by the culture and value systems of the dominant Mexican population but also by similar factors in the United States population. Many shop and work in El Paso and watch television shows broadcast from stations in the United States. Often the women who were receiving prenatal care from TBC came across the border for exams on "shoppers' passes," and some arrived for the first time in labor, having literally crossed the river border in the middle of the night. After delivering, a number of the mothers and infants were never seen again for postpartum care, a fact presumably related to difficulties in crossing the border. Occasionally, another person would bring an infant to the center for an examination when the mother herself could not cross the border.

Consistently, the sociocultural background (as indicated by primary language spoken) emerged as a factor affecting maternal behavior, as will be discussed in the following chapters. Since ethnicity was also related to income, occupation, and education, however, it is likely that the primary factors influencing behavior were due to poverty, low education levels, and a lower standard of living rather than to differences in cultural background as described by the terms "Mexican culture" or "Anglo culture." The Mexican women were from a lower socioeconomic class as indicated by occupation and income, were more likely to choose TBC because it cost less to have a baby there than in any other maternity care arrangement, and had fewer years of formal education than the Anglo women who participated in the study. These variables are reflected in Table 2.3. This was independently confirmed by the women of Mexican background who were also fluent speakers of English. These women had a high school or more education, tended to have incomes higher than $3000, and most often chose TBC for philosophical reasons. In addition, their behavior during the immediate

TABLE **2.2.** Characteristics of Women in the Bonding Study

Variable	N	Frequency (%)
Language		
Spanish	83	75.5
English	20	18.2
Both	7	6.4
Marital status		
Married	87	82.1
Single	15	14.2
Wid/Div	4	3.7
Age (years)		
<18	15	14.0
19–25	64	59.8
26–30	22	20.6
31–40	6	5.6
Previous pregnancies		
None	50	45.5
One	28	25.5
Two	11	10.0
Three	9	8.2
Four or more	10	9.3
Education		
None	4	4.1
Primary	42	42.9
Secondary	40	40.8
College	12	12.2
Preparation		
No classes	9	9.1
Some classes	23	23.2
All classes	67	67.7
Income		
< $3,000	57	67.9
$3,000–$5,000	15	17.9
$5,000–$10, 000	7	8.3
> $10,000	5	6.0
Occupation		
Labor	57	58.2
White collar	13	13.3
Professional	11	11.2
Other	11	11.2
Student	6	6.1
Why center chosen		
Expense	40	51.3
Philosophy	31	39.7
Religion	1	1.3
Reputation	6	7.7

TABLE **2.3.** Comparison of the Hispanic and Anglo Women

Variable	Hispanic	Anglo	X^2	Significance
Income				
< $3,000	55 (80.9%)	2 (12.5%)	24.72	$p<.00001$
> $3,000	13 (19.1%)	14 (87.5%)		
Occupation				
Labor	54 (68.4%)	3 (15.8%)	15.30	$p<.0001$
Other	25 (31.6%)	16 (84.2%)		
Education				
Primary or less	45 (57.7%)	1 (5.0%)		
Secondary	29 (37.2%)	11 (55.0%)	26.46	$p<.00001$
Some college	4 (5.1%)	8 (40.0%)		
Why center chosen				
Financial	42 (67.7%)	5 (31.3%)	5.63	$p<.02$
Philosophical	20 (32.2%)	11 (68.8%)		

postpartum period more closely resembled the behavior of the Anglo mothers than the other Hispanic mothers.

In general, however, there were a number of examples of maternal behavior that were probably due to the Mexican cultural influence rather than to socioeconomic and educational factors. In Mexico and other nonindustrial, non-Western cultures, the concepts of a woman regarding birth and motherhood are largely shaped by her mother and other older women. This was evidenced in the current study by the 43 (48% of all Hispanic women) mothers who were with their daughters during labor and delivery. A number of other relatives came to visit during the first hour after birth, indicating the importance of the new member to the extended family. In the traditional Mexican culture, childbirth is regarded as a natural event, and medical supervision is not deemed necessary in most circumstances. *Parteras,* or midwives, are called to aid in delivery, and a *curandero* (traditional medical practitioner) is rarely consulted. Because of these attitudes, the type of care provided at TBC was not very different from the way birth had been handled in previous generations of the Mexican women who participated in the study. Most of the women had themselves been born at home or in a *clinica* with *parteras.* Perhaps the practice that required most adjustment for these women was the encouragement by the midwives of the husband's participation in childbirth education classes and in the delivery itself. Very rarely did husbands accompany their wives to the childbirth preparation classes, and they were present at the deliveries in only 43% of the cases.

Counter to this attitude toward childbirth, women in the dominant United States culture are much more heavily influenced in their concepts of maternity by books, professionals, and peers. The tendency is to follow whatever is the current trend, whether it be complete pain-free birth, Dr. Spock's advice on child care, or back-to-earth, natural, organic, additive-free childbirth and child care. Rather than seek advice from mothers and older women, such advice, if offered, is often regarded as old-fashioned and not worthy of consideration. The current trend emphasizes husbands and siblings at birth and little emphasis is placed on any social group beyond the nuclear family. Husbands were present at every Anglo birth in the current study, and siblings were usually nearby, although they were not necessarily present for the actual birth. At only two of these births was there an older woman: one mother of the parturient and one mother-in-law. One new grandmother visited within an hour of birth. There was, in addition to these three, a single exception to the nuclear family group: one young, primiparous woman was accompanied in labor and delivery by her husband, her parents-in-law, her grandparents, her two brothers, her parents, and several friends. Fifty minutes after birth, the entire childbirth education class of which she had been a member came in for a visit.

As mentioned previously, childbirth in the United States is considered an illness appropriately handled in the hospital. This accounts in part for the lack of visitation by older family members who are often opposed to or unaware of the fact that their daughters are giving birth in the attendance of lay midwives. The high mobility of the Anglo population explains this in part, also, although it is not uncommon for mothers to come from elsewhere to assist their daughters upon their return from the hospital after childbirth. The border population of Mexicans may be as mobile as members of the United States population, however, so mobility is not so likely an explanation for who attends births as are attitudinal factors.

Swaddling of the infant is a common practice in Mexican and several other cultures, as is bathing the infant soon after birth. TBC midwives believe that olfaction and tactile contact are important for bonding and, thus, neither bathe the infant nor dress it until the newborn examination, 3 hours after birth. These practices were never commented upon by the Anglo women, but they were almost always challenged by the Hispanic women. Approximately two-thirds of the latter group attempted to keep their infants covered during the first hour compared to fewer than one-half of the Anglo women. One Mexican woman, in particular, after a midwife had uncovered the infant to examine it, got up out of bed, searched for and found a dry towel, and determinedly wrapped her infant tightly in it.

Many of the Mexican infants were brought to the center for follow-up care wrapped in several layers of clothes and blankets, even in the hottest summer months. A scolding by the midwife seemed to have little effect, since the infants would often return 2 weeks later as tightly wrapped. This reflects the Mexican tendency to follow the "old ways." The Anglo women were anxious to follow all of the suggestions of the midwives and usually asked many more questions at the follow-up examinations. This is, of course, partly due to the language differences, but it is also suggestive of the Mexican inclination to seek advice from relatives and the Anglo inclination to seek advice from professionals and books. Although most of the books in the TBC lending library were in English, the few that were written in Spanish were rarely consulted by literate Hispanic women. Almost every Anglo woman had consulted or read one of the popular books on birth and child care.

A common practice followed by the Hispanic women was to give the infant "manzanilla" tea (*Matricaria chamomilla*). The women who gave birth at TBC were repeatedly advised against any supplemental feeding until breastfeeding was fully established, and they were particularly cautioned against the tea, which tends to make the infants somewhat lethargic. When home visits were made on the day following birth, the midwives often found that the tea was being given despite their admonitions. Stronger negative sanctions were usually reiterated at that time; they were often ineffective, as well as could be determined at the 5-day visit. Again, this is evidence that cultural norms outweigh professional advice.

While the Hispanic women may be representative somewhat of the border culture from which they were derived, the same cannot be said of the Anglo women who participated in this study. This further accentuates the differences between the Hispanic and Anglo women in the current study. Most of the Anglo women had planned their pregnancies, all were married and accompanied by their husbands, most chose to give birth at "home" for philosophical reasons, and they were highly motivated to bond to their infants and to do all the "right" things in the first few hours and days after birth. This is the source of criticism of studies of home births in general: home births seem to have better outcomes than hospital births (Mehl, 1976) but only because home birth women are better prepared physically and emotionally, are more cooperative, and are highly motivated for success of the delivery and subsequent bonding. Fortunately for the objectives of this study, many of the women who delivered at TBC did not fit the foregoing description and, therefore, may be more representative of parturient women in general.

One other factor should be considered when examining behavioral differences in the Hispanic and Anglo women: most of the midwives were from the Anglo culture and few spoke Spanish fluently. Thus, some of the differences observed may be accounted for by the different cultural background of the Hispanic women and the midwives who attended them.

METHODOLOGY

Techniques for recording maternal activities in this study were modeled after naturalistic observations of free-ranging primate species and other mammals. Observations were made behind a one-way mirror situated at the end of the bed on which most of the deliveries took place (Figure 2.1). Each mother was observed for 1 hour following birth, the hour beginning at the officially recorded birth time. A master check list was used for keeping track of individual behaviors.

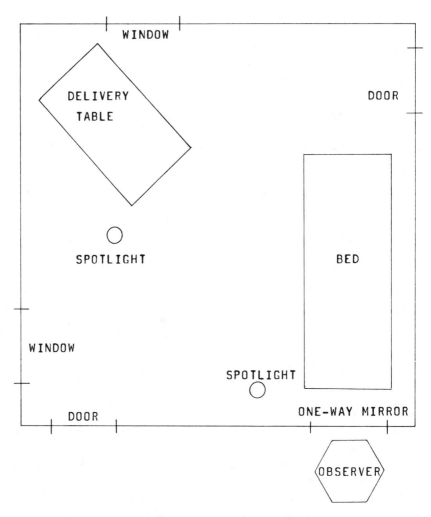

FIGURE 2.1. Diagram of the setting in which observations of mother–infant interaction were conducted. Reproduced from *Developmental Psychobiology* 14:549–558 with permission of John Wiley and Sons, Inc., New York. Copyright, 1981.

In addition, time sampling techniques were used to provide a continuous record of maternal behavior in one 10-minute segment of the first hour. A 10-second time unit was used as the basis of analysis, with observations beginning as soon after birth as the mother was able to devote most of her attention to her infant and I could see well enough to make accurate observations. An attempt was made to begin within 10 minutes of birth whenever possible, but the actual range of tape beginnings was from 1 to 50 minutes after birth. The mean beginning time was 11.3 minutes, and 41 were actually begun in the first 10 minutes.

At each 10-second observation point, the mother's visual and tactile behaviors were recorded. For the visual mode, she was described as (a) looking at her infant, (b) looking at another person or at her own body, and (c) looking away at nothing in particular or with eyes closed. For the tactile mode, her behavior was recorded in terms of what she was doing with her hands in interaction with her infant. These were subsequently transcribed (original observations were made with a tape recorder) and grouped into nine discrete categories: (a) holding the infant with both hands; (b) holding the infant with one hand; (c) not holding or touching the infant although he or she is with her; (d) fingertips stroking the infant's face; (e) fingertips stroking the infant's extremities; (f) fingertips stroking the infant's trunk; (g) palmar massaging of the infant's extremities; (h) palmar massaging of infant's trunk; and (i) infant not with the mother. Although these categories are not all mutually exclusive, a division into discrete categories was necessary for comparisons among the mothers. Thus, a system of precedence was established, and a mother who was holding her baby in one arm and stroking its face with her other hand was recorded as stroking the infant's face. The "holding" categories were recorded only when the mother was doing nothing active with her hands and reflect a more passive interaction with the infant. Since the mother was usually the only one available to hold the infant, doing simply that in the absence of any visual contact with the infant may indicate, in some instances, no more interest in the infant beyond keeping it from falling onto the floor.

The checklist observations were maintained during the 10-minute recording of behavior. Notes on other activities beyond the categories described on the tapes were also made. Thus, when the mother was looking at another person, a record was made of the identity of that person (husband, friend, midwife). Infant-directed behaviors such as smiling at, talking to, kissing, rocking, patting, and nursing were also recorded. These behaviors have been described as attachment behaviors and help to describe the bonding process for each mother–infant dyad.

For the visual mode and the tactile mode behaviors, there were 60 recorded observations. These were important in describing the percentage of total time spent in each activity, but equally important for the purposes of this study was the sequence in which the various behaviors occurred. Thus, the order of activities was preserved as well as the actual number of instances each occurred. In most cases, the 10-minute observation period began with the first exploration ventures of the mother. In more than 55% of the cases, this initial involvement and the taped observations began before the delivery of the placenta. The remainder of the time it began after the woman had been cleaned up and left alone.

A stopwatch was used to record the number of minutes and seconds that a woman spent looking into the infant's face during the first hour. Timing began with the very first eye contact, was recorded in 10-minute segments, and ended exactly 1 hour after birth. When she was looking at the infant below the head, the time was not recorded.

A tape recorder was activated at the moment the infant's head was born and continued until 10 minutes after the actual birth time. The primary purpose of this was to record the mother's voice when talking to or toward her infant, with particular interest in pitch and verbal content.

The newborn examination was given by the midwives 3 hours after birth when the infant was first weighed and dressed. Eye prophylaxis (silver nitrate) for protection from gonococci, which can cause blindness in the infant, was administered at this time. The substance is irritating to the eyes, so the midwives chose to delay its administration until the latest recommended time. In hospitals it is usually administered within a few minutes after birth.

During labor and delivery, a second set of variables was collected that were later tested for effects on attachment and mothering behaviors during the first hour postpartum. These included time of birth, mother's reaction to labor, duration of labor, difficulty of the delivery, presentation, and whether or not artificial oxytocics were administered postpartum. Additional information concerning the infant included Apgar scores at 1 and 5 minutes postpartum, gender, weight, amount of vernix, and time of initial nursing.

Five days after birth, the mothers and infants returned to the center for an examination that included a PKU (phenylketonuria) test on the infant. At this time, the infant's weight and health were noted, and two observations of maternal behavior were made, including her reactions to the PKU test itself and her reactions to the infant's crying. This phase of the study was modeled after the Case Western Reserve study reported by Klaus *et al.* (1972). In the original study, however, the infant was simply examined by the physician, and there is no evidence that pain was inflicted on the infant. The PKU test, performed at 5 days at TBC, required that a midwife puncture the infant's heel with a lancet and squeeze it hard enough to draw sufficient blood for the test. In all instances, pain was apparently felt by the infant and vigorous crying ensued.

The mother and infant returned for a second physical examination at 2 weeks, when again the infant's health and weight were recorded and inquiries were made about breastfeeding. The mothers were also asked about postpartum depression or *demasiado*. At 4 months, letters were sent to all women using addresses recorded on the birth certificates. They were asked to answer questions that were printed on a stamped, self-addressed envelope including questions about the infant's health and breastfeeding status.

ONTOGENETIC AND PROXIMATE FACTORS INFLUENCING MATERNAL BEHAVIOR AT BIRTH AND IMMEDIATELY POSTPARTUM

Although most of this book is concerned with phylogenetic aspects of human parturition, it is important that ontogenetic and proximate factors influencing maternal reactions to birth not be overlooked. Influences on the outcome of pregnancy and the mother's behavior toward her child begin even before conception. Since entire books can be and have been written on these factors, I shall concern myself here only with those that I specifically noted for the women who delivered at TBC. A number of the variables selected for further study were those that previous studies had suggested had an influence on the birth experience. Each of these will be reviewed and their relationship to parturition behavior for the women in the present study, when appropriate, will be elaborated upon in following chapters.

Childbirth Preparation Classes

Numerous studies have reported that taking childbirth preparation classes results in reduced anxiety and more positive feelings about labor and delivery for the woman (see Newton, 1971, for a review of some of these studies). It has been pointed out that, in most cases, women who choose to enroll in childbirth education classes have initially different attitudes toward birth. Since childbirth preparation (a series of seven classes) was required by the midwives in the current study, regardless of the desire for such on the part of each woman, it was reasoned that the actual amount of preparation would be independent, to some extent, of initial motivation. A greater percentage of the Anglo women completed the series (83%) when compared with the Hispanic women (64%), but the differences were not statistically significant.

Reason for Choosing Care with Midwives

Perhaps a better indicator of initial attitudes toward childbirth is the basis for choosing to deliver with midwives. Those who chose such for philosophical reasons would, perhaps, be more highly motivated toward a positive birth and bonding experience than those who came for financial reasons. Total costs at TBC are about 15% of costs for prenatal care and delivery with local physicians. In effect, since there is no collection agency to force payment, the care is free for some women. Also, most of the women who deliver at TBC have no health and maternity insurance coverage. The primary reason that the center was chosen by most of the women in this study was financial. Not surprisingly, however, since income and occupation have some effect on why TBC was chosen for the birth, this factor was not independent of sociocultural background ($X^2 = 5.63, p <$ .02). One motivating factor for the Mexican women may have been desire for the child to be born in the United States, but that was an issue I chose not to raise with these women.

Attitude toward Childbirth

The mother's attitude toward childbirth, whether frightened, somewhat apprehensive, or excited with no fear, was expected to have some effect on her birth experience. Attitude toward childbirth was independent, in this sample, of sociocultural background and parity.

Obstetrical Medications

Obstetrical medication results in depression of respiration, decreased activity, lowered temperature, and poor sucking response in the neonate in the immediate postpartum period. This means an infant is less responsive to his mother's attention, which, in turn, may result in a decrease in her mobilization to form attachment (Brazelton, 1961). Reciprocal interactions are important in forming attachment, and a mother who receives little or no response from her newborn is unlikely to continue her efforts at interaction. Klaus and Kennell (1976:79) refer to this principle as "you cannot fall in love with a dishrag." The infant, who, when maternal medication is not used, is in the quiet alert state for 45–60 minutes of the first hour after birth (Desmond *et al.*, 1966) may not enter that state for several days after a medicated birth.

Medication was not used during labor and delivery for any of the births that took place at TBC during the time of the current study. An artificial oxytocin was administered intramuscularly postpartum by the midwives if the mother was in danger of losing too much blood. The administration of this hormone appeared to be associated with reduced time spent looking at the infants *en face* and reduced time spent in such activities as patting, rocking, stroking, talking to, rubbing, and encompassing the infant. The hormone produces more than the usual cramping, which would draw the mother's attention away from her infant. Because the hormone was only administered for excessive bleeding, however, the apparent association actually may indicate the effects of heavy bleeding on visual and interactive behavior rather than the effects of the hormone itself.

Parity

Parity has a potential impact on maternal behavior through several channels. For primiparas, labor and delivery are usually longer, uncertainty is probably greater, and there is no previous experience with neonates upon which to draw. Many observers of nonhuman primate deliveries note significant differences in behavior and reactions to neonates in primiparas compared to multiparas. Neonatal mortality is generally much greater for first-borns because of their mothers' inexperience with young infants.

Thoman *et al.* (1971, 1972) found that multiparous human mothers are more sensitive to their infants' needs than are primiparous mothers. Their studies revealed that, although primiparous mothers spend more time in feeding and nonfeeding activities with their infants, they are less successful than multiparous mothers at getting their infants to feed and recognizing when their babies are ready to nurse. Experience undoubtedly enhances confidence in caretaking ability, perhaps enabling the mother to be less uncertain in her early interactions with her infant. De Chateau (1976) noted, however, that several minutes of "extra contact" with the newborn can result in a primiparous mother behaving in a way similar to that of a multipara with more experience. Thoman's subjects did not have this "extra contact." In the current study, maternal parity (primiparity or multiparity) was related to amount and pattern of touching and timing of initial breastfeeding. Amount of time spent *en face* and verbal interaction were independent of parity.

Gender of the Infant

There is evidence that maternal behavior varies with gender of the infant. Moss (1967) found that mothers held and attended male infants about 35 minutes more per 8 hours when the infants were 3 weeks of age and 11 minutes more per 8 hours at 3 months of age when compared with mothers of female infants. Leiderman *et al.* (1973), however, report no differences in maternal confidence in caretaking relating to gender of the infant. De Chateau (1976) found that there were marked differences in maternal behavior directed at boys: mothers spent more time smiling at and maintaining close body contact with male infants than with female infants. Lewis (1972) reports similar results from his study of 32 infants. Newborn males seem to have greater muscular strength and vigor and are larger and sturdier (Garn, 1958), perhaps making their mothers less hesitant to handle them.

In the present study, infant gender was related to tactile behavior in that mothers of males spent more time in exploratory touch than did mothers of females (see Chapter 5). Visual and verbal behavior were independent of gender.

Information was obtained from the women before birth regarding the desired gender of the child. Some of the women had no stated preferences, but of the 54 who did, 31 (57.4%) desired a boy and 23 desired a girl. The only variable that was significantly associated with gender desired was parity. Of the primiparas, 15 wanted a boy, whereas only 4 expressed a desire for a girl. Of the multiparas, 16 desired a boy while 19 desired a girl ($X^2 = 4.29$, $p < .05$). There were no differences in gender preferences according to the mother's sociocultural background.

One of the philosophical goals of TBC midwives was allowing the mother or another family member to discover the gender of the child. Often the mothers asked about the gender shortly after birth, but the midwives, having been advised not to tell, usually responded that they did not know. Even when the gender of the infant differed from that desired, the mother seemed excited when she first determined the child's gender. The sense of discovery may be an important part of the bonding process.

The time that the mother first noted the gender of the infant was determined in 87 cases. Of the mothers, 32 (37%) noted the gender immediately (within 1

TABLE **2.4.** Mother's Immediate Reaction to Her Newborn Infant

	Present study		Newton and Newton, 1962	
	N	Frequency (%)	N	Frequency (%)
Greatly pleased	30	27.5	157	31.9
Smiles a little	45	41.3	263	53.5
Indifferent	32	29.4	65	13.2
Disgusted	2	1.8	7	1.4
Total	109		492	

minute) after birth. Between 1 and 5 minutes after birth, 38 (44%) did so, 13 (15%), between 5 and 15 minutes after birth, and 4 did not seem to know their infants' genders until more than 15 minutes after birth. The time when she first noted the infant's gender was significantly associated with sociocultural background. Two-thirds of the Anglo women noted the infant's gender immediately, while less than one-third of the Hispanic women were aware of the gender within 1 minute of delivery ($X^2 = 10.56$, $p < .05$).

Birth Environment and Location

Newton and Newton (1962) observed that the birth environment and the course of labor and delivery influenced the attitudes of a mother toward her newborn. They studied the immediate postpartum reactions of 634 women, 159 of whom were judged to be greatly pleased at the sight of their infants and 72 of whom were judged to be indifferent or disgusted. These two groups were then compared using 50 social, psychological, and medical factors and were found to differ in 13 ways that were statistically significant. Of importance to the current study, women who experienced a calm, relaxed labor, with emotional and physical support from hospital personnel, showed far more joy at the sight of their infants than did women for whom labor was painful and frightening.

The measures I used of the mother's immediate reaction to her infant were derived from the study by Newton and Newton (1962): Mothers were described as "greatly pleased," "overwhelmed but smiles a little," "overwhelmed and seems uninterested," or "disgusted." The frequencies for the four categories in this study are somewhat different from those in the Newton's study as shown in Table 2.4. The categories "indifferent" and "disgusted" were collapsed into a single category for analysis in both studies. Following the Newtons' example, the groups showing the maximum contrast were studied (i.e., the "greatly pleased" group was compared with the "indifferent" or "disgusted" group with regard to other variables).

The Newtons found that women who were calm and cooperative during labor were more likely to be greatly pleased at the first sight of their infants than were

TABLE **2.5.** The Effects of Presence of Family Members on the Mother's Immediate Reaction to Her Infant

Variable	Greatly pleased	Indifferent or disgusted	X^2	Significance
Husband present	24 (71%)	10 (29%)	14.41	$p<.0001$
Husband absent	6 (20%)	24 (80%)		
Family members present	27 (55%)	22 (45%)	4.36	$p<.05$
Family members absent	3 (20%)	12 (80%)		

women who moaned, squirmed, and were uncooperative. In the study done at TBC, the mother's reaction to her child was independent of her reaction to labor (i.e., calm, average, upset). The Newtons also found that women who established good emotional rapport with attendants were more likely to be greatly pleased at first sight of their infants. In the current study, a related phenomenon was noted: The presence of the husband and other family members significantly affected a woman's first reaction to her infant, as can be seen in Table 2.5.

Duration of labor, the presence of a midwife fluent in the mother's language, and the degree of difficulty of the birth, all variables that were expected to affect her immediate reaction to her infants, actually had no significant effects on that reaction. A number of other background variables, most of which were related to sociocultural background, appeared to be related to her immediate reaction. For the 13 Anglo women on whom a judgment was made, all seemed greatly pleased at first sight of their infants. Two-thirds of the Hispanic women, however, were judged to be indifferent or disgusted ($X^2 = 15.91$, $p < .0001$). Such a difference immediately suggests that the rater, myself, was more likely to report the socially approved behavior of "greatly pleased" when the women were more like me, a problem pointed out by the Newtons who had white observers rating black women on these same points. Thus, the same analysis was performed using only Hispanic women. For this group alone, presence of the husband ($X^2 = 4.46$, $p < .05$) and choosing the maternity center for philosophical rather than financial reasons ($X^2 = 17.50$, $p < .01$) continued to be significantly associated with immediate reaction to the infant. In addition, the presence of a midwife fluent in Spanish was positively associated with the mother's immediate reaction to the infant ($X^2 = 3.79$, $p < .05$).

Jordan (1985) has recently pointed out that the expectation that a woman and her attendants experience joy at the birth of the infant may not be common in most cultures. She suggests that an immediate reaction of joy (greatly pleased) may be the result of cultural training in the United States. In her observations of births in France, Germany, Holland, and Yucatan, the more common reaction seems to be a period of indifference while the woman recovers from the exertion of the delivery. We can perhaps conclude, then, that the Anglo women I observed had been culturally well trained and thus exhibited more signs of joy at birth. The Hispanic women were more variable in their reactions: One group reacted positively, perhaps in response to the culturally appropriate sounds of joy emitted by the Anglo midwives; another response was the period of indifference that Jordan suggests is more likely the "natural" response.

The Father's Role in Labor and Delivery

Westbrook (1978) found that women who had positive marital relationships were more likely to have positive childbearing experiences and feel greater maternal warmth than women with negative marital relationships. The participation of the father in labor and delivery is a fairly recent phenomenon in our culture and is somewhat uncommon throughout the world. Today, primarily due to consumer pressure, it is usually possible in the United States to find a physician and hospital that will allow a husband to be with his wife throughout labor and delivery. A number of childbirth preparation methods, including Lamaze and Bradley's Husband-Coached Childbirth, encourage the husband's presence at birth as a way of alleviating pain, anxiety, and complications. Several studies support the notion that attendance of fathers at birth facilitates delivery and enhances bonding between mother and child, and, in addition, provides optimal opportunity for fathers to bond to their infants. Fathers who participate in birth also participate more in later caretaking of infants (Manion, 1977). In today's highly mobile nuclear families, child care by the father may be the only relief the mother has; thus, it is adaptive to enhance his interest and confidence in infant caretaking by allowing him to attend the birth of the child. In other cultures where female relatives are nearby, there are many others to assist the mother, and paternal care may not be so critical. This was probably true in the past, as well.

In the current study, husbands were present at 53% of the births and were absent or nonexistent (in the case of unmarried women) for the remainder. Although husbands were always encouraged to attend births, many chose not to be present. Of the variables that were associated with husband's presence or absence during delivery, the most significant was sociocultural background. All of the Anglo fathers were present at delivery, while fewer than one-half (43%) of the Hispanic fathers were present [it should be noted that all of the Anglo women were married, while 15 (14%) of the Hispanic women were unmarried]. Women who had chosen to deliver with midwives for philosophical reasons and those who described their relationship with the father of the child as "good" were more likely to have their husbands with them at delivery than those who chose TBC care for financial reasons and those who had problems in their relationship with the father of the child (Table 2.6). These associations are not

TABLE **2.6.** Factors Associated with Father's Presence or Absence at Birth

Variable	Present	Absent	X^2	Significance
Education				
Primary or less	16 (35.6%)	29 (64.4%)		
Secondary	25 (62.5%)	15 (37.5%)	11.36	$p<.01$
Some college	10 (83.3%)	2 (16.7%)		
Language				
Spanish	38 (42.7%)	51 (57.3%)	19.30	$p<.00001$
English	20 (100%)	0		
Income				
<$3,000	23 (40.4%)	34 (59.5%)	10.86	$p<.001$
>$3,000	22 (81.5%)	5 (18.5%)		
Why Center chosen				
Financial	20 (42.6%)	27 (57.4%)	4.98	$p<.05$
Philosophical	22 (71.0%)	9 (29.0%)		
Relationship with father of the child				
Good	43 (66.2%)	22 (33.8%)		
Some to many problems	10 (35.7%)	18 (64.3%)	6.21	$p<.05$

surprising in light of the evidence that in much of Mexico, maternity, related events are primarily female activities, and, even in the United States, the emphasis on family bonding during and immediately after delivery is a product of the well-educated, highly motivated parturient population.

In the current study, the presence or absence of the father appeared to have an effect on the mother's attitude in the first hour after birth (positive or negative) and the time at which the child's gender was first noted. Women whose husbands were present were more likely to have immediate reactions to the child that were described as ''positive'' and were more likely to note the gender of the child within 1 minute after birth (Table 2.7). There was no evidence that the presence of the father contributed to an easier delivery or more relaxed labor, as previous studies have suggested.

Apgar Score

The infant Apgar score, developed by Virginia Apgar (1953), is a method of quickly evaluating infant well-being immediately after birth. It is usually determined at 1 minute and at 5 minutes after birth and was done routinely at TBC. Five vital signs are evaluated and scored according to the technique in Table 2.8. A score of 7–10 indicates a vigorous infant, a score of 4–6 indicates a depressed infant, and a score below 4 is cause for concern. Normally the Apgar at 5 minutes is higher than that at 1 minute. Table 2.9 lists the Apgar scores at

TABLE **2.7.** Associations between Father's Presence or Absence at Birth and Labor and Delivery Variables

Variable	Present	Absent	X^2	Significance
Mother's reaction to labor				
Calm	17 (42%)	19 (53%)		
Average	31 (66%)	16 (34%)	5.86	$p<.05$
Upset	10 (39%)	16 (62%)		
Mother's attitude in first hour after birth				
Positive	51 (58%)	37 (42%)		
Negative	5 (28%)	13 (72%)	4.32	$p<.05$
Atmosphere in room				
Calm, quiet	9 (30%)	21 (70%)		
Moderate	35 (66%)	18 (34%)	10.07	$p<.01$
Tense, loud	14 (56%)	11 (44%)		
Noted child's gender				
Immediately	24 (75%)	8 (25%)		
1–5 minutes	16 (42%)	22 (58%)	11.70	$p<.01$
Plus 5 minutes	5 (29%)	12 (71%)		

TABLE **2.8.** Apgar Scoring Technique

Sign	0	1	2
Color	Blue, pale	Body pink, extremities blue	Completely pink
Heart rate	Absent	Slow and <100	Over 100
Reflex irritability	No response	Grimace	Cry
Muscle tone	Flaccid	Some flexion of extremities	Active motion
Respiratory effort	Absent	Slow, irregular	Good, crying

1 and 5 minutes for the 110 infants in this study. Although these scores are not technically at the interval level of measurement, the mean for 1 minute was 7.4 and the mean for 5 minutes was 8.9 for the infants in this study.

SUMMARY

The reproductive and parenting strategies inherited by the hominid female have been discussed in Chapter 1. In Chapter 2, I have described a sample of 110 contemporary hominids delivering infants under conditions that only imperfectly approximate those under which human females have given birth for

TABLE **2.9.** One-and Five-Minute Apgar Scores

Score	Apgar 1 minute		Apgar 5 minute	
	N	Frequency	N	Frequency
1	6	5.5	0	
2	5	4.5	0	
3	3	2.7	2	1.8
4	1	.9	1	.9
5	2	1.8	2	1.8
6	5	4.5	2	1.8
7	11	10.0	3	2.7
8	31	28.2	14	12.7
9	39	35.5	51	46.4
10	7	6.4	35	31.8

the last several thousand years. Observations of these women provide clues to the behavior of females giving birth without medication and with minimal technological intervention. Because mothers and infants were not separated at birth, observations of their behaviors during the first hour postpartum also provide clues to what human mothers and infants may typically do when they meet each other for the first time. The next chapters include, among other things, the results of these observations.

3
THE PROCESS OF PARTURITION

In order to elucidate the differences between birth in human and nonhuman primates, a brief survey of physiological, biochemical, and behavioral aspects of labor and delivery in representative species will be presented. These cross-species comparisons will facilitate the development of an evolutionary perspective on human birth. Cross-cultural comparisons will also be offered to present the universal and particularistic aspects of birth in the human species.

PHYSIOLOGY AND BIOCHEMISTRY OF LABOR AND DELIVERY IN HUMAN BEINGS

Labor in human beings is defined as the entire process, beginning with noticeable uterine contractions, that leads to the delivery of the infant and the placenta. It is usually divided into three stages: The first stage is the period during which cervical dilation takes place. It begins with the onset of uterine contractions and ends at full dilation when the cervix is no longer felt as distinct from the lower uterine segment. The cervical diameter at complete dilation is arbitrarily given as 10 cm, although the actual range may be from 7.5 to 13 cm. In general, cervical dilation proceeds slowly at first (sometimes referred to as the "latent phase") and progresses rapidly during the last few hours of the first stage (sometimes referred to as the "active phase"). The average rate of dilation during this phase is 1.2 cm per hour for primiparas and 1.5 cm per hour for multiparas. In primiparas the length of the entire first stage is usually given as 11 hours and in multiparas, as between 6.5 and 7.2 hours (Friedman, 1978).

During the second stage of labor, the fetus completes its descent through the pelvis and is expelled from the uterus. Contractions are stronger and more frequent, and a woman usually feels the urge to push or bear down, involving abdominal muscles and the diaphragm in the expulsive effort. The second stage usually lasts from .75 to 1.1 hours for primiparas and .32 to .39 hours for multiparas (Friedman, 1978; Myles, 1975). The third stage begins at delivery and ends when the placenta is expelled. Its usual duration is about 15 minutes.

It is uncertain what signals the start of labor in mammals, although it is likely related to a complex of events and factors including hormonal changes, pressure of the presenting part of the fetus on the cervix, irritation of the uterus, placental changes, and signals from the fetus itself. Three systems mature during the process of gestation: the maternal system, the fetal membranes, and the fetus itself. In normal pregnancy, there is likely a complex interdependency among these three systems, so that labor begins when all have reached maturity. In sheep, it is known that the fetal system dominates, and that signals from the fetal pituitary and adrenals initiate labor. Which of these three systems is dominant in human beings? Does labor begin with changes in maternal hormones? Does the fetus itself signal its readiness to be born? Or do the fetal membranes mature to the point that labor is triggered? Unfortunately, although a great deal of research has been done, there does not appear to be an easy answer to the question of what triggers normal labor in our species.

Irregular uterine contractions occur in all mammals in late pregnancy, but the contractions of true labor are distinctive in their regularity and synchrony. This synchrony, which leads to the expulsion of the fetus, is possible because, at the time of labor onset, gap junctions between myometrial cells are completely formed, resulting in communication pathways throughout the uterus (Fuchs and Fuchs, 1984). The role of estrogen in initiating labor appears to be a facilitatory one in that this hormone plays an important role in formation of these gap junctions. Estrogen, the Greek root of which means "mad desire to produce," is also responsible for maintaining growth of the myometrium and, once labor has begun, is a factor in stimulating contractions of the myometrium. The term actually refers to three separate hormones, estradiol, estrone, and estriol, with similar functions and properties. They are secreted by the ovaries and are active during the menstrual cycle and pregnancy. High levels of estrogen are found at ovulation and at the very end of pregnancy and appear to greatly reduce pain sensitivity (Sadow, 1980). The increased production during late pregnancy is a product of the placenta.

Along with estrogen, the hormone progesterone (Greek, "in favor of gestation") acts to keep the uterus in a quiescent state during pregnancy. The hormone is produced at all times in the normal ovulating female and ranges in amount from 3 to 20 mg per day in the nonpregnant state, rising at ovulation. By midpregnancy, production reaches 75 mg per day, increasing to 250 mg per day in late pregnancy; most of the increase is due to production by the placenta. Before delivery, progesterone production drops precipitously in most women, thus withdrawing its inhibitory effect on estrogen and suppression of uterine contractions. Presumably, these hormonal changes play a role in determining the end of gestation, and yet they are not essential for triggering labor since they do not occur in all women.

Women with twins or excessive amniotic fluid (polyhydramnios) often begin labor earlier than those with normal single infants, suggesting that the simple stretching of the uterus may be responsible for the initiation of labor contractions. Other candidates for the trigger include placental aging, any emotional or physical disturbance at term, and the biorhythms of the menstrual cycle: labor begins 40 weeks or 10 cycles after conception.

The role of the fetus in initiating labor has been argued, based on laboratory studies in which the fetal pituitary has been removed, resulting in a delay in the onset of labor. Further evidence of the initiation role of the fetal pituitary under natural circumstances comes from observations of a herd of sheep in which birth was delayed considerably so that many of the ewes died attempting to deliver oversized lambs. The lambs were subsequently found to have underdeveloped adrenal glands and malformed or absent pituitaries. The cause was traced to skunk cabbage or false hellebore (*Veratrum californicum*), an item in the diet of the ewes, that was found to contain a chemical responsible for the maldevelopments (Hogarth, 1978).

When the lower uterine segment and cervix are stimulated, nerve impulses are sent to the posterior pituitary, and oxytocin (in the Greek, "swift birth") is released into the bloodstream. Its primary purpose during parturition is the stimulation of uterine contractions that lead to delivery of the fetus. It has a similar role in other mammals and is responsible for expulsion of the egg in birds and the spawning reflex in some fish. Blood levels of oxytocin in chickens appear to reach a peak just before an egg is laid. This hormone and progesterone act to stimulate muscle contractions in the uterus and vagina, usually resulting in the laying of an egg. In one experiment, obstetrical oxytocin was injected into a hen inducing her to lay an egg prematurely in less than 4 minutes, likely as a result of the hormone's ability to induce uterine contractions.

Although there is no doubt of the major role of oxytocin in stimulating and maintaining uterine contractions, evidence of its role as a trigger of labor has only recently been gathered. It was expected that if oxytocin was the trigger, a rise at the onset of labor would be detected; in humans, that expected rise does not occur (Hogarth, 1978). Characteristically at the beginning of labor, however, the number of oxytocin receptor sites reaches its maximum, suggesting that, although there has not been a dramatic increase in maternally produced oxytocin, there are now enough receptors so that minimal increases trigger contractions. It appears that oxytocin-induced uterine contractions are not sufficient for dilation of the cervix without prostaglandins, the production of which may itself be stimulated by oxytocin. The effects of prostaglandins are in turn enhanced by the production of prostaglandin receptor formation facilitated by progesterone. Prostaglandins, particularly $PGF_{2\alpha}$, appear to be important in maintaining uterine contractions during labor.

Recently, the role of the fetus in initiating human labor has been reaffirmed by the study of oxytocin concentrations in the umbilical cord. At delivery, the oxytocin levels in the umbilical artery are consistently higher than those in the umbilical vein, indicating greater passage from the fetus to the mother than vice versa (Hogarth, 1978). In anencephalic births, there is no oxytocin in the vein or arteries of the umbilical cord. It has been suggested that the sequence of events leading to regular uterine contractions begins with this fetally produced oxytocin which, at term, finds a sufficient number of oxytocin receptors in the myometrium (Fuchs *et al.,* 1982).

A summary of the current view of the endocrinology of labor as seen by Fuchs and Fuchs (1984) is as follows: Progesterone and estrogens play facilitatory roles in the development of oxytocin receptor sites, in the formation of gap junctions between myometrial cells, and in the formation of prostaglandin receptors. Once these three developments have reached appropriate levels, oxytocin present at existing concentration triggers regular, synchronous uterine contractions. $PGF_{2\alpha}$, in sufficient concentration, is necessary for the continuation of labor contractions and for cervical dilation. The fetus may play a role as coordinator of these processes through its mechanical effects on the uterus, leading to increased production of placental estrogen. In addition, it is likely that secretion of neurohypophyseal hormones by the fetus stimulates prostaglandin synthesis. Labor is a positive feedback mechanism: once it has begun, it must continue, building up progressive speed. This process is depicted in Figure 3.1.

The uterus is the largest muscle in the human female body, exerting an average of 30 pounds of force during contractions of labor. When a woman begins to push with contractions of the second stage, her efforts can double that pressure. Before labor, the uterine muscle is about equal width from the fundus to the cervix. During pregnancy, the cervix is thick and closed, but toward the end it becomes shorter and begins to efface, or thin. At the beginning of labor, it is said to be ''ripe'' if it is soft, less than .5 inches long, admits a finger, and is dilatable. During the latent phase of labor, cervical softening and effacement occur, but dilation is slow. When the rate of dilation increases and progresses steadily, usually from 4 to 10 cm, the parturient is said to be in the active phase of labor.

During contractions, the uterus gradually thickens at the fundus and thins at the cervix, resulting in dilation and effacement. The contractions are longest and hardest in the fundal region and move down to the cervix. They occur approximately two to five times every 10 minutes, becoming more frequent as labor progresses. Intensity also increases, but the duration of each contraction changes very little, varying from 45 to 90 seconds. In general, the stronger the contraction, the longer it lasts.

If the stages of labor significantly exceed the limits given above, labor is said to be abnormal. Labors less than 3 hours are often referred to as ''precipitate''; the acceleration usually takes place during the active phase. Abnormally long labors may be due to a prolonged latent phase, slow dilation during the active phase, or arrested dilation or fetal descent. Prolonged labors appear to be related to, among other things, early rupture of the membranes and excessive sedation. There is little evidence of correlation between prolonged labor and maternal age or size of the newborn. Arrested dilation (2 hours with no progress during the active phase) in multiparas is more likely among older women with larger babies. No such associations have been observed in primiparas with arrested dilation (Friedman, 1978).

The factor that has the most consistent influence on the length of the first two stages of labor is maternal parity. In general, the length of the first stage

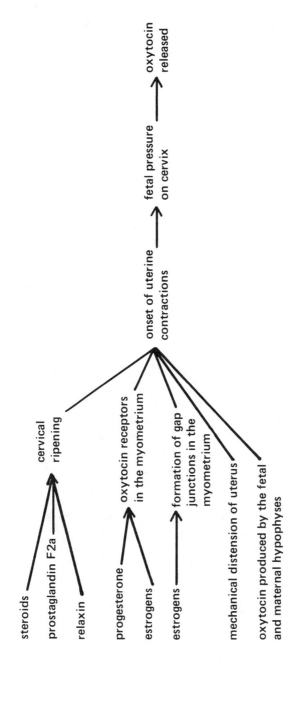

FIGURE 3.1. Current view of the process of labor in the human female (after Fuchs and Fuchs, 1984).

decreases with increasing maternal parity as does the length of the second stage. The third stage appears to be independent of parity. Table 3.1 presents a summary of data describing labor length in a typical hospital population (Friedman, 1978) and in an out-of-hospital sample from TBC. The trends are similar, although the length of the first stage of labor was longer and more variable in the out-of-hospital sample than it was in the hospital sample. For primiparas, the second stage was shorter in the TBC sample than it was in the hospital sample; for multiparas, the lengths for the two samples were comparable. The differences in the length of the second stage for primiparas may be accounted for in part by method used for pushing. In a 1982 study (Barnett and Humenick, 1982), it was found that prolonged (more than 10 seconds), forceful pushing while holding the breath resulted in a mean second stage length of 14.6 minutes (range 9–37 minutes), while open glottis pushing (exhaling while pushing less than 6 seconds) averaged 43.6 minutes (range 19–80 minutes). There is no information on method of pushing in Friedman's study. At TBC, women were encouraged to use the first method. Another factor that may account for the differences observed is the position assumed by the woman for delivery. Although it is not stated in Friedman's work, it is likely that most of the women that make up his sample were supine during delivery. The women who delivered at TBC were seated or semi-reclining during the second stage; perhaps the more upright position contributed to shortening the length of that stage.

Other factors that may have contributed to the differences observed include pharmacological (in the hospital sample, medication was used on many of the women with the effect of shortening the first stage of labor, whereas in the TBC sample, no medication was used), nutritional (the TBC sample included women whose nutritional status and hemoglobin levels were very low), and technological (intervention to shorten the length of labor was rarely done at TBC, whereas in a typical hospital population, if the first stage exceeds what is deemed a safe limit, intervention, including oxytocin stimulation and cesarean section, often occurs).

As noted previously, the beginning of the second stage of labor is marked by complete dilation and retraction of the cervix, usually accompanied by strong expulsive contractions. If the membranes of the amniotic sac have not already ruptured, they usually do so soon after the second stage begins. Contractions become stronger and more frequent because the fetus is in closer contact with the cervix and vagina.

The location of the presenting part (usually the head) in relation to the level of the ischial spines is designated "station," and indicates the degree of advancement through the pelvis (Figure 3.2). Stations are expressed in centimeters above (minus) and below (plus) the level of the ischial spines (zero). The fetus is said to be engaged if the largest presenting diameter has passed through the pelvic brim and is approximately at zero station. In head or vertex presentations, the largest diameter is the head breadth or biparietal; in breech presentations, it is the hip, or intertrochanteric. Engagement usually takes place

TABLE **3.1.** Labor Length by Parity in Two Sample Populations

Stage	Friedman ($N = 10,293$)	TBC sample ($N = 1,312$)
First		
Parity 1	13.5 hr	16.4 hr
Parity 2	7.6 hr	12.5 hr
Parity 3	7.6 hr	11.7 hr
Parity 4	7.0 hr	10.4 hr
Second		
Parity 1	57.0 min	36.3 min
Parity 2	16.2 min	17.6 min
Parity 3	12.0 min	14.0 min
Parity 4	12.0 min	13.5 min

during the thirty-eighth week of pregnancy for the primigravida; if it has not occurred by the beginning of labor, there is often, although not always, cause for concern. A common cause is cephalopelvic disproportion. Usually, if the fetus is not fully engaged at the onset of contractions, labor will be longer.

The second stage can also be subdivided into two phases: the first, or descent phase, ends when the presenting part reaches the pelvic floor, approximately 4 cm below the ischial spines or $+4$ station. Occasionally, a fetus is at $+4$ at the beginning of the second stage, and a woman may not experience a descent phase. The second phase ends with delivery of the infant.

Most babies enter the birth canal with the occiput anterior, usually lying to the left or right of the midline of the mother's body. As the infant meets resistance on descent, the head flexes, pushing the chin toward the chest. With the occiput presenting first, the smallest diameter of the fetal head is accommodated. At this point, the infant is lying on the left or right side with the head in a position transverse to the mother's pelvis, which is wider left to right at the pelvic inlet. Once the infant reaches the pelvic outlet, which is widest front to back, the head rotates again, usually to an occiput anterior position. Once the head has crowned by passing under the pubic symphysis, it emerges from the canal through extension. (See also Figure 1.7.)

After the head has been born, the baby rotates back to its original position, bringing the shoulders to a position perpendicular to the plane of the mother's body. On the next contraction, the anterior shoulder is born, followed by the posterior shoulder. The trunk follows fairly quickly.

BEHAVIORS ASSOCIATED WITH PARTURITION

Although the physical and physiological changes that take place during parturition are important to our understanding of the evolution of this process,

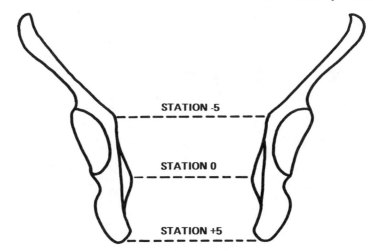

FIGURE 3.2. Frontal view of the human female pelvis indicating stations of descent of the fetal presenting part.

the primary focus of this chapter is behaviors associated with birth in human and nonhuman animals. The next section is initially a survey of birth-related behavior in selected mammals, with special emphasis on primates, including human beings. Cross-species comparisons and evolutionary significance of some of these behaviors will be presented following the somewhat cursory descriptions. A serious limitation to these comparisons is the paucity of recorded observations of birth under natural conditions for primates in general, including humans.

Parturition in Nonhuman Mammals

Observers become aware that the laboratory rat is near parturition when she begins nest-building. She also becomes more lethargic and increases genital licking. Finally, active contractions begin, and she lies on her stomach in the nest, hindlimbs stretched back and up. During delivery she stretches her body full length, arches her back downward, and pushes her hind legs against the floor, pressing her stomach down to aid expulsion of the fetus. She also keeps her mouth open and her head and neck forward. When the fetus emerges, she puts her head between her legs while sitting on her lower back, hindlimbs spread widely. As a contraction propels the fetus out, she pulls it with her mouth. All of this occurs in a matter of seconds and does not appear to require the same amount of energy as that expended by a human parturient (Rosenblatt and Lehrman, 1963).

Mice have been observed using their paws to assist delivery by holding apart the vulval folds until a fetal head emerges. Infants are usually then pulled out by their mothers' teeth or paws, and they are invariably licked. Placentas are completely consumed (King, 1963).

In the domestic cat, the approach of parturition is also marked by increasing anogenital licking. She also becomes more lethargic and rests more often as her attention is focused on her own body. With obvious abdominal contractions, she flexes and raises her legs somewhat sporadically. Other behaviors include squatting, crouching, and straining as if defecating. Occasionally she will scratch at the ground as if she were covering feces or urine. Behaviors usually associated with mating (rolling, rubbing, and lordosis) are also seen. The kittens emerge in two contractions: one brings the fetus into the vulva, and one expels it. They are often enclosed in the amniotic sac and appear to emerge with little straining on the part of the mother. She usually licks them completely and consumes the placenta and related fluids (Schneirla *et al.*, 1963; personal observation).

The Mount Kenya hyrax (*Procavia johnstoni*) usually gives birth to two or three young in inaccessible (to humans and other large animals) crevices and holes, so observations of parturition behavior in these animals are rare. Sale (1965) observed parturition in seven captive females and noted a number of behaviors not usually seen in small mammals. These are normally social animals, and it appears (although not confirmed by field reports) that pregnant females isolate themselves from the group and form temporary nursery groups. Nests are apparently not created, although, even in captivity, the female will seek the most remote corner available for delivery.

Squeaking noises usually accompanied contractions in the births observed by Sale. During a contraction, the females remained still, but in between contractions they moved around in a small area. Length of labor in the animals observed by Sale ranged from 10 to 105 minutes (this last delivery took place under artificial camera lights, so it may not be a normal length at all). No genital licking was observed nor did the mother attempt to rupture the amniotic sac in which the infant was born. None of the females consumed the placenta or membranes, and none made any attempt to break the umbilical cord. This lack of action on the part of the mother at birth is possible only because of the degree of precociality of the infants at birth. They begin moving and attempting to crawl immediately after birth, a process that results in the breaking and removal of the membranes and cord. Once this movement has begun, the mother responds by licking the neonate. Eventually, within a few hours after birth, the young climb onto the mother's back.

Most herd mammals separate themselves from the rest of the group when parturition approaches. Increased position changing and restlessness have been observed in ungulates. Cows often kick at their abdomens and look repeatedly at their flanks during labor. They give birth lying down accompanied by fairly powerful expulsive contractions. Contractions with straining occur about four times an hour and may continue for several hours. Once the anterior part of the calf has emerged, the cow usually rises to a standing position and the rest of the calf is born, breaking the umbilical cord in the process. As it is for humans, the passage of the fetal head through the birth canal is the most difficult part of parturition in many ungulate species, and once this has occurred, expulsion is completed quickly. During labor, most other domesticated ungulates behave in ways similar to that described for the domestic cow. Mares frequently alternate between standing up and lying down, but they lie on their sides for actual delivery. The foal's movements rupture the amniotic sac, and its mother does not begin to lick it until about 30 minutes after birth (Fraser, 1968).

Frenzied nest-building marks the early part of labor in the domestic and feral sow. The female usually lies down for actual delivery of the piglets but may stand between births. The entire expulsive process usually takes about 3 hours with 15-minute intervals between births. Consumption of the placenta (placentophagy) is common.

David (1975) observed parturition in a South African bontebok (*Damaliscus dorcas dorcas*) who delivered, lying down, after 20 minutes of labor. In this case, the female did not separate herself from her group, which included an adult male, two other adult females, and three immature animals. During labor, she alternately lay down and stood up, depending on the intensity of contractions. During what appeared to be the most powerful contractions, she lay on her side. When she finally delivered the calf, she was on her side, surrounded by other members of her group, who were also lying down. The calf was unable to rise and follow its mother for about 1.5 hours after delivery. The mother ate the fetal membranes and licked the infant, who did not nurse until it was about 3 hours old. The placenta was delivered about 4 hours after birth but was not eaten.

Townsend and Bailey (1975) describe parturition in captive white-tailed deer (*Odocoileus virginianus*). Otherwise atypical pacing and restlessness preceded parturition and served as a signal to the observer that birth would occur within approximately 24 hours. Tail elevation usually accompanied pacing. Noticeable contractions were recorded approximately 2 hours before birth. During a contraction, the doe would arch her back or assume the posture usually taken for urinating. Intervals between contractions ranged from 14 minutes early in labor to less than 4 seconds before birth; contractions increased in duration from 6 to 51 seconds. As described for other ungulates, the white-tailed doe lay down during intense contractions and stood between them. Actual delivery took place while she was lying on her side and took approximately 21 minutes from appearance of the head and forelegs to complete expulsion. Presentation of the fetus was usually occiput posterior ("dorsosacral position"). Typically, the parturient doe stood after the head and forelegs had appeared, and the fetus dropped to the ground, breaking the umbilical cord in the process. The mother immediately licked her newborn fawn, continuing until the amnion was removed and the fawn was dry.

Twins are often born in this species. The entire second delivery, in the cases observed by Townsend and Bailey, occurred while the mother was lying down. Contractions were less severe, and the second fawn presented in the same position as the first. Nursing by both young commenced an average of 36 minutes postpartum. Placentas delivered an average of 82 minutes after the last birth (after nursing had begun) and were completely and "urgently" consumed by the does.

In the wild and in captivity, sheep and goats tend to isolate themselves from the rest of the herd as parturition approaches. As with most species, the first sign that birth is near is increased restlessness and frequent licking of the perineal area. Ewes in labor alternate between lying down and standing up, but Fraser (1968:124) notes that many show "extreme dullness" and remain "stationary with the head drooping." For the actual delivery, all ewes he observed lay on their sides. The entire process, from the onset of labor to expulsion of the fetus, lasted an average of 82 minutes. In deliveries observed by Hersher and colleagues (1963), the young were born, head first, while the mother stood or sat. The interval between emergence of the head to complete expulsion ranged from 30 minutes to 3 hours, although it is likely that the longer period is an artifact of domestication. Presumably a wild female caught in such a compromising position would quickly fall prey to nearby predators. Almost invariably, the ewe licks her young until it is dry, consuming the membranes and often the placenta in the process.

The first signal that parturition will occur in a few days in captive dolphins is the attempt by the mother to isolate herself from the rest of the group. In deliveries observed by McBride and Kritzler (1951), abdominal contractions were noted about 20 minutes before birth, during which time the mother made unusual "barking sounds." Typically, the tail of the fetus emerged first. In the dolphin, the critical part of delivery is the passage of the upper trunk with the pectoral and dorsal fins. During this passage, the abdominal contractions appear to be very forceful, and the mother attempts to enhance expulsion by dorsal flexion of her trunk. Any delay at this point could result in a stillbirth, not an infrequent occurrence, at least in captivity. Immediately after expulsion of the fetus, the mother whirls around sharply to face the infant, a movement which breaks the relatively short umbilical cord, and thus, one that McBride and Kritzler interpret as purposeful. Since the delivery occurs under water, it is important that the infant be free to seek air; in fact, its first movement is to the surface where it takes its first breath. Searching for the teat begins soon after birth, but in many instances nursing does not actually begin until 2–4 hours later. The placenta may not be expelled for up to 10 hours after delivery of the fetus. In one observation, the fetus rapidly moved its tail when delivery was arrested, probably by one of the pectoral fins becoming caught in the maternal pelvis. Eventually this movement ceased, and the infant was stillborn. Interestingly, the mother's behavior, normal to that point, became erratic, suggesting to the observers that she sensed that the delivery had become abnormal.

Female elephant seals (*Mirounga angustirostris*) give birth in close proximity to other females in their harem. Restlessness precedes parturition, but the signal that birth is imminent is her assumption of a "U-shaped" posture, head and tail extended in the air while she lies on her stomach. This position is assumed each time she has a contraction during the expulsion stage. The fetus emerges in a caudal or cephalic position after less than 3 minutes of second-stage labor. Once the pup has been expelled completely, the mother turns toward it, breaking the umbilical cord in the process, as was described for the dolphin. The placenta is delivered within an hour after birth but is not consumed by the mother. Suckling begins within 2 hours (Le Boeuf *et al.*, 1972).

Tree shrews (*Tupaia* species) begin nest-building 4 or 5 days before delivering. Most species come into estrus at the time of parturition, so males in the vicinity attempt copulation. Females usually become more aggressive at this time, and most copulation attempts are unsuccessful until after delivery. Labor in tree shrews is said to last from 1½ to 21 minutes, with the mean being about 10 minutes per offspring. In a delivery described by Harrisson (1963, cited in Brandt and Mitchell, 1971) the mother delivered on all fours, spreading her hind legs, arching her back, and tucking her head down between her front feet. Unfortunately, in this delivery as in most captive tree shrew deliveries, the young were cannibalized by the mother or another group member (Brandt and Mitchell, 1971). Even when successful caretaking follows birth, the tree shrew mother is notable for her system of "absentee mothering"; in one species, she attends and nurses her young for only a few minutes once every 48 hours.

Parturition in Strepsirhine Primates and Monkeys

Two or 3 days before parturition in the slender loris (*Loris tardigradus*), changes in the vulva are noticed, and there is a mucus-like secretion from the vagina. The animal exhibits heavy breathing, becomes uneasy and aggressive, and begins frequent licking of her ano–genital region. A typical labor can be divided into three phases before actual delivery (Doyle *et al.*, 1967): during the first, the animal is very active and teases nest material. Intense grooming of herself and others occurs during the second phase along with increased restlessness, frequent position changes, and genital examination. Finally, during the third phase, she grooms her genitals almost constantly until the birth of the infant. In one loris delivery observed by Doyle and colleagues, the expulsion of the fetus took only about 30 seconds (Doyle *et al.*, 1967).

Observers of another loris delivery noted that after the amniotic fluid had passed through the vagina, contractions lasting about 1 second each occurred, three every 5 minutes. These apparently severe contractions were accompanied by low moaning and increased vaginal licking. They lasted less than 12 minutes before the fetal head appeared, occiput posterior. It took approximately 4½ minutes for delivery to be completed once the head had emerged. Contractions during the expulsion stage lasted 3–5 seconds each and occurred at the rate of five or six per minute. Maternal assistance was limited to holding the head and licking. Even in a breech presentation, the infant pulled itself out in a "somersault-like movement" (Kadam and Swayamprabha, 1980:569).

As with tree shrews, cannibalism of young has been reported for lorises and galagos in captivity (Brandt and Mitchell, 1971). A pair of galagos (*Galago senegalensis zanzibaricus*) in a Polish zoo, however, successfully produced 12 young with no evidence of cannibalism. The female gave birth in a nest box during the day, and, in the one delivery observed, the process lasted about ½ minute. All group members showed interest in the newborn infants, and it was, in fact, this interest that signaled to the observers that young had been born (Gucwinska and Gucwinska, 1968).

A female free-ranging sifaka (*Propithecus verreauxi*) observed by Richard (1976), followed her usual routine until less than 1 hour before delivering an infant. This she did seated on a horizontal branch of a tree. No contractions were observed, and the infant apparently was expelled and climbed up to its mother's nipple (in the armpit) with no assistance on her part. The placenta was delivered 15 minutes after birth and was consumed by the mother.

Restlessness also preceded the onset of labor in marmoset (*Callithrix jacchus*) deliveries described by Rothe (1974). Other behaviors included stopping all movement and lifting the abdomen, a posture that was assumed while the female closed her eyes and breathed heavily. This was likely a response to a contraction, and the observer used it as a marker for the onset of the first stage. In two deliveries, this stage lasted 37 and 91 minutes. The beginning of the second stage was marked by the parturients assuming a squatting posture. One female required 21 minutes to expel her singleton fetus, while another expelled triplets in 46 minutes. The singleton presented the vertex, occiput posterior, while the triplets were, in order of appearance: (1) vertex, occiput anterior; (2) vertex, occiput posterior; and (3) breech. The last infant did not survive, but the others climbed to the nipples, unaided, between 19 and 35 minutes after birth. The third stage lasted 14 minutes for the mother who gave birth to a single young, and she consumed the placenta herself. The placenta (all marmosets have fused placentas) was delivered in less than 1 minute after birth for the mother of three, and it was consumed by the other members of the group. Group members showed great interest in the neonates, some (fathers and an uncle) trying to take the infant away from the mothers right after birth.

Stevenson (1976) describes as Stage 0 that period before the first stage onset of contractions during which the parturient captive marmoset exhibits increased restlessness, straining, perineal exploration, and increased defecation. Alternating strains and pauses accompanied the contractions of the first stage in the seven deliveries she observed. Erection of the tail and hair occurred during contractions, and unusual grunting sounds were emitted. In six of the seven deliveries, the first stage lasted between 14 and 105 minutes. The seventh lasted 5 hours and resulted in a stillborn infant. The amniotic sac ruptured spontaneously between 5 and 15 minutes before birth.

A squatting posture was assumed for the second stage expulsion process, and in all births observed by Stevenson, the fetus was born in a vertex occiput posterior position. Manual assistance was limited to cradling the infant's head during delivery. The total length of the second stage ranged from 3 to 30 minutes. The placenta took from 10 to 24 minutes to deliver, and was consumed by all females if the infant was born alive. Other group members also participated in placentophagy. In several cases, the adult male took an infant away from the mother soon after it was born and licked it until it was dry. Infant carrying by other group members was common as early as the first day.

Observers of squirrel monkeys (*Saimiri* species) know that birth is near when there are sudden changes in the eating or sleeping patterns of the females. Urination also increases. Labor always begins between dusk and dawn, and if delivery does not occur before morning, contractions stop and begin again in the evening (Brandt and Mitchell, 1971). Labors typically last between 1 and 2 hours. In one observed labor, 28 minutes before birth the female cried out and strained while clinging to the wire netting of her cage. She stretched up and down on her hindlimbs, repeating this sequence several times. Between contractions, she sat or walked around the cage. During actual expulsion, the female was on all fours, and total emergence of the head took about 5 minutes (Takeshita, 1961–1962). This length of time is on the slow side for most primates but is a typical head-delivery speed in humans. The similarity in times in squirrel monkeys and humans is not surprising since the two species have among the largest neonatal dimensions, relative to maternal pelvic dimensions, in the order.

Typical squirrel monkey behavior during contractions includes freezing position, arching the back, opening the mouth, and drawing the thighs together. The second stage usually lasts about 15 minutes, the mother squatting for delivery. When the infant's head appears, typically with the occiput posterior, the mother usually licks it, and the infant often vocalizes. In several cases, the infant, once the shoulders were freed, reached up onto the mother's abdomen and pulled itself out (Hopf, 1967). Before the placenta delivers, the mother licks her infant, and within minutes it is crawling around her body, eyes open, searching for the nipples.

The third stage in the delivery observed by Takeshita (1961–1962) lasted 7 minutes, and the mother consumed the placenta within 3 minutes of its appearance. The observers counted a total of 11 contractions during the entire birth process.

Bowden *et al.* (1967) described a breech delivery in one squirrel monkey that required 900 contractions over a 3-day period. Although the cervix was completely dilated on the second day, expulsion of the stillborn fetus did not occur until Day 3. Again, the death of the breech is not surprising, considering how close the cephalopelvic dimensions are in this species. In another, more normal delivery, observed by these same authors, the infant presented the vertex, occiput posterior, after 11 observed contractions in 42 minutes. The placenta emerged 11 minutes later, and the mother consumed it before she paid much attention to the infant.

Sekulic (1982) observed no signs of labor in two free-ranging howler monkeys (*Alouatta seniculus*) until just before the fetal head emerged. The total delivery took less than 2 minutes. Among few primate species is there as much "room to spare" in the birth canal as there is in howlers. Perhaps this ample space results in fairly easy, stress-free labors and deliveries for this genus. The deliveries observed by Sekulic occurred in trees, and the placenta was consumed.

Restlessness and constant movement were observed the evening before delivery in a female *Colobus guerza* who had isolated herself from the rest of the group. She experienced obvious labor contractions for at least 4½ hours before giving birth. Posture changes during labor were systematic alterations between arching her back and forming a concavity with her back, movements which Wooldridge (1971:481) attributes to "forcing an expansion of the birth canal opening." Although I could not locate maternal pelvic and neonatal cranial dimensions for *Colobus*, it is likely that they are similar to those observed in *Nasalis* in which cranial dimensions are from 90 to 95% of the sagittal and transverse diameters of the female pelvic inlet (Schultz, 1949; Leutenegger, 1981). Thus, the fit is likely close enough that any behavioral adaptations in labor that would help to increase the pelvic opening would be favorably selected in this or any colobine species.

As with other primate species observed, the parturient colobus monkey observed by Wooldridge (1971) frequently touched and examined her perineum during labor. No vocal sounds were heard by the observer. Contractions intensified 20 minutes before delivery. For delivery, the monkey squatted on a branch and spread her legs apart, bringing her vaginal area forward between her legs. She used her hands to assist delivery of the infant who began to cling to her abdomen immediately and was nursing within minutes. Wooldridge noted that "she licked him almost continuously for the first several hours of life, especially on the tail, and constantly rearranged him in her lap" (p. 482). The placenta was delivered a few seconds after the infant but was ignored by the mother until it was removed by a keeper a day later.

One field report of a Hanuman langur (*Presbytis entellus*) delivery suggests that in some cases these normally arboreal animals come to the ground to deliver. A female lay on her left side during contractions while two other females observed. After 21 minutes of labor, the fetal head emerged at which time the mother sat up; the rest of the infant's body followed 4 minutes later. As she suckled her newborn 5 minutes after birth, the two females who had previously been absorbed in the delivery began to look around nervously. Several minutes later all three animals climbed back into the trees. Their interest in the delivery is not surprising in a species in which interest in infants is high, but it is uncertain whether or not coming to the ground with "attendants" is part of normal delivery behavior for these langurs. Placental consumption was not observed (Oppenheimer, 1976).

Captive guenons (*Cercopithecus* species) react to labor by stretching and pulling on cage walls, grunting, scratching, self-grooming, and vaginal inspection. Shaking of the body often occurs with contractions, and the animals usually assume a squatting position for delivery. In one observed delivery of a captive guenon, the mother punctured the amniotic sac with her fingers after about 30 minutes of active labor. While she squatted and pushed, the head crowned a few minutes later. It took about 15 minutes for the head to emerge fully, at which time the mother licked her infant, and it vocalized. The whole body emerged 8 minutes later. Total delivery time from onset of contractions was 1 hour, and 26 contractions were counted. The third stage lasted 32 minutes, and the placenta was consumed by the mother (Rosenblum and Rosenblum, cited in Brandt and Mitchell, 1971).

The alternate arching of and forming a concavity with the back that has been described for several species during labor has also been observed in deliveries of captive Java macaques (*Macaca fascicularis*) reported by Kemps and Timmermans (1982). Unlike the colobus monkey, which assumed these postures while standing, the Java macaques made the alternating movements while standing, hanging, sitting, squatting, and walking. Use of the hands in inspection and manipulation of the perineum, infant, placenta, and umbilical cord was also observed in these monkeys during and immediately after delivery.

As in colobus, the posture changes may serve to increase the size of the pelvic opening. Pelvic and newborn cranial dimensions are recorded for *Macaca mulatta,* showing that the cephalopelvic fit is very close in that species and, perhaps, for the entire genus. The newborn fetal head averages 98–99% of the maternal sagittal and transverse pelvic dimensions (Schultz, 1949; Leutenegger, 1981). Kemps and Timmermans (1982:79) suggest that arching the back is associated with contractions. At the time of delivery, squatting was the most common position for all females and is probably associated with pushing or bearing down during the second stage. During this stage, reaching for support with the arms was also a common behavior. Most delivered on branches, and only one of five females observed made any vocal sounds during labor and delivery. The female who vocalized considerably (and also was the only one not to deliver in the branches) delivered a breech presentation, requiring intervention from the keepers.

Touching the infant's head during expulsion was observed in three of the four macaques delivering normally. All four manually assisted in delivering their young. The female with a breech presentation attempted to pull her infant out with her hands and mouth. All infants delivering normally did so with the occiput posterior, the face emerging toward the mothers' abdomens. All infants were able to cling immediately; even the infant delivering by the breech attempted to grasp with its legs before it died, unborn.

For the first several minutes after birth, there were apparently no contractions since no associated postural changes were observed. Expulsion of the placenta was associated with back arching, grasping of branches, and squatting, behaviors indicative of uterine contractions. All females ate their entire placentas, focusing complete attention on this activity. Licking of themselves and of their infants was common, although more attention was focused on the former than on the latter.

Until 1930, only seven published reports of parturition in primates were available in Western scientific literature. Most of these had been the results of fortuitous observations and, in most cases, the animal in late stages of labor gave the first sign of pregnancy. Tinklepaugh and Hartman (1930), whose observations on parturition in 17 rhesus macaques were published that year, noted that it was usually impossible to distinguish pregnant from simply fat females who were caged alone and had little opportunity for exercise. The animals they observed in 1929 were housed together in a large enclosure and were much more active. Pregnancy was obvious in this colony because of noticeably protruding abdomens, unlike those of the nonpregnant females.

Labor in these macaques was first noted when the females began alternating arching and extending their backs, posture changes that have been described previously in other species. Straining and sudden grasping of stationary objects were also noticed. As contractions became more intense toward the end of the first stage of labor, the monkeys usually assumed a squatting position and pulled and pushed against the cage walls with their arms. They occasionally removed the mucus plug manually and usually assisted the emerging fetus in delivery. The apparent need to consume great quantities of water was observed in most of the parturient females. Vocalizations are rare in this species as in others during labor and delivery.

One female, whose labor lasted more than 32 hours, experienced 30 or more contractions per hour for the first 8 hours, was free from contractions during hours 9–12, and then had 19 contractions in the next 3 minutes, although examination revealed that the fetal head had not yet engaged. Pituitrin was administered, resulting in an increase in contraction severity and duration, although no progress in delivery was made. For especially severe contractions, the monkey assumed a squatting position. Finally, a stillborn infant was born, weighing 660 g. The large size of the fetus (most rhesus infants weigh between 300 and 500 g) and the prolonged labor in this 14-year-old female suggest cephalopelvic disproportion.

For the rhesus deliveries described in detail, one can see a range of behaviors from great discomfort and exhaustion to frantic, energetic action. Other observers have noted that primiparas, in particular, seem confused and bewildered by parturition. Pain was evident from facial expressions, behavior, and physiological symptoms in all, but none of the monkeys made any vocalizations other than soft grunts or sighs. An exception occurred whenever an observer touched a laboring female during a contraction, even for gentle palpations, when sharp cries and shrieks ensued.

Manual assistance in delivery was provided by all of the mothers, and the placenta was consumed in most cases. Exceptions to this behavior will be noted and discussed later. Labor length, from onset to the end of the third stage, ranged from 23 minutes to 34½ hours. This last figure was recorded for a breech delivery in which the observers intervened to provide assistance. The female, whose infant was already dead, was placed on the floor on a white lab coat, her arms and legs held down by the observers. The fetus was gently pulled out as the mother bore down. She was then released into her cage to deliver the placenta unassisted. In this case, the monkey submitted to being caught without protest, although under normal circumstances, she was difficult to touch (Brandt and Mitchell, 1971).

In 12 rhesus deliveries observed by Brandt and Mitchell (1971), labor lasted from less than ½ hour to more than 5 hours. The former figure was typical for multiparous monkeys, while the latter figure was recorded for a breech delivery in which the observers intervened to provide assistance. Normal primiparas delivered in 1–3 hours.

Adachi *et al.* (1982) describe parturition in seven captive rhesus macaques. They noted that a characteristic sequence of posture changes was common in the deliveries of these animals. First the monkey stood up, arched her back, and grasped the floor mesh of her cage. This was followed by squatting while abducting the thighs and then crouching, pressing her chest to the floor. Since it is difficult to judge when uterine contractions begin in these monkeys, these authors suggest that the initiation of these otherwise abnormal posture changes should signal the beginning of the first stage of labor. According to that measure, the first stage averaged 71 minutes with a range from 35 to 210 (SD 63) in these seven females. Stage two, actual expulsion of the infant, lasted no more than 1 minute in any of the seven deliveries. Few vocalizations were recorded for any of the females during these two stages. The third stage ranged from 1 to 43 minutes. A single exception was noted for a female who had had two previous cesarean sections and did not deliver the placenta until almost 12 hours after birth of the infant.

Rawlins (1979) describes delivery behavior in a rhesus macaque on Cayo Santiago. Previously described behaviors such as exploring the genitals, crouching and stretching during contractions, squatting to deliver, and attempting to use the hands to facilitate delivery were all observed. The only unusual thing about this delivery was that the placenta was delivered more than 8 hours after birth. There did not appear to be any negative consequences resulting from this delay.

A captive stumptail macaque (*M. arctoides*) observed by Gouzoules (1974) began actively exploring her vaginal area 2 weeks before delivery. This behavior intensified a day before delivery and was associated with restlessness and sleeplessness. What was probably an early strong contraction resulted in a sharp vocalization. Rapid pacing back and forth and inhalation vocalizations occurred as labor apparently intensified. Birth occurred 13 minutes after the first sharp vocalization. The infant was licked briefly, but the mother spent most of her time consuming the placenta, which delivered 3 minutes after the infant. Most group members paid more attention to this process of placentophagy than they did to labor and delivery of the infant. The mother did not pick the infant up until she had consumed the placenta, 25 minutes after birth.

Two days before the onset of noticeable contractions, a caged female baboon (*Papio anubis*) became restless and apparently uncomfortable (Love, 1978). Noticeable contractions began 67 minutes before delivery. During this period, the female spent most of the time during a contraction squatting on a bar and pulling up on it with her arms. Between contractions, she walked around the cage, but whenever a contraction caught her off guard she "would throw out an arm to try to grasp anything" (Love, 1978:304). At the birth of the head, the mother ran her fingers around the head, clearing the fetal membranes from around the mouth and nose. With the next contraction, she pulled on the head and delivered the rest of the infant. As with macaque deliveries observed, the mother paid more attention to the consumption of the placenta, which was delivered 4 minutes after the infant. Then she devoted her attention to the infant.

Howell *et al.* (1978) report observations of parturition in feral anubis baboons in Gombe National Park, Tanzania. In one, obvious contractions began 42 minutes before birth, and reactions to the contractions included the commonly reported behaviors of arching and stretching the back and genital exploration. Soft grunts ("gecks") accompanied contractions for the last 17 minutes before birth. The mother delivered her infant in an unusual position with her chest pressed to the ground and her haunches stretched up into the air. Similar posture was observed in a female who delivered her infant in a tree. Wild hamadryas females typically squat during delivery (Kummer, 1971; Abegglen and Abegglen, 1976).

Gillman and Gilbert (1946) observed parturition in a captive chacma baboon (*P. ursinus*), which lasted a total of 7 hours, 23 minutes, from the onset of contractions to the delivery of the placenta. In the sixth hour of labor, contractions occurred at 3-minute intervals, each lasting 15–20 seconds. The infant emerged, occiput posterior, and the mother provided manual assistance in the delivery.

Jeanne Altmann (1980) describes parturition in free-ranging yellow baboons (*P. cynocephalus*) in Amboseli National Park, Kenya. One began labor in the evening and remained lying on her side on the ground long after other members of her group had climbed into the trees for the night. She jerked her limbs frequently, a behavior likely associated with contractions. Finally, she ascended into the trees, where she apparently delivered an infant during the night. Another female delivered her infant while the group was moving during the day. She was away from the group for about an hour for the delivery but afterward continued traveling with the group until the end of the day. In a second daytime delivery, the female remained behind, as the group traveled, to deliver her infant after 1½ hours of labor. Jerky movements were noted in this animal, and she occasionally grasped and strained against a log, likely during contractions. She consumed the placenta after delivery.

Dunbar and Dunbar (1974) observed a birth in a herd of wild gelada baboons (*Theropithecus gelada*). One minute before delivery, the female was grooming another female, fully involved in normal social interaction. She suddenly stood up, crouched, and vocalized as an infant was born in one contraction. As reported for other primates, she licked the infant intermittently until the placenta was delivered 7 minutes later, when her entire attention turned to its consumption. Once done, she devoted more attention to cleaning her neonate.

Parturition in Great Apes

After a 263-day gestation period, a captive orangutan (*Pongo pygmaeus*) observed by Graham-Jones and Hill (1962) exhibited noticeable abdominal contractions to which she responded by reaching out with both arms to grab bars above and beside her. Posture changes, slight gruntings, and shuddering accompanied the contractions. Close to the time of delivery, the contractions increased in duration and frequency. Once the fetal head had delivered, the mother assumed a crouching position, leaving the left arm free to aid in delivery of the body. The fetal head emerged at a 45° angle toward the mother's left leg, indicating an emergence position of right occiput posterior. The mother turned it with her hands to orientation in her sagittal plane. Total time from the onset of contractions to delivery was about 25 minutes.

Although observations were hindered by rain, dark, and natural vegetation, assistants to Galdikas (1982) were able to observe events surrounding parturition in two wild orangutans in Borneo. In one, labor appeared to last approximately 2 hours, judging from agitated behavior of the female. At one time, she was observed tightly "hugging" the trunk of the tree in which she had made her nest. The delivery occurred in this nest, 22 m above the forest floor. The placenta was not consumed in this case, although in a second delivery described by Galdikas, it was consumed by the mother. The delivery of the infant in this second case was not actually witnessed, but it also took place in a nest, approximately 10 m above the ground.

Galdikas emphasizes the variability in behavior related to birth in these two females and suggests that it may be due to the fact than one was a primipara, the other a multipara. (The two were mother and daughter.) The primipara, for example, showed a notable decrease in physical activity just before birth and remained for a longer time in the nest where parturition occurred. The multipara exhibited behaviors not unlike those that characterized her normal life. This included remaining solitary for most of the time before and after parturition, a behavior that is fairly typical of adult orangutans. The younger primipara associated more frequently with other orangutans before and after parturition, a behavior that was common for juveniles and adolescents. Both animals increased consumption of animal protein (specifically termites and other insects) in the month before birth, indicating increased nutritional needs.

Stewart (1977; 1984) describes parturition in three wild mountain gorillas. The first sign that any were in labor was restless changing of positions occurring less than 3 hours before birth. During noticeable labor, which lasted from 18 to 30 minutes, nest-building activity was prominent. The animals assumed various positions, alternately sitting or lying on their sides, and frequently touching the perineum. Delivery appeared to occur while they were in squatting positions, and they probably used both hands to assist the process. In two of the births, the females made unusual screaming sounds that were apparently associated with the expulsion of the infant. One female appeared to experience a painful labor as indicated by these screams during the 30 minutes preceding delivery (Stewart, 1984).

Nadler (1974) describes parturition in a captive female lowland gorilla. Labor was first ascertained by the restlessness she exhibited and the frequent changing of position, alternating reclining, sitting, and pacing. Also accompanying the behaviors were a discharge from the vagina and apparent contractions. About 2½ hours after the judged onset of labor, the female tore the amniotic sac; the infant delivered completely less than 20 minutes later. During this time, the mother reclined on her forearms, knees, side, or back, changing positions frequently. Emergence of the infant's body occurred while she was lying on her side. Licking of the infant and birth fluids followed birth, but the mother did not consume the placenta, which was delivered seconds after the infant.

Delivery behavior in a captive lowland gorilla observed by Beck (1984) included pacing quadrupedally, lying down during first stage contractions, and squatting for the expulsive contractions. She ruptured the amniotic sac with her finger and caught the infant as it was delivered. The time from first pacing to delivery was slightly less than ½ hour, although she had been unusually restless for several hours before and had attempted to isolate herself from the rest of the group. After the birth of the placenta (3 minutes after the infant), she devoured it and then licked the infant until it was dry. Some of her licking movements appeared to clear mucus from the mouth and nose.

Goodall and Athumani (1980) describe parturition for Winkle, one of the females in the Gombe Stream Reserve study area. Winkle made several nests, appeared to be restless, and spent more than the usual time lying down. The first contraction was noted 1 hour and 52 minutes before delivery. During contractions, she was observed to bear down in a crouching position while emitting fairly loud grunts. Between contractions, she usually lay in her nest. The amniotic fluid was released 1 hour before delivery; after that she began to devote much of her attention to her genital area. She put her finger into her vagina and appeared to feel around 15 minutes before delivery. Her body trembled during the 25 obvious contractions she experienced in the first stage. She assumed a crouching position for the second stage, and once the head emerged, she pulled the infant out while pushing with the contraction. The placenta emerged 8 minutes later, and she consumed it immediately, eating leaves with it as chimpanzees usually do when consuming animal prey. Most of the chimpanzee births described for captive animals have lasted less than 30 minutes (Brandt and Mitchell, 1971), suggesting, as Goodall and Athumani do, that Winkle's delivery was unusually difficult.

Parturition in the Human Primate

Descriptions of labor and delivery in human beings are usually restricted to physiological and physical processes, such as those reviewed at the beginning of this chapter. At the end of their extensive review of parturition in primates,

Brandt and Mitchell (1971) note that "there have been very few truly naturalistic or seminaturalistic studies of human behavior that have been handled in the same manner as have nonhuman primate field studies or observational studies in the laboratory" (p. 208). Although they suggest that human beings should also be subjected to such scrutiny, they define natural parturition as that occurring "without medical or midwife aids." By this definition, natural childbirth is virtually nonexistent in our species, except in accidental or rare circumstances. As I have previously argued, attendance at childbirth has been part of the heritage of our genus for at least 1 million, perhaps two million, years. I shall further argue that birth with manual (but not medical) assistance *is* natural in our species. There is a major difference, however, between human and nonhuman primate birth. That difference, as Brandt and Mitchell point out, is the degree to which the brain, and I would add "culture," interfere with the process in humans. An important component of this is the use of language to communicate feelings and experiences that in nonhuman primates can only be inferred from postural changes, grimaces, and rare vocalizations.

The following description of behavioral aspects of parturition in the human female is derived from the more than 200 midwife-assisted deliveries that I have observed at TBC and in the homes of parturients since 1977. Descriptions will be limited to the kind of data that have been obtained from observations of nonhuman primates, as described previously.

As with most species, increased restlessness marks the approach of labor in the human female. Difficulties in sleeping, increased activity, and even "nest-building" have been observed and reported. Mild, irregular contractions may be felt for several days before labor begins, but when they become more regular, occurring approximately once every 15 minutes, they serve as markers for the onset of true labor. Sometimes the first stage of labor begins with spontaneous rupture of the membranes, but more commonly this occurs late in the first stage or during the second stage of labor. Another common sign of early first stage labor is persistent backache. Discharge of the cervical plug ("bloody show") may occur before, at the onset of, or after labor has begun.

In some cases, the first regular contractions may be alarming to a woman, in which case she usually seeks assistance or advice immediately. For a multipara or a well-prepared primipara, the early contractions may be merely distracting, and she may choose not to interrupt her normal routine at all. In fact, an observer is not aware that labor has begun unless the women *says* something about it: her behavior gives no clues, unless one is especially attentive to pauses.

When contractions intensify, occurring once very 5 minutes, she pauses often enough and freezes her actions for long enough that it is obvious to observers that she is in labor. Her breathing rhythm also changes at this time, and a common behavior is rubbing the abdomen. By this time, however, several hours may have passed since she first began experiencing regular uterine contractions.

Usually, when contractions begin occurring every 5 minutes, the woman has sought assistance, and there are other people with her. These may include the father of the child, a birth attendant, relatives, and friends. With each contraction, the woman grimaces, clutches anything or anyone that is near, and occasionally moans or groans. Between contractions, however, she often talks and laughs and walks around as if nothing unusual is happening. Pacing is a common behavior between contractions, and lying down or leaning against a support are common behaviors exhibited during contractions. Some women perform practiced breathing exercises; others seem to breathe as the moment demands. Some women cry, complain, or vocalize loudly in conjunction with contractions. Occasionally, clinched fists, writhing, and other behaviors indicative of fear and pain are observed. In almost all cases, it appears that the woman is experiencing intense discomfort and pain during the later contractions of the first stage.

At one point in labor, as contractions become stronger and closer together, most women exhibit changes in behavior that include shaking, vomiting, difficulty in talking, anxiousness, and a state that can only be described as "spaciness." This marks transition and indicates that the first stage is drawing to a close, although it may last another 1–2 hours for primiparas. At times, women seem to lose control of themselves during the intense contractions of transition. Crying and whimpering increase.

Finally the woman begins to make straining motions as she attempts to push the fetus out, marking the beginning of the second stage of labor. At this point, she may assume a variety of postures including squatting, standing, lying down, crouching on hands and knees, or, most commonly, reclining in a semi-sitting position. The contractions of the second stage are described as expulsive, and they are usually accompanied by straining and exerted pushing efforts on the part of the parturient. Muscle spasms and cramps are not uncommon with these contractions. Usually the woman holds her breath during the pushing contractions, and often exhalation commences with a sharp cry or "yelp." The woman does not appear to experience so much pain as was obvious in the late first stage contractions, but she is expending far more effort. It is during the second stage that "labor" with its meaning as "work" is most evident. She usually appears exhausted between contractions, but she seems to be more in control of her body and emotions than she was during transition. In most cases, a birth attendant has her hands at the perineum and a husband, friend, or another support person is near the woman's head or sitting behind her, providing something for her to push against. During a contraction of the second stage, she pushes against something or someone with her legs and pulls up with her arms. It appears that all muscles in her body are devoted to the task of pushing the baby out.

If the membranes have not already ruptured, they usually do so early in the second stage. As the head begins to crown, the birth attendant becomes more actively involved in the delivery as she attempts to guide the head slowly out of the birth canal. The woman is no longer pushing, expulsion being accomplished solely by uterine contractions. Once the occiput (the usual presenting part) passes under the pubic symphysis, the head is born by extension. In some cases, the perineum will tear, especially if delivery of the head has been too rapid. Delivery of the head is almost always accompanied by a vocalization from the mother.

After rotation of the fetal head to put the shoulders in the transverse dimension of the pelvic brim, the anterior shoulder emerges on the next contraction. Again, the attendant provides guidance or the mother herself may reach down and complete delivery of her child. Tearing of the perineum may occur at this point if the shoulders emerge too quickly. Once the shoulders have passed the perineum, the body is born very quickly. The cord is cut when it stops pulsating, and the third stage ends with expulsion of the placenta, usually within 30 minutes after birth. The placenta is not consumed.

COMPARISONS OF BIRTHS IN HUMAN AND NONHUMAN PRIMATES

An obvious difference between births in most mammals and those in primates is the use of the hands in assisting delivery of the infant. This has likely been an important adaptation for arboreal animals who usually give birth in trees and on bare limbs (not in nests); infants born without manual assistance from their mothers would likely fall. For some species, the infants are coordinated enough at birth so that they can pull themselves out of the birth canal.

Nonhuman primates also use their hands to explore the genital area just before and during labor. In a number of instances previously described, the parturient used her hand to rupture the amniotic sac. Rubbing the abdomen is commonly seen in human parturients, but there are no reports of women exploring their vaginal areas with their hands. To some extent, this relates to cultural proscriptions about such behavior, but it is also physically difficult for a pregnant woman to get herself in a position that would enable effective exploring. Perhaps the counterpart to this in the human is the occasional practice of manual exploration of the abdomen or vaginal area by the birth attendant.

A common practice followed by birth attendants in the United States is to check for cervical dilation when a woman reports that she is in labor. Other things that will be noted during vaginal examination are the state of the membranes, the fetal station and presentation, the stage of cervical effacement, and any abnormalities. Likelihood of infection increases when any object, including a gloved hand, is introduced into the vagina. Thus, most people strive to keep vaginal examination to a minimum.

One common concern worldwide is that a desire to push may come before complete cervical dilation. If a woman begins to push prematurely, the result can be laceration of cervical and perineal tissue, excessive bleeding, infection, and perhaps hypoxia and intracranial injury for the infant. Many birth attendants thus make an effort to ascertain the extent of cervical dilation and effacement when a woman announces that she has the "urge to push." Occasionally, the amniotic sac will be ruptured manually if cervical dilation is perceived as too slow, but in most cases it is left intact because it provides a cushion for the fetal head. Rupture too early also increases the risk of infection.

Presentation of the Infant

In many of the primate deliveries already described, the fetus emerged in a vertex position with the occiput posterior (i.e., against the mother's sacrum). This position was specifically noted for the slender loris (Kadam and Swayamprabha, 1980), marmoset (Rothe, 1974; Stevenson, 1976), squirrel monkey (Hopf, 1967), Java macaque (Kemps and Timmermans, 1982), chacma baboon (Gillman and Gilbert, 1946), and orangutan (Graham-Jones and Hill, 1962). Human fetuses rarely emerge with the occiput posterior, although many enter the birth canal in that position and rotate to the more common position of occiput anterior. Persistent posterior positions, those that do not rotate, are considered abnormal in humans.

Among the problems associated with posterior delivery in humans are an increased likelihood of perineal lacerations, prolonged delivery because a broader part of the fetal skull must pass through the pelvis, arrest at the perineum, and more extensive molding of the cranial plates. Myles (1975) notes that the fetal head in an occiput posterior position does not fit so well against the cervix leading to lowered stimulation of nerves in that area and, thus, weaker uterine contractions. Anything that retards progress of the second stage increases risks to the infant. On the mother's part, severe backache is much more common in persistent posterior presentations.

Oxorn and Foote (1975) suggest that posterior presentations are more common in android and anthropoid pelves (see Figure 3.3) in which the anterior portion is usually narrow. With these pelvis types, "there is a tendency for the back of the head with its long biparietal diameter to be pushed to the rear, so that the front of the head with its short bitemporal diameter can be accommodated by the small forepelvis (p. 133)." The anthropoid pelvis receives its name from its resemblance to the pelves of monkeys and apes and occurs in approximately 25% of women (Oxorn and Foote, 1975). Compared to the normal or gynecoid pelvis (50% occurrence), the anthropoid pelvis is longer in the sagittal dimension and shorter in the transverse dimension. In most cases, it can be described as "adequate" for delivery, although engagement of the fetal head may be altered, as already noted.

Presumably, a change in normal orientation of the fetus thus has occurred with the evolution of the more gynecoid female pelvis associated with bipedalism and encephalization. This change also affected the entire emergence pattern of the fetus and, thus, the mother's response to that emergence. In nonhuman primates, the fetus usually emerges with its face toward that of its mother (Figure 3.4).She may then reach down and pull it up toward her along the normal flexion of its body. In other cases, the infant may pull itself out of the birth canal by climbing up along the mother's abdomen. If the occiput emerges in an anterior position,

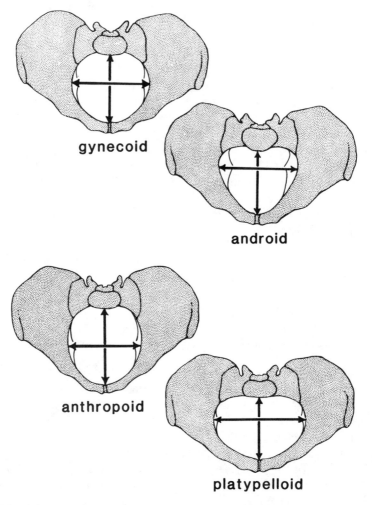

FIGURE 3.3. Classification of the human pelvis. Reproduced from *"Human Labor and Birth,"* Third Edition by H. Oxorn and W. R. Foote. By permission of Appleton-Century-Crofts, New York. Copyright, 1975.

with the face away from the mother, she will tend to pull the infant backward, risking injury to it in the process. All other things being equal, it is therefore advantageous for an infant to emerge facing its mother if she is likely to use her hands in pulling the body out.

In humans, however, all other things are not equal: The close equivalence of cephalopelvic dimensions has resulted in the usual process of an infant being born facing away from its mother. In this position, the use of her own hands to assist delivery before the shoulders have emerged could result in pulling the

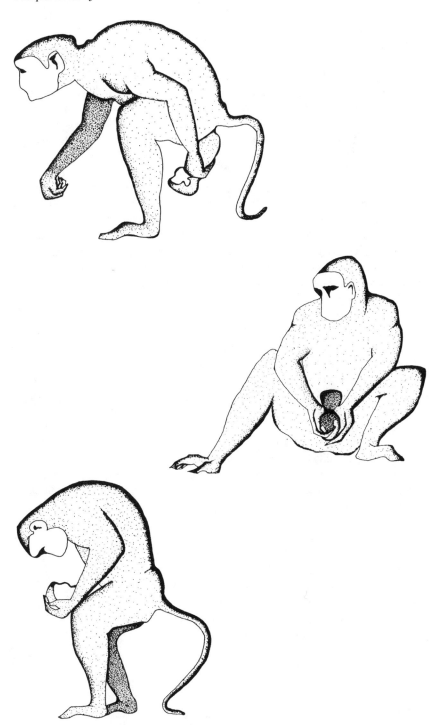

FIGURE 3.4. Schematic illustration of a monkey delivery. (Drawings by Bryan McCuller.)

infant against the normal flexion of its body, again with the risk of injury, particularly to the nerves of the neck. In most human births, an assistant is present who helps to "catch" the infant after delivery of the shoulders.

Mortality appears to be high for primate infants who attempt to deliver in a breech presentation. Nash (1974) describes a stillborn breech delivery in a feral anubis baboon who carried the dead infant around with her for two days. Breech deliveries have also been recorded for the squirrel monkey (Bowden *et al.*, 1967), Java macaque (Kemps and Timmermans, 1982), and rhesus macaque (Brandt and Mitchell, 1971), all of which resulted in stillborn infants. In two cases, intervention by the human observers was necessary to remove the fetus from the birth canal. This suggests that breech deliveries in the wild may increase the risks for the mother, as well. Breech deliveries occur in approximately 3–4% of all deliveries in contemporary human females (Oxorn and Foote, 1975). The fetus may present the buttocks first (in a "complete," legs flexed position, or a "Frank," legs extended position), one or both feet first, or knees first (Figure 3.5). Breech presentations are often associated with prematurity, hydrocephaly, excess amniotic fluid, and placenta previa (Oxorn and Foote, 1975). Often, in multiple pregnancies, one or both infants will present breech. There does not appear to be an association with pelvis type, but many women habitually deliver breech infants suggesting that their pelves may favor breech over vertex presentation; alternatively, there may be other genetic factors affecting the tendency to deliver breech babies. Oxorn and Foote (1975) note that abnormalities are twice as common in breech as in cephalic presentations.

Even today, in Western nations with modern medical technology, mortality for infants who are born with a breech presentation is high, between 10 and 20% (Oxorn and Foote, 1975). Of breech presentations, 60–90% are delivered by cesarean section in the United States, according to a recent estimate, reflecting this fear of mortality associated with vaginal delivery (Marieskind, 1979). In fact, the expectation that breeches will be delivered by cesarean section is so great that many medical schools do not teach their students how to deliver a breech vaginally (Marieskind, 1979). As a result, mortality associated with vaginally delivered breeches has actually increased recently, because many of those who are managing them have had little or no experience with the procedure.

There are numerous problems associated with breech presentations in humans, many of which are probably common in nonhuman primates as well. The buttocks, feet, or knees are poor dilators of the cervix, and, thus, labor and delivery are often prolonged. A common problem is that women feel the urge to push before the cervix has dilated completely. This could result in the fetal head being held too long at the cervix.

Early rupture of the membranes is also common in breeches, and since the fetus does not fit fully in the pelvic brim, prolapse of the umbilical cord may result. Probably the greatest danger is that the head cannot be easily compressed in a breech delivery, and it may be held too long by the pelvic outlet, resulting

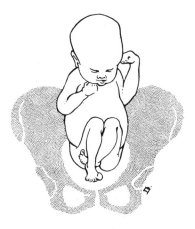

A. Complete breech.

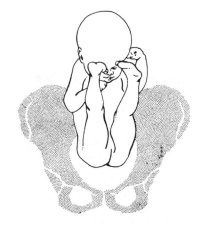

B. Frank breech.

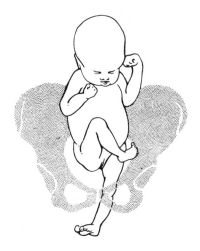

C. Footling breech.

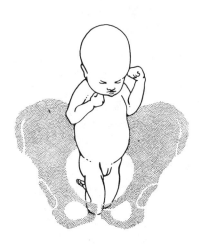

D. Kneeling breech.

FIGURE 3.5. Types of breech presentations in human births. Reproduced from "*Human Labor and Birth*," Third Edition by H. Oxorn and W. R. Foote. By permission of Appleton-Century-Crofts, New York. Copyright, 1975.

in hypoxia in the fetus. When the fetus experiences the rapid cooling of its lower body upon emergence, attempts at breathing may begin; asphyxia and aspiration of amniotic fluid are likely outcomes. This is apparently what often happens in breech deliveries in nonhuman primates. As already noted, Kemps and Timmermans (1982) record that a Java macaque delivering in a breech presentation attempted to grasp its mother's hair as its hindlimbs emerged. It succumbed before birth of the head, however, probably as a result of asphyxiation.

In a normal cephalic presentation in humans, molding of the cranial plates takes place slowly, over several hours. In breech deliveries, however, the skull is subjected to very rapid compression and decompression, occasionally resulting in injury to the brain or fracture of the skull. If the attendant is not skilled in delivering a breech, further complications could result, including fractures of the neck and long bones, paralysis of cervical or brachial plexes, damage to the abdominal organs or liver, and injury to the spinal cord (Oxorn and Foote, 1975).

Proper delivery of a breech requires many fine movements and close coordination between the attendant's actions and the bearing down efforts of the mother. Episiotomy is usually recommended to prevent further delay in emergence of the head. Once one-half of the infant's body has emerged, it is important that delivery be completed in the next 5 minutes. Usually the head rotates to an occiput anterior position (face to the sacrum) and the body is lowered so that the occiput passes under the pubic symphysis. The body then must be raised so that the face passes over the sacrum and perineum. At any point in the passage of the head, arrest can occur requiring further intervention, including instrument delivery.

Given the skill required in delivery and the maneuverings that are necessary for successful birth of a breech, it seems highly unlikely that a woman could deliver a breech entirely alone. I would suggest that mortality has been close to 100% for unassisted breech deliveries. This in itself would argue for selection favoring assistance at childbirth and, if there is a genetic component to breech presentations, powerful selection against that tendency.

Time of Birth

Another common trend seen in primates is that diurnal species most often give birth at night, and nocturnal species deliver more often during the day. In 1972, Alison Jolly published a compilation of birth times recorded in published accounts of primate deliveries. In 1973, she followed that with the results of a survey of time of birth in primates housed in 72 zoos around the world. To these data, I have added birth times recorded in selected publications that Jolly did not examine and in those published since 1972. Of 75 births in nocturnal prosimians, 45 or 60% occurred during the day. Among diurnal prosimians 328 births are recorded, 203 or 62% of which occurred during the night.

For the one species of nocturnal New World monkey, there were eight recorded birth times, seven of which were during the day. Of the 161 delivery times recorded for diurnal New World species, 143 or 89% occurred at night. There were recorded birth times for 846 Old World monkeys, 702 or 83% of which were nocturnal deliveries. It appears that selection has favored nocturnal deliveries in these diurnal species, particularly for those that move often in search of food or depend on a social group for their survival. A female who stops to deliver an infant during the day risks being left behind by the social group, further jeopardizing her already vulnerable position. This is particularly true for the Old World species that spend much of their day foraging on the ground.

Dunbar and Dunbar (1974) suggest that giving birth at night provides both the mother and infant with a few hours to recover from delivery and adjust to a new relationship. Most monkey infants have poor motor control, initially, but are strong enough to cling unaided after a few hours. For species in which other group members have great interest in newborn infants, the mother and infant have time alone before they are discovered, if she delivers at night. It is especially critical for the infant to have an opportunity to nurse before juveniles take it away from its source of nourishment.

The exceptions to this trend toward nightime births in diurnal species are informative. Chism and colleagues (1978) report that most patas monkeys in two captive groups (one in California, one in Kenya) deliver during daylight hours. They suggest that this is adaptive in a species in which members spread out to sleep alone at night but come together in a social group during the day. Thus, the patas monkey females tend to deliver when they are in proximity of other group members on whom they depend for safety.

Another exception to the trend is the howler monkey. Sekulic (1982) notes that these monkeys are relatively immobile all the time so that there may not be a particularly opportune or inopportune time to deliver. They also appear to have the least difficult and fastest deliveries of all primates, in which case recovery time may not be so great. Interest in infants is high among other females in the patas and howler monkeys, but the mothers apparently do not let others hold their newborn infants (Mitchell, 1979).

There is also a statistical bias toward nocturnal births in three of the ape species. For hylobatids, chimpanzees, and gorillas, 219 birth times are recorded. Of these, 149 or 68% took place at night. The orangutan is an exception to this trend: of 99 deliveries, 55 or 56% occurred during the daylight hours. The great apes have few predators other than human beings, so it is unlikely that predator pressure has affected the distribution of birth times in the same way that it has for the smaller monkeys. Adult orangutans are rarely social, eliminating another factor that potentially may affect birth times. Thus, in this species, births are distributed more randomly throughout the day and night.

Like most other haplorhine primates, the human birth hour is not random either. There is a statistical bias toward deliveries occurring at night, although it is not so strong as it is in other primates. In one study of 601,222 births that occurred in the United States and Western Europe between 1848 and 1960, there was a peak between 0300 and 1200 and a trough between 1300 and 2000 (Kaiser and Halberg, 1962). A similar trend was observed in deliveries that took place at TBC between June 1978 and May 1982 (Figure 3.6). Jolly (1972) has suggested that this nonrandom distribution reflects a time in our past when it was advantageous to deliver at a time when fellow band members were available to

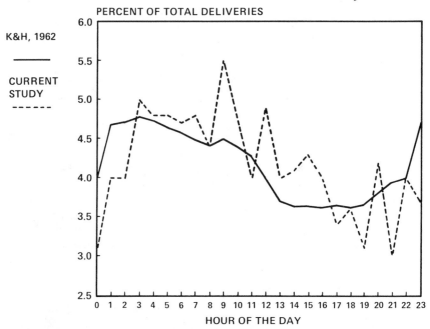

FIGURE 3.6. Time of birth in two studies.

assist and provide protection. Mothers who delivered in the afternoon ran the risk of being away from camp and other adults while they foraged alone for food.

Labors that terminated between 0600 and 1200 were shorter in the TBC sample than those that terminated during any other 6-hour period (Table 3.2). This may also reflect past adaptations. Certainly being relaxed contributes to shorter labors; our ancestors who labored throughout the night in the presence of close friends and relatives were undoubtedly more relaxed than women who labored alone during the day while other band members were foraging. Perhaps that tendency continues today as women find themselves more readily able to relax during the night when others are quiet and sleeping, and family members are nearby.

Length of Labor

It appears that the length of labor in human beings is three to four times as long as that in other mammals (see Table 3.3). Burns (1978) suggests that lengthened labors can be attributed, in part, to alterations in the utero–vaginal angle resulting from postural modifications for bipedalism. Other contributing factors cited include the irregularly arranged bands of uterine smooth muscle, the cervical band of fibrous tissue, and heightened sympathetic innervation. Certainly the large size of the human fetus also plays a role. Although normal labor may be longer in humans than in any other species described, that may be, to

TABLE **3.2.** Labor Length by Time of Birth (6-Hour Units)

Time of birth	Percentage of total	First stage (hr)[a]	Transition (min)	Second stage (min)
0000–0600	25.6	13.7	55	20
0600–1200	28.2	12.1	58	23
1200–1800	24.6	13.5	63	23
1800–2400	21.6	14.0	56	20

[a]$p<.01$.

TABLE **3.3.** Length of Labor in Selected Primate Species

Species	First stage (min)	Second stage (min)	Third stage (min)	Source
Sifaka	ca. 42		15	Richard, 1976
Marmoset	30–300	10–30	10–24	Stevenson, 1976; Rothe, 1974
Langur	21	4		Oppenheimer, 1976
Colobus	240	20		Wooldridge, 1971
Guenon	30	30	32	Brandt and Mitchell, 1971
Macaque	23–210	1–2	1–711	Adachi *et al.*, 1982; Rawlins, 1979; Tinklepaugh and Hartman, 1930
Baboon	42–67	4	4	Love, 1978; Howell et al., 1978
Orangutan	120	30		Graham-Jones and Hill, 1962; Galdikas, 1982
Gorilla	18–155	1–18	2	Nadler, 1974; Beck, 1984; Stewart, 1977
Chimpanzee	ca. 120	7	8	Goodall and Althumani, 1980
Human beings	37–2400	2–385	1–98	TBC data

some extent, an artifact of the ability of human females to communicate the onset of contractions even though they may not show overt signs of its onset. In other words, most women do not give observable signs that they are in labor until they reach the active phase, when the remaining time in labor is only 2 or 3 hours; this puts human labor more in line with the other mammalian data (Lindberg and Hazell, 1972).

Ashley Montagu has suggested that labor is longer and harder in human beings than it is in mammals because it replaces licking of the newborn in providing skin stimulation (Montagu, 1971). Most mammals lick their young immediately and for several days after birth; humans are the rare exceptions. Licking of infants appears to be necessary for proper functioning of the digestive tract and the respiratory system. Animals who have not been licked are often unable to breathe, defecate, or urinate properly. Licking also provides warmth and serves to remove odors that would be attractive to predators. In some species, it appears to be important in forming a mother–infant bond. Montagu suggests that unlicked human infants would also suffer complications were it not for the stimulation provided by prolonged uterine contractions. As evidence, he notes that respiratory and digestive problems and poor control of the bladder and sphincter are common ailments in prematures and those born by cesarean section, infants who experience brief labors or none at all. Later we will examine immediate postpartum stroking and massaging of the newborn infant as a selected replacement for licking.

Several of the accounts of deliveries in nonhuman primates suggest that labor is longer for primiparas than for multiparas. Brandt and Mitchell (1971), for example, note that labor in rhesus deliveries lasted about ½ hour in multiparas, while more typical of primiparas were labors lasting 1–3 hours. This was noted earlier in this chapter as a factor that influences the length of labor in human beings as well. There also appear to be differences in length of labor in humans when age is considered as a factor. Following Friedman (1978), the women delivering at TBC were divided into three groups by age: those under 18, those between 18 and 35, and those over 35. For primiparas, there were no significant differences for any of the three groups except for the length of the second stage: younger women had significantly shorter second stages than those 18 and above ($F = 5.33$, $df = 2,421$, $p < .005$). Multiparous women between the ages of 18 and 35 had shorter second stages than older or younger women ($F = 3.36$, $df = 2,417$, $p < .05$). This is somewhat different from the labors reported by Friedman: in his sample, the length of the second stage increased with each age group increase. Age was not noted as a factor in deliveries described for nonhuman primates.

Medication is often cited as a factor affecting length of labor and outcome in human deliveries. In much of the twentieth century, providing obstetrical medication for human females in labor and delivery was a normal part of giving birth in a hospital. Some, such as barbituates and tranquilizers, are administered simply to help the woman relax. Others help to relieve perception of pain and include amnesics, analgesics, and anesthetics. Finally, exogenous oxytocics help to induce or augment labor. Use of medication in labor has been curtailed in many places, however, because of potential problems they cause for the fetus (this will be discussed later) and the desires of many women today to deliver without medication.

After several years of supervising births at TBC, the director began to note a trend toward longer labors in women who had previously been administered exogenous oxytocin in labor. (In many Mexican clinics, oxytocin is administered routinely during labor, regardless of indications of need for the hormone.)

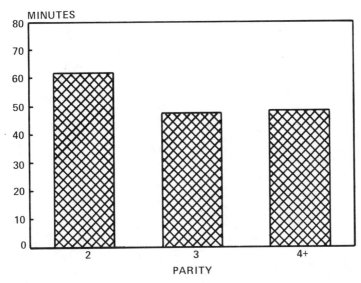

FIGURE 3.7. Length of active labor for multiparas with no previous exogenous oxytocin.

Previous history of exogenous oxytocin use during labor and delivery was known for 704 of the multiparous women: 358 (51%) had never received it at previous deliveries, 225 (32%) had received it once, 64 twice, and 57 three or more times. There was no significant variation between the length of the first stage or the second stage. The length of the transition phase, however, appeared to be related to previous use of exogenous oxytocin ($F = 3.20$, $df = 3,700$, $p < .02$).

Analysis of all multiparas who had not recieved oxytocin at previous deliveries indicates that the length of transition decreases from parity two to parity three or more as can be seen in Figure 3.7. Almost the opposite effect is noted for multiparas who had received exogenous oxytocin at three or more previous deliveries (Figure 3.8). In other words, for labors analyzed in this and other studies, the expectation is that length of transition decreases or remains the same as parity increases. For women who have used exogenous oxytocin before, the length of transition goes against expectation.

As further illustration, Figure 3.9 depicts transition length for 133 women of parity five or greater. The length of transition increases slightly for those with exogenous oxytocin once or twice before and makes a sharp increase for those who received the hormone at three or more previous deliveries.

Why should the length of transition increase for women who have received oxytocin at three or more previous deliveries? Certainly underlying factors requiring exogenous oxytocin are likely to repeat their effect at subsequent deliveries. It is possible, however, that some women, after receiving it for several deliveries, develop a dependency on exogenous oxytocin and cease to

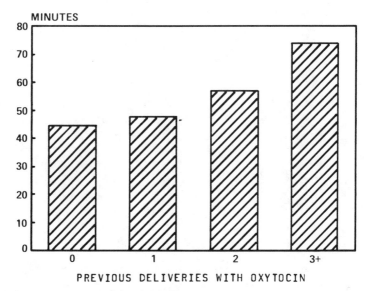

FIGURE 3.8.   Length of active labor for multiparas with exogenous oxytocin at previous deliveries.

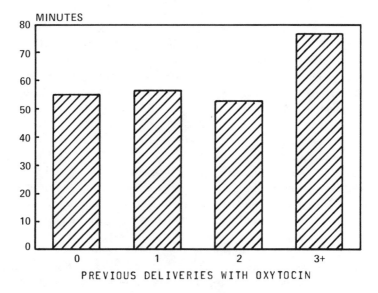

FIGURE 3.9. Length of active labor for multiparas of parity five or greater.

produce enough to maintain normal contractions and progressive cervical dilation.

As already noted, there is much variation in the time of spontaneous rupture of the membranes. In both human and nonhuman primates, the membranes may rupture long before, at the onset, or during the first or second stage of labor. Several accounts of nonhuman primate deliveries note that the female ruptured the amniotic sac with her fingers just before delivery (guenon: Brandt and Mitchell, 1971; gorilla: Nadler, 1974; Beck, 1984). In the medical model of human birth, if the membranes rupture and labor does not begin for several hours, labor will be induced. Risk of infection to the fetus and the mother increases with premature rupture of the membranes. In some hospitals, if labor is perceived as progressing too slowly, the membranes will be ruptured artificially in the (mistaken) belief that it will hasten delivery.

Time of rupture of the membranes was known for 1208 of the women who delivered at TBC: 24 (2%) ruptured before labor begin, 341 (28%) during the first stage, and 843 (70%) during delivery. Only during the second stage were membranes occasionally ruptured artificially; at all other times, rupture occurred spontaneously. The first stage, transition, and the second stage were longest for women whose membranes ruptured during the first stage of labor. These results are similar to those of Friedman (1978) who found labor shorter for women whose membranes ruptured before labor began or at delivery, when compared with women whose membranes ruptured during labor.

For primiparas, rupture during the first stage was associated with more time in labor and delivery; however, the differences were significant only for transition ($F = 3.21$, $df = 2,333$, $p < .05$) and the second stage ($F = 6.51$, $df = 2,378$, $p < .01$). For multiparas, first stage, transition, and second stage were all significantly longer for women whose membranes ruptured during labor (Table 3.4). Women whose membranes remained intact until delivery were more likely to be older ($F = 6.13$, $df = 2,1204$, $p < .01$), to be of greater parity ($F = 17.24$, $df = 2,1201$, $p < .0001$) (two factors that are themselves associated), and to have experienced greater weight gain during pregnancy (($F = 4.25$, $df = 2,897$, $p < .01$).

Jacklin and Maccoby (1982) found, in a study of 320 deliveries, that labor was longer for women giving birth to boys than for those giving birth to girls. The differences were similar for primiparas and multiparas. They suggest that their finding of longer labors for mothers of boys compared to mothers of girls may explain some of the differences in behavior observed in male and female neonates. For the women who delivered at TBC, however, there were no significant differences for any phase of labor associated with the gender of the infant, for the total sample or among primiparas or multiparas. I would argue that, although Jacklin and Maccoby controlled for medication in labor and birthweight in their sample, it is likely that the out-of-hospital sample presented here more closely approximates the "natural" conditions, suggesting that labor does not normally differ according to gender of the infant. One possible

TABLE **3.4.** Length of Labor and Rupture of the Membranes (ROM)

Variable	ROM Before labor	During labor	During delivery	Significance
First stage				
Total sample	10.8 hr	15.5 hr	12.7 hr	***
Primiparas	12.5 hr	17.5 hr	16.1 hr	NS
Multiparas	9.2 hr	13.0 hr	11.6 hr	*
Transition				
Total sample	50 min	74 min	53 min	***
Primiparas	61 min	77 min	61 min	***
Multiparas	41 min	71 min	51 min	***
Second stage	.			
Total sample	20 min	31 min	18 min	***
Primiparas	29 min	43 min	32 min	**
Multiparas	10 min	21 min	13 min	***
Third stage				
Total sample	9 min	10 min	9 min	*
Primiparas	8 min	11 min	9 min	**
Multiparas	10 min	9.5 min	9 min	NS

$*p<.05; **p<.01; ***p<.0001.$

explanation for the differences found in the previous study is differential effects of labor medication on the genders.

Pain, Position, and Place

Several of the observations of delivery behavior in nonhuman primates and other animals report that contractions were obviously causing pain to the female experiencing them. Indications of such in primates included grimacing, moaning, grasping ''blindly'' at objects, unusual postures, and occasionally loud cries. Nissen and Yerkes (1943) note that pain and distress were indicated in all nine chimpanzee deliveries they observed. Others have noted that some females seemed to experience a great deal of pain, whereas others did not seem affected. Fraser (1968), observing that pain is associated with parturition in domesticated ungulates, offers the suggestion, first presented by Walser (1965, cited in Fraser, 1968), that pain serves to signal to the animal that birth is imminent and results in her giving undivided attention to the event. Although it is difficult, if not impossible, to measure degree of pain perceived by an animal, it is evident that human beings are not unique in interpreting birth as a somewhat painful experience.

Labor contractions are recognized as painful stimuli for human parturients in all parts of the world, and there are numerous remedies for alleviating the pain, including herbal medicines, sympathetic magic, heat, and massage. Analgesics and anesthetics have been the twentieth-century answer to the need to alleviate pain, but with concern for their effects on the neonate, many women have begun to rely on psychoprophylaxis or have been willing to accept the pain as part of the natural process of delivering an infant.

In some parts of the world, women are encouraged to walk during labor; in others they remain seated or lying down. Most of the evidence suggests that remaining active in labor helps to speed the first stage and enhances the delivery of oxygen to the fetus. In a series of studies done in Central America, for example, it was noted that labor was 36% shorter in primiparae and 25% shorter in multiparae who remained ambulatory, compared to those those who labored in a supine position (Caldeyro-Barcia, 1979). The upright position increases the strength of the contractions and increases the pressure of the fetal head on the cervix, resulting in faster cervical dilation and shorter labor. All primates whose deliveries were described previously moved more or less constantly between contractions.

Position changes during labor in nonhuman primates that include alternately arching the back and crouching forward have been interpreted by several observers as serving to increase the size of the birth canal. The pelvic opening of the human female also appears to widen slightly when she is in an upright position. Crouching and squatting are the most common positions for delivery in nonhuman primates. This is in part due to the necessity of using the hands for delivery of the infant. The position that the human female assumes for delivery depends on various factors, including her own feelings of comfort and effectiveness, the norms of her culture, and the position prescribed by the birth attendant. An upright position appears to be optimal because the woman's expulsive efforts work with the force of gravity in expelling the fetus. When a woman is upright (sitting, squatting, or standing) the presenting part, the occiput, bears most of the force of the infant's body. The occipital bone is the most developed of the cranial plates at birth and can more adequately withstand this stress. When a woman is lying down for delivery, the force of the infant's body must be absorbed by the more fragile frontal bones which lie against her sacrum. If the fetus is lying in a posterior position, the stress will be applied to the base of the skull, close to the spinal cord.

The most common position for delivery cited in the ethnographic literature is a seated or semi-reclining position. This has the advantages of providing some comfort for the parturient, being a fairly good position in which to push, and providing opportunities to rest between contractions. The birth attendant can easily see the delivery process, as can the mother. Other common positions cited include squatting, kneeling, standing, and left lateral or Sims' position. The lithotomy and dorsal positions, those most commonly used in the United States until recently, are rarely used in other cultures.

Throughout the world, birth most commonly takes place in the home, often the home of the parturient's family. In some groups, special houses for birth are designated or built for the event. Also common are deliveries out-of-doors, although rarely do births take place "in the field" as the woman is conducting her daily chores. There appears to be an association between the location of birth and the attitude women have toward the event. In cultures where birth takes place in an unfamiliar setting, women usually fear delivery; when it takes place in the home and in the presence of family and friends, women are less fearful.

Although the delivery process itself is virtually the same for all women with vertex presentations and normal pelves, the things that are done to aid that process in human beings range from no intervention, even in complicated deliveries, to complete manipulation and control. Massage of the abdomen, which helps to stimulate labor, is common during the second stage. Occasionally, heavy fundal pressure is applied to speed delivery, sometimes resulting in premature separation of the placenta. Internal and external versions of breech presentations are commonly performed, and in a few cultures cesarean sections are done, although this more commonly occurs after death of the mother to remove the fetus. Vaginal stretching, perineal massage, episiotomies, and manual dilation of the cervix are mentioned in various ethnographic reports. Techniques for dealing with complications include ignoring them, calling in a shaman or other special practitioner, and applying of herbal medicines, magico–religious procedures, and physical manipulations. Inducing vomiting is common. Occasionally, intercourse or other forms of sexual stimulation are advised, a practice which induces the release of oxytocin.

Placentophagy

An obvious distinction can be made between human and nonhuman primates as concerns disposal of the placenta; nonhuman primates usually consume the organ in part or wholly; humans rarely consume the placenta. In nonhuman primates, it is such a normal and expected part of parturition that some reviewers propose a fourth stage of labor: that time from expulsion of the placenta to its consumption by (usually) the mother. Placentophagy is not restricted to primates; it is common in almost all mammalian species, including those that are otherwise exclusively herbivorous.

Several observers have noted that the process of placenta consumption is one of compulsion rather than of eating a preferred food. Typically, while the placenta is being consumed, the mother ignores everything else, including her newborn infant and special food delicacies that are usually attractive to her.

Placentophagy almost always accompanies parturition in strepsirhine primates and monkeys, both in captivity and in the wild. In almost all cases, it is a behavior limited to the parturients, although in Callitrichidae it is not uncommon for other group members to eat all or part of a placenta (Stevenson, 1976; Rothe, 1974). The pattern is more variable in the pongids: only about one-half of the gorilla and chimpanzee births observed have been followed by consumption of the placenta. This may relate to a suggested function of placentophagy:

avoidance of detection by predators. The smaller, more vulnerable species routinely consume the placenta and all fluids associated with birth, while the two least-preyed upon primate species are as likely not to consume the placenta as they are to do so.

Fraser (1968) has noted that ungulates that do not eat their placentas after delivery are those that move their young away from the birth site soon after parturition. Those that remain at the birth site for several hours or days normally consume the placenta and all birth fluids, suggesting that need to avoid detection is a factor distinguishing the two behaviors. For example, mares, which usually give birth at night, move away from the birth site with their young in the early morning, leaving behind the unconsumed placenta. As further support of his argument that placentophagy is related to predator avoidance, Fraser notes that fetal membranes have been found undigested in stomachs several weeks after consumption. This appears to argue against any nutritional consequences of placentophagy.

The hormonal significance of placentophagy has been suggested by the urgency with which the placenta is consumed by most species. The organ is rich in hormones, particularly oxytocin, which stimulate uterine contractions and inhibit postpartum bleeding. (Oxytocin can be absorbed into the body through the digestive tract.) It may also function in stimulating the mammary glands for earlier milk production.

Despite evidence to the contrary cited previously, the nutritional consequences of placentophagy have also been argued as a function of that behavior. Labor and delivery are energetically demanding processes that leave little time for foraging. Immediately after delivering, a mother has a newborn infant whose physical and nutritional requirements must be met, again leaving little time for foraging. By consuming the placenta, a parturient female receives an energy-rich package of protein, vitamins, and minerals that can satisfy her nutritional needs for several hours. The placenta is especially high in iron, a mineral important for an animal that has depleted its blood supply. Hafez (1968, cited in Townsend and Bailey, 1975) suggests that the birth fluids are sources of salts that may be critical for restoring endocrine and osmotic balance in the parturient.

Finally, consumption of the placenta and birth fluids may facilitate the mother–infant bonding process, particularly in animals that depend at all on olfactory cues for infant recognition.

Interestingly, placentas are often not consumed following abnormal deliveries and stillbirths. This was noted for captive marmosets (Stevenson, 1976), squirrel monkeys (Bowden *et al.*, 1967), and rhesus macaques (Brandt and Mitchell, 1971). Nash (1974), however, observed placentophagy following birth of a dead infant by a wild anubis baboon. In most of these cases, labor and delivery were longer and perhaps harder than usual, suggesting that exhaustion may be partly responsible for the failure to consume the placenta. Supporters of the bonding and predation arguments would argue perhaps that a dead infant obviates the need to consume the placenta.

A clear exception to placentophagy in the primate order is the contemporary human species. In a survey of more than 300 cultural groups in the Human Relations Area Files (HRAF) and other sources, I found no evidence that placentophagy was a normal part of the immediate postpartum period. The placenta, or parts of it, may be dried and retained for medicinal purposes (e.g., among Miao, Vietnamese, Burmese) or for use as an eye wash (e.g., among Siwans and Mixtecans). One source notes that, among the Kol, a childless woman may eat some of the placenta in hopes that it will help her to bear a child (Griffiths, 1946, HRAF). Hart (1965) says that, occasionally, a Filipino midwife will add placenta blood to a rich porridge she feeds the mother after birth in the belief that it will help her regain her strength. Much more commonly found in the ethnographic literature are prohibitions against placentophagy, as among the Lepcha who, according to Gorer (1938, HRAF) believe that eating the placenta will cause skin eruptions.

An exception to this practice of not consuming the placenta can be seen among some contemporary home-birth populations in the United States. Janszen (1980) estimates that placentophagy accompanies 1–2% of home births in the eastern United States and about 5% of those along the West Coast, especially California. She concludes that the practice is part of the "back to nature" movement and is founded, to some extent, on the belief that placenta consumption is common in other cultures and is part of the human heritage. Many of those who participate in placentophagy are otherwise vegetarian but believe that placentas are "unkilled" meat and therefore appropriate for consumption (Janszen, 1980).

Perhaps the most important thing to note about the practice of placentophagy in the United States is the fact that the organ is recognized as having spiritual, emotional, or ritual significance. Although placentas are not normally consumed by contemporary human beings, they are rarely ignored or treated as rubbish, as they are in most of Western society. In fact, if there is a childbirth practice that comes close to universal incidence, it may be concern with the proper disposal of the placenta and umbilical cord. Of 200 cultures in the HRAF that specifically mention disposal of the placenta, only 7 report that it is thrown away without regard. By far the most common method of disposal is burial (130 of 200 cases). Often it must be buried in a special place, usually under the house or not far from it. Trees may be planted over it or it may be buried under a tree. For those contemporary home-birth parents in the United States who do not participate in placentophagy, burying the placenta in the garden or in association with a tree is a common way of recognizing the special significance of the organ.

The disposal of the placenta is believed by many to affect a child's later life. A potpourri of examples from the HRAF follows: in Okinawa, children are supposed to laugh as the placenta is buried so that the infant will be happy. The placenta is well washed by the Thai and placed in a pot with salt so that the baby will not get pimples. According to the Trobrianders, burying the placenta in the garden ensures that the child will be a good gardener. In Iran, if a placenta is put in a mouse hole the child will be smart. In parts of Mexico, placing the placenta in a tree will make the child able to climb trees. If the Nootka want a child to be a good dancer, they sprinkle the placenta with down and spin a top on it four times.

The disposition of the placenta may also reflect sex roles. In the Marshall Islands, a boy's placenta is thrown into the sea so that he will be a good fisherman, and a girl's placenta is hung in a pandanus tress so that she will be a good weaver. The Aymara bury the placenta with miniature farm implements for a boy and cooking utensils for a girl.

In some cultures, the disposal of the placenta is tied to future childbearing by the mother. For example, the Pawnee midwife wraps it in leather and grass and hangs it in a tree with requests that the next birth to that woman be easy. The Tzeltal will bury the placenta deeply if they do not want more children. The Cherokee father, charged with burying the placenta, crosses one, two, or three mountain ridges in doing so, depending on the number of years he wants to pass before the next child is born.

A belief in a supernatural or otherwise special relationship between an infant and its placenta is common. For example, the Yoruba believe that the child is supernaturally tied to the placenta and that he or she will always look back toward the father's house where it is buried. This belief is so strong among the Mam that if a birth occurs away from home, the placenta must be cooked until it is dry so that it can be brought back and buried in the home. Upon death, according to Egyptian mythology, a person's soul returns to his *ka,* a double or twin personality; some scholars believe that the *ka* is actually the placenta.

One reason for concern about the placenta in several cultures is ascription of "personess" to it. For example, in Tibet the placenta is called *dartsendo* or "birth friend." Terms with similar meanings are used among the Kurd and Trukese. The Thai believe that it is part of the child and must be disposed of quickly so that it will not fall into the hands of someone who wants to do evil to the child. The placenta is considered to be the younger sibling of the child in cultures of Malaysia, Jordan, and Java. Among the Fellahin and Ganda, it is called by a term that means "second child."

Even in contemporary sociobiological writing, the placenta has been referred to as the sibling of the fetus (Mackey, 1984). According to Mackey, the placenta has its own metabolism, its own life span, and it can live in the absence of a fetus. Since it cannot reproduce itself, however, it is by definition "celibate" and, according to Mackey, can be used to test sociobiological models of altruism, inclusive fitness, and parental investment. He argues that since the placenta and fetus share 100% of their genes, while the placenta and mother share only 50% of their genes, it would be expected that the placenta would evolve a strategy that favors the fetus. Since both fetus and placenta are dependent on the mother, however, her survival is, of necessity, also favored. Furthermore, any future offspring of the mother are related to the placenta by at least 25% of their genes, so the placenta should, given a choice, favor the mother's life over that of the fetus, its identical "twin." In other words, if the placenta favors the fetus to the extent of jeopardizing the life of the mother, its inclusive fitness is far lower (perhaps 0) than it would be if the placenta favors the life of the mother over that of the fetus (if the mother has future offspring, the placenta's fitness would be far higher than 0). Mackey (1984) proposes a testable hypothesis deduced from sociobiological theory: "Maternal deaths in humans associated with pregnancy should be significantly lower than fetal deaths as indexed by spontaneous abortion and still-births" (452). Analysis of fetal and maternal death rates in the United States from 1950 to 1980 supported his hypothesis, a conclusion that should surprise no one.

Birth Attendants

Perhaps the most significant difference between parturition in human and nonhuman animals is that birth is routinely performed with assistance in our species. There are several reasons for this, most of which have been reviewed previously.

Probably the primary importance of having attendants at birth is that they provide security and emotional support for females of a species in which degree of intellectual development is such that they are more aware than most mammals of their vulnerability at the time of labor and delivery. There are also mechanical or physical reasons that having assistance at birth has been favored in our species. These include: the close correspondence between fetal head size and maternal pelvic size brought about by bipedalism and encephalization; the risks of injury to and infection of the perineal area resulting from too rapid delivery of the head and shoulders; the tendency for the fetus to present the occiput in a position anterior to the mother's pubic symphysis, risking injury and paralysis in the infant if it is brought forward too rapidly by the mother herself; and the helplessness of the neonate and associated greater difficulties in establishing respiration, nursing, and thermoregulation. Despite all of these difficulties, women can and have given birth unassisted for millennia, but mortality increases significantly in those cases.

In few species other than human beings does assistance and solicitude by others during parturition approach that observed in dolphins. Brown (cited in Russell and Russell, 1975) describes a three-female, three-species interaction wherein one female was giving birth to a stillborn infant whose fin was caught in the maternal pelvis. One female from another species pulled the fetus out and helped the mother hold it at the surface. A second female pulled out the placenta. In other cases, a second female has been observed chasing intruder males away from a new mother and infant. Occasionally a mother, helper, and infant will be surrounded by other group members if an outside danger is present. All of these observations were made on captive dolphins, but it suggests that the potential for assistance at parturition is part of the behavioral repertoire of this family.

Typically in nonhuman primate births in captivity, other group members, especially females and juveniles, are interested in the delivery process and the newborn infant. Actual assistance to the mother is rare, however. Doyle *et al.* (1967) report that a female loris was observed grooming the perineal area of a laboring cagemate. Marmoset males appear interested in the delivery process and often try to interfere, but their assistance is usually limited to curious touching of the crowning fetal head and cleaning of the neonates (Caine and Mitchell, 1977). Others have reported interest in the delivery process on the part of animals other than the mother in captivity (e.g., Gouzoules, 1974; Mitchell and Brandt, 1975).

Occasionally the mother is afforded protection by other members of her group, both in captivity and in the wild, but rarely is there interference in the birth process. Examples include the two female langurs who came to the ground with a laboring troopmate and remained with her until delivery was complete (Oppenheimer, 1976). They were most likely motivated by curiosity, but their presence, for whatever reason, probably added a measure of protection and security to the mother and infant. In general, macaque and langur births attract attention from other females and juveniles who are often so persistent in their desires to see and touch the infant that they pose hazards to the mother and her infant. This attention is not necessarily maladaptive, however, because it enhances the likelihood of adoption in the event that something should happen to the mother.

Abegglen and Abegglen (1976) report an incident during parturition observed in a wild hamadryas baboon that suggests that intervention and assistance may occur in unusual circumstances. In this case, a female was delivering what was probably her first infant, while squatting over the edge of a cliff. When the infant was expelled, it thus fell over the cliff, dangling by its umbilical cord. Her male harem leader had been watching nearby throughout her entire labor but had made no attempt to interfere or to touch her. When the infant fell over the edge of the cliff, he jumped up and attempted to catch it. The mother had already grabbed it before the male got to them, however.

Perhaps the closest thing to a midwife-attended delivery in primates was observed in a pair of captive orangutans. The male of the pair became sexually aroused as parturition approached, but as soon as the head appeared he seated himself behind the female and assisted her in giving birth by pulling the infant gently with his mouth over the infant's head. Once the head was out, he used his hands to complete the delivery and handed the infant to the mother when she turned around to receive it (Ulrich, 1970, cited in Caine and Mitchell, 1977). This report is particularly interesting in connection with the Bornean Iban myth that knowledge of midwifery skills was obtained by a man who watched an orangutan assist his mate in delivery (Jensen, 1967).

For caged animals, there is little control over animals being attracted to the parturient and neonate, although females will often attempt to separate themselves from the group. In the wild, it may be more common to seek isolation before giving birth. Goodall (1971) notes that chimpanzees become more solitary as parturition approaches; Galdikas (1982) reports the same thing for orangutans. In more vulnerable species, such as gelada (Dunbar and Dunbar, 1974) and hamadryas (Kummer, 1968) baboons, isolation may not be adaptive, and birth usually takes place in the midst of group members. In most circumstances, for mammals other than human beings, it is probably best to have no interference during parturition. The mother and infant are particularly vulnerable to infection at this time, and newborn infants could be stepped on or eaten by overly interested birth watchers. Thus, if assistance is not necessary, it is adaptive to deliver in isolation to reduce the risks of infection and injury. These are also risks for human mothers and infants, but in this case the benefits of assistance outweigh the risks of having a few other people present.

Assistance at childbirth has probably been a normal part of parturition in human beings for more than a million years. I would argue that the obstetrical problems confronting human females today originated with encephalization in our lineage that began that long ago. As with modern humans, it was likely possible for *Homo erectus* females to give birth without assistance, but having that assistance and support would have made the difference between life and death for many mothers and infants in that grade. Even a slight reduction in mortality would lead to selection for the behavioral characteristic of seeking companionship during parturition. Today, it is almost universally distributed in our species.

In a few cultures, under special circumstances, women may choose to give birth alone. In all of these cultures, however, marriage rules require that a woman mate with a member of her own group, often with a distant relative. Thus, mother and father would be similar in genotype and body size and shape, and their offspring would be compatible with the mother's genotype and pelvis. Of the 296 groups that I surveyed where mention is made of attendance at childbirth, ethnographers for 24 of them mention that delivery may and often does take place unattended. Among the Igbo of Southeast Nigeria, for example, the first birth is always supervised, but if that one is easy, subsequent births may take place alone (Uchendu, 1965). Women of the nomadic Pitjandjara tribe of Australia may also drop behind the group to deliver alone if no problems are anticipated (Tindale, 1974). !Kung San primiparae give birth in the bush alone, according to Estermann (1976), but an older, experienced woman watches nearby and assists if difficulties arise. Shostak (1981) notes that a woman giving birth alone aroused consternation in the !Kung group she studied. Howell (1979) reports that although giving birth alone is the cultural ideal for !Kung women, most have their mothers, sisters, or other women with them when they give birth.

More commonly, the ethnographic literature reports the presence of a birth attendant at parturition. In general, there are three major categories of birth attendant found throughout the world. The first, and probably the most ancient, is an older female relative who has received no training in midwifery other than having given birth herself. In a number of cultures (26), it is required that a woman's mother attend her; in a few (5), the mother-in-law is the primary attendant. Only on Yap and Easter Island is the father the normal attendant at birth.

A second category, which is probably the most common, is the traditional or village midwife, a woman who is not necessarily a relative of the parturient woman but who has attended many births so that the habit of calling her for assistance has developed in the local area. Usually she herself must also have given birth, and there are a number of cultures that forbid any childless woman from attending births. An exception are the Samoans who prefer that their midwives be barren.

In the third category are the professional midwives. These women have received formal training or have attended so many births that their expertise is widely known. They usually call themselves midwives and often receive compensation for their services. Often these women began practicing as traditional midwives but sought further formal training or apprenticed themselves to another, more experienced midwife. In some countries, programs have been set up for training and licensing midwives, usually attracting younger and better educated women. Despite the evidence that formal training results in better pregnancy outcomes, however, the licensed midwives are not always preferred by the village people. This is in part because the professional midwives do not always adhere to the cultural traditions surrounding childbirth. For example, in India, traditional midwives come from the Untouchable caste, and they are thus inferior to the women of the castes they serve and have no sanctions against working with the blood and fluids of childbirth. Government-trained midwives, who come from higher castes, will not cut the cord, clean up after a birth, or return to change bandages; instead they call upon an Untouchable woman to perform these duties. Since this means that two fees must be paid at birth, many Indian women prefer to call on the traditional midwife because she is cheaper, although usually less skilled (Gordon *et al.,* 1964, 1965).

Most traditional midwives are simply attendants and do very little to interfere with the birth process unless complications arise. Providing prenatal care is rare, although postpartum care of mother and child is a duty of many midwives. The term that is used for midwife is often indicative of her primary function. In many languages, it can be translated roughly as "one who receives the child." For example, the southern Chinese midwives are *tan-min*, "women who catch birth." Among the Tiv of Nigeria, the midwife is "she who seizes the child." The Navajo term for midwife is *awe-xai-zi-si*, "the woman who pulls the baby out." The Tikopia midwife is *te fafine o tesiki*, "the woman of the catching."

Massage during the last weeks of pregnancy and during labor is part of the practice of many midwives around the world. In a number of cases, massage is used effectively to turn a breech. Often the midwife's claim to fame is her expertise in herbal remedies, although administration of concoctions during labor and delivery is far from universal. Vaginal stretching is done by midwives in several cultures, and perineal tearing (episiotomy) is performed by some, when necessary. Manual dilation of the cervix is practiced by some, and fundal pressure may be provided if necessary.

Aggressive midwives are not uncommon, and in some cultures it is believed that labor must be very short and delivery hastened. Moller (1961:77) says of the Bahayas that, "The principle of 'masterly inactivity' on the part of the midwife is unknown." The Iban midwives are said to use a great deal of force, according to Jensen (1967). Among the Thonga of South Africa it is desirable to have the baby and the placenta expelled at the same time, so violent pressure is often applied to the abdomen.

Midwives usually take responsibility for the newborn infant and will try several procedures to get it to take the first breath. This may include holding it upside down by the feet, dipping it in cold water, shaking, rubbing, or massaging it, or artificial respiration. Most often it is the midwife who cuts the cord and bathes and dresses the child, while simultaneously keeping an eye on the mother, watching for delivery of the placenta and excessive postpartum bleeding. Although herbs with oxytocic effects are known and used and bimanual pressure on the uterine artery is practiced by midwives in various parts of the world, postpartum hemorrhage is probably the greatest single cause of maternal mortality in childbirth today and in the past.

In summary, there is a great deal of variation in the qualifications, experience, and practices of midwives throughout the world. But, the practice of having some form of assistance at birth is one of the best candidates for that elusive human phenomenon, the cultural universal.

Participation by Adult Males in Birth

Highly variable in the primate order is the role of the father, or adult males in general, in birth and parenting. As has been noted, males of many species take an active interest in parturition and neonates, especially in species that are socially organized in such a way that the father is somewhat determinable. Males are not likely to invest time and energy in offspring that are not certainly their own. Not surprisingly then, we find more paternal care and interest in pair-bonded species such as gelada and hamadryas baboons, gibbons, and callitrichids. On the other end of the continuum in primates are those species in which males show intolerance of or open hostility toward young. In some cases, hostility is evidence that the adult male is likely not the biological father. In fact, although it may be difficult to determine who the father *is* in some primate groups, it is occasionally a simple matter to guess who the father is *not*.

The prime, and by now familiar, example of this are the Hanuman langurs observed by Sugiyama (1966) and by Hrdy (1977). Under certain conditions, such as high population pressure and scarce resources, members of this species may organize themselves in one-male heterosexual groups and all-male "bachelor" bands. The adult male in the heterosexual group is usually the only one who mates with the females in that group; thus, his paternity is assured. Occasionally a bachelor band will attack a heterosexual group, driving off its resident male who is replaced by a male from the marauding band. In such instances, the new leader male has been observed killing young that are still nursing. This stress or some associated factor appears to induce spontaneous abortion in some of the females carrying the offspring of the previous male leader. They then come into estrus, the new male mates with them, and the resulting offspring contain his genetic investment. This is one of the clearest examples known of intrasexual competition among males of a mammalian species. Obviously it is disadvantageous for the females and young, and indeed females in a band will often unite in their effort to protect their young from the infanticide-intent male. Once things have settled down, however, the females may perhaps benefit from the greater genetic and protective potential of their new leader.

On the other end of the continuum are marmosets and tamarins, the males of which take active interest in young even at parturition. Stevenson (1976) reports that in captivity, males will lick neonates and will carry them as early as the first few hours of their lives, behaviors that are otherwise almost universally restricted to mothers. Paternal care usually continues beyond the birth day, with the male carrying the offspring (commonly twins) a great percentage of the time, although other members of the social group also perform caretaking roles, especially after the first month (Epple, 1975; Vogt *et al.,* 1978).

In most other nonhuman primate species, males show various degrees of tolerance toward and interest in newborn infants. In some species, such as gibbons and siamangs, caretaking by the fathers does not begin until several months after birth of the infant, often coinciding with the return of estrus in the mother. Overall, paternal interest in very young infants is highly variable among all primate species. Within a single species, particularly in captivity, male behavior may range from infanticide to active caretaking. There are no clear trends within the order, suggesting that ecology, ontogeny, and idiosyncratic variables have stronger effects on paternal behavior than phylogeny (Mitchell and Brandt, 1975). Mackey (1976) reinforces this view by arguing that the human adult male–child bond is not a product of our primate heritage but rather derives from the behavioral–ecological role of food sharing and is, thus, a bond convergent with that in social carnivores.

The within-group variation in paternal care is nowhere so clear as it is in our own species. The social definition and role of fatherhood ranges from almost nonexistence to our current emphasis on equality of parenting roles for mothers and fathers. (Thus Margaret Mead's frequently quoted statement that fathers are a biological necessity but a social accident.) An equivalent range can also be found regarding paternal participation in childbirth. On Manus, not only is a man forbidden to be present at the birth of his child, he is not permitted to see it for 1 month (Mead, 1930). After this, however, he participates extensively in child care. On Yap, Easter Island, and among some contemporary Western couples, fathers actually assist in the delivery of their offspring.

Of the more than 300 cultures that I surveyed in the HRAF and other sources, only 159 make any mention of men being allowed to attend or being prohibited from being present at childbirth: in 31, husbands are encouraged to attend and are given specific tasks to perform; in 42, husbands may attend but they do so rarely or they are called in only when complications arise; in 86 societies, it is stated that all men, including husbands, are forbidden at childbirth. Among the reasons cited for prohibiting males at childbirth are that it is polluting, unclean, or dangerous for men to participate. Modesty may also be a reason for preventing males from viewing the delivery of a child, and some simply state that men do not want to or should not see their wives in such extreme pain. Where husbands do participate in delivery, their role is to provide physical, emotional, or ritual support for their wives. In some cases, their participation is so great that they undergo restrictions and participate in activities similar to those of the parturient herself, such as in the couvade practiced in parts of South America. By most interpretations, this process and other rituals of childbirth practiced by males help to assure the social paternity of the father (Paige and Paige, 1981).

In the United States, the father's role in childbirth has fluctuated with the location of labor and delivery. When it was common for delivery to take place at home, the father usually remained with his wife during birth, occasionally serving as midwife himself. When hospital births became the norm, the father was often excluded altogether and could see his child only through nursery windows. Today, primarily due to consumer pressure, it is common for men to participate in labor and delivery, even in hospitals. A number of childbirth preparation methods, including Lamaze and Bradley's Husband-Coached-Childbirth, encourage the husband's presence at birth as a way of alleviating pain, anxiety, and complications. Henneborn and Cogan (1975), for example, found that women whose husbands attended delivery reported less pain and more positive feelings about the total birth experience than did those whose husbands did not attend delivery. They were also less likely to receive medication than the women whose husbands were not present. Given current concerns about the effects of obstetrical medications on neonates, this renewed behavior is adaptive if it does serve to reduce their usage.

The rationale of enhancing bonding between father and child is commonly given for encouraging fathers to be present at birth. John Bowlby (1958), who did some of the pioneering work on infant–to–mother attachment, stated that the father is not important to the infant except as a source of economic and emotional support for the mother. There is now a great deal of research that argues that fathers have a predisposition to bond to their infants in the same way mothers do, but it is obscured by cultural roles and expectations. McDonald (1978) describes a typical paternal reaction to birth and the newborn that includes hovering above the mother and infant, prolonged gazing at the infant, face-to-face interacting, fingertip exploring, and palmar massaging of the infant. The fathers he observed were with their wives at home deliveries. We will see later that many of these behaviors are those that have been described as ''species specific,'' and perhaps genetically mediated, in human mothers.

Greenberg and Morris (1974) describe a paternal behavior they call ''engrossment'' and define as a sense of preoccupation, absorption, and interest in the infant. They found that fathers express eagerness to look at and to touch their infants, are aware of distinctive characteristics in their newborn, and describe a magnetic attraction to their infants and a ''high'' feeling when they interact with them. These behaviors and feelings appeared in fathers, regardless of whether or not they had attended the delivery of their child. Those who had been present at the delivery felt more confident that they could recognize their own in a room full of newborn infants, felt more comfortable holding their infants, and felt more certainty about their paternity.

Several studies have found that fathers who participate in birth also participate more in later caretaking of infants. This new trend is adaptive in a highly mobile society characterized by neolocal family organization, where fathers are often the only other persons available to help the mother with child care. In the past and in most other cultures today, female relatives live near enough to provide occasional relief for the mother from caretaking duties.

Greenberg and Morris (1974) have hypothesized that the engrossment they describe for fathers is a basic, innate potential in all fathers and that problems with the father–infant dyad and with the family unit may develop when engrossment is not allowed to develop fully. If they are correct, the behavior was most likely selected very recently in human evolution (unlike mother–to–infant attachment, which is likely several million years old) and may help explain the origin of the human pair-bonded family, Thus, if infants are elicitors of attachment and engrossment in fathers, the males are more likely to remain in a family unit with their young and their mothers and are more likely to provide for and protect them if engrossment is allowed to develop fully.

An alternative view, and one that has the cross-cultural evidence behind it, is that since fathers have not normally participated in birth and neonatal care until recently, the nurturing behavior exhibited by many fathers is a learned reaction. Perhaps, then, early contact with infants is even more important for fathers because unlike mothers, they are not biologically or culturally primed to be responsive to infant cues. The birth experience appears to be a powerful releaser of nurturing behavior in observers of all ages and both sexes, a factor that may assure that a bond will form between the infant and participants at delivery who have genetic or emotional investment in him.

Alice Rossi (1977) is a proponent of the foregoing view and notes that as we become freer to chose to have offspring or not, the mother–child relationship may become even stronger, perhaps to the exclusion of the father. She concludes that,

> If a society wishes to create shared parental roles, it must either accept the high probability that the mother–infant relationship will continue to have greater emotional depth than the father–infant relationship or institutionalize the means for providing men with compensatory exposure and training in infant and child care in order to close the gap produced by the physiological experience of pregnancy, birth and lactation. Without such compensatory training of males, females will show added dimensions of intensity to their bonds with children (p. 18).

There have been a number of theories about the origin of the human family and the pair bond, most of which allude to the importance of sexual division of labor as a major contributing factor. At some point in human evolution, one argument runs, it became selectively advantageous for males to forage more widely than females who had young infants and to provision those females and young. This shift from every-individual-for-itself to sharing of food accompanied changes in hominid morphology, in the ecosystem occupied, and in increased helplessness of the hominid infant (Lovejoy, 1981).

Owen Lovejoy (1981) has pointed out that pair-bonding and male parental care are adaptive in the callitrichids because of the high protein and calorie requirements of these small animals with their high metabolic rates. Gestation and lactation place heavy burdens on the female, a disadvantage usually compensated for by smaller body size in most primate species. Among callitrichids, however, males and females are almost equal in body size. Thus, by carrying the infants while the pair forages, the male helps to equalize their burdens. By extrapolation to our species, Lovejoy argues that males, foraging widely and provisioning females and young who stay closer to the home base, also help to equalize parental burdens. A male is unlikely to provision young that are not his own, so it follows that pair-bonding and certainty of paternity were necessary components of this adaptive strategy. By becoming bonded to one female, a male could be relatively assured of paternity of her offspring. If he were a good provider, she would in turn be able to provide better care to his offspring, reduce chances of accidents resulting from traveling long distances in unfamiliar territory, and perhaps reduce her energetic requirements so that the period of postpartum amenorrhea was shortened. This would mean that she could conceive sooner after birth and that, over their lifetimes, the pair-bond would have greater numbers of offspring. More young infants, of course, meant further decrease in female mobility and further dependence on male providers. Lovejoy continues his argument by stating that it was the origin of the nuclear family that enabled the hominid species to embark on a reproductive strategy that resulted in increased population and in our becoming the dominant species on earth today. Fisher (1975, 1982) and Alexander and Noonan (1979) have developed similar arguments, expanding on the importance of loss of estrus and concealed ovulation in the females as an enhancement of male–female bonding. Tanner and Zihlman (1976) add that, although the mother–infant bond is the fundamental core of sociality in our and other primate species, hominid females have tended to favor males who contributed not only economically to the family unit, but socially as well. Thus, caring and sharing are characteristics of most human fathers today, and the potential for high interest in childbirth and neonates is inherent. Furthermore, if males were attracted to the birth of an infant in times past, they were more likely to provide assistance and protection to the mother and infant at an especially vulnerable time. In the long run, males who assisted their mates at birth would have more surviving offspring. Such a behavior could become fairly well established in several hundred generations in a species as dependent on assistance and emotional support at birth as are hominids.

SUMMARY

In this chapter, we have added a number of other characteristics that are part of the human reproductive strategy and that help distinguish human behavior at birth from that of most other primates. The endocrine activity and mechanical actions of labor and delivery are somewhat similar among all primates. Sensations of pain in labor are apparently felt by females in most primate species as well. Distinguishing characteristics in humans are the tendency to deliver the fetus in a face-to-sacrum position, the tendency not to consume the placenta, although ritual disposal is common, and, perhaps most important of all, the very common and apparently unique practice of having assistance at birth. We have also seen that the human neonate is more helpless at birth than neonates of other haplorhine primates. As has been argued and will be argued in the next chapter, this places a number of demands and restrictions on human mothers that make her behavior at birth somewhat different from that observed in most other female primates.

CHAPTER
4

THE NEWBORN
INFANT

In Chapter 1, I argued that, in some ways, the human neonate is an exterogestate fetus, in that many of the physiological and biochemical processes necessary for normal functioning are not fully developed at birth. As I and others have suggested, this state of incomplete development results from selection for birth to occur in humans at a time when the expanding brain can still emerge through the narrow pelvis of the bipedal human female. The result is a finely tuned balance between the maximum stage of development that can be passed successfully through the birth canal and the minimum stage of development that can allow the neonate to survive without placental support. Expanding cultural and behavioral supports over the last two million years have been critical for the success of that adaptation. Still, the balance is often not achieved as evidenced by incidence of prematurity, postmaturity, and growth retardation due to placental insufficiency. A review of the challenges faced by the neonate in the immediate postpartum period may help us appreciate the difficulties encountered as selection favored encephalization in a bipedal animal.

At birth, the infant faces dramatic changes in every aspect of its environment: sound, light, temperature, humidity, gravity; everything in the external world becomes different and a challenge to meet. Even more dramatic, however, are the changes in the internal environment that must occur before the infant can even begin to respond to the new world outside its mother's body.

We think of neonates as extremely vulnerable organisms, and indeed they are, but they apparently tolerate far more stress at parturition than the older infant or adult could endure. For example, neonates tolerate more hypoxia than older individuals can, and their response to rapid cooling at delivery is moderate enough that excessive strain is not placed on energy metabolism (Stave, 1970). Newborn infants also have great tolerance for low blood glucose levels and drastic changes in plasma pH values that take place at birth. Stave lists the precursors of shock in the adult was described by Selye in 1956 (e.g., hypothermia, hypotension, depression of the CNS, decrease in muscle tone, hemoconcentration, generalized tissue catabolism acidosis) and notes that, although all of these stresses are associated with parturition, the normal infant does not exhibit symptoms of shock that would be expected in the adult. Because

119

shock would likely be lethal to neonates, selection has favored neonatal tolerance to these stresses that essentially makes them ineffective. Such tolerance is not exhibited in adults, who, if faced with the stresses that an infant experiences during parturition, would certainly experience shock and, likely, death.

While *in utero,* the placenta performed many of the functions that the infant at birth must assume for himself. The placenta was the organ of respiration, digestion, and excretion. A fetus could lack entirely or have serious defects of the lungs, liver, kidneys, and neocortex and survive until birth when the placenta is no longer available as a substitute for these organs.

The most immediate need at birth is establishment of respiration. While *in utero,* the fetal lungs are partially filled with fluid, and the rest is compressed so that there is no air in them. Pressure on the chest walls during the birth process prepares the lungs for breathing, and it is probably that the sudden impact of cool air on the face makes a baby gasp and take its first breath. At that time, an infant usually cries, a behavior that is likely reflexive in response to the rapid filling of the lungs and the air passing over the vocal cords for the first time. Birth is undoubtedly stressful, but this first cry is unlikely a cry of distress. In fact, for those present at a birth, this first cry is a joyful sign that the infant has met its first challenge to survival. Initial respirations for most infants are shallow and irregular. Regular respiration, with peaks of about 85 breaths per minute, is established 15–30 minutes after unmedicated deliveries, 90 minutes after medicated ones (Desmond *et al.,* 1963).

In response to the change in the source of oxygen, there is a change in the delivery system. Four channels through which oxygenated blood flowed during fetal development close at birth, or shortly thereafter, as the lungs, rather than the placenta, become the source of oxygen. For a few minutes after birth, the placenta continues to supply oxygen to the infant. Since even a few minutes without oxygen can result in brain damage, it appears that among our adaptations to the birth process is a brief period of time during which oxygen is supplied both by the placenta and through the lungs. The placenta ceases to supply the oxygen, and the cord stops pulsating within a few minutes after birth, when, presumably, the transition is complete.

In the United States, the umbilical cord is usually cut immediately after birth. The argument supporting this controversial practice is that an excess of blood transfusion from the placenta will put extra stress on the neonatal circulatory system which is already stressed to its limits. Excess blood also results in a higher than normal hematocrit which could lead to polycythemia, a condition that in turn can result in respiratory and neurological problems. Late clamping may also result in transfer of higher than normal levels of placental steroids which could, in turn, affect neonatal state changes and other behaviors (Theorell *et al.,* 1973).

Those who argue for late clamping of the cord note that richer blood gives the infant a head start, especially if the mother's hemoglobin has been low during pregnancy. It has been suggested that clamping the cord too soon prolongs the third stage because the placenta remains engorged with blood. The argument about a backup source of oxygen is probably the most cogent one: without oxygen, the infant is certain to die or suffer brain damage; with too much blood, the chances of survival may be reduced, but not by so much. Perhaps in recognition of the advantages, very rarely is the cord cut immediately after birth in most societies of the world.

While *in utero,* the fetal production of red blood cells is higher than that produced after birth. Most of it is fetal hemoglobin (HbF) rather than normal adult hemoglobin (HbA), and it is not until several months after birth that infant blood has the same composition as adult blood. The primary function of hemoglobin is transport of oxygen, so it is likely that the greater number of red blood cells produced *in utero* facilitates greater oxygen transport to the developing brain. One of the consequences of high production of red blood cells just before birth is that there are a great number of them that must be broken down and stored or excreted. Normally this takes place in the liver, but the neonatal liver does not function fully until several months after birth (Crelin, 1973). Hemoglobin thus breaks down, one of its products being bilirubin, but the products cannot be stored or excreted. The increased concentration of bilirubin results in a normal state known as ''physiologic jaundice of the newborn,'' which appears about 3 days after birth. Rapid build-up of excess bilirubin, which results in jaundice on the day of birth, is usually cause for concern. The infant also produces too much bilirubin when it is ABO or Rh incompatible with its mother. In serious cases, this results in hemolytic disease of the newborn.

As mentioned previously, a fetus can completely lack kidneys and still develop normally until birth. Since fetal urine contributes substantially to the amniotic fluid, especially late in pregnancy, there will be almost no amniotic fluid surrounding a fetus lacking kidneys. Otherwise, the kidneys begin functioning at birth, although they do not reach adult level of filtration until about 6 weeks after birth (Crelin, 1973). Blood urea levels are higher than normal until this time.

The immature state of the neonatal liver and kidneys is one of the reasons why obstetrical medication is so dangerous for an infant. The mother's liver can detoxify the drugs she is administered during labor, and her kidneys function to excrete the by-products of this process. With an undeveloped liver, however, the infant has more trouble processing the medications that enter its body through the placenta, and the kidneys are not functioning at levels sufficient to pass them completely. For this reason, medications from which the mother can soon recover may stay in the neonatal system for weeks. The undeveloped CNS is the target for most of the drugs administered to the mother during labor, so it is no wonder that infants whose mothers received high doses of medication (narcotics, barbituates, tranquilizers) perform more poorly on tests of neuromotor functioning at birth than do those whose mothers labored without drugs.

Just before delivery, the fetal heart rate tends to drop but increases immediately at delivery. Desmond *et al.* (1963) found a mean heart rate of 180 beats per minute at peak acceleration which occurred 3 minutes after birth for babies whose mothers received medication during labor and at 2 minutes for babies whose mothers labored without medication. Typically the rate drops to 140 by '30 minutes after birth. For most infants, the heart rate becomes labile, and thus responsive to activity levels, by 2–3 hours after birth.

The newborn lacks the immunity to infections that characterize later life. While *in utero,* maternal antibodies, particularly immunoglobulin G (IgG), passed to the infant through the placenta and provided protection from most infectious agents. Some of the immunities remain for several days to several weeks; additional protective agents are derived from colostrum. The newborn also has a deficient inflammatory response and a poor ability to localize infections (Wennberg *et al.,* 1973).

Once the infant has adapted appropriately to extrauterine sources of oxygen, regulation of body temperature now becomes critical. While *in utero,* the fetus is kept at a fairly constant temperature of about $37.6°C$, through no effort of its own. The cooling experienced at birth is probably adaptive in that it stimulates breathing, but the human neonate is an "imperfect homiotherm" (Sinclair, 1978). Although the fetal hypothalamus is mature at birth, the challenge to maintaining a constant body temperature is greater than that facing normal adults. This is largely due to the greater amount of surface area of the newborn infant compared with that of the adult. In addition, the infant has far less body fat than the normal adult, resulting in what Bruck (1962) estimates to be a heat loss per unit body weight of about four times that seen in adults.

Other factors affecting heat loss include environmental temperature, gestational age of the infant, asphyxia, injury, and anesthesia. Typically, newborn infants born in hospitals are placed under radiant heaters. Concern about a drop in neonatal temperatures has been one of the reasons that mothers and infants have been routinely separated following hospital deliveries. A series of recent studies has revealed, however, that there are no significant differences in rectal temperatures of infants held by their mothers and those placed under radiant heaters (Phillips, 1974; Hill and Shronk, 1979).

As noted in Chapter 2, infants born at TBC were held by their mothers during the first few hours following birth. Rectal temperatures were obtained from 1168 of the infants at 5, 15, and 30 minutes after birth. Mean temperatures were as follows: $37.4°C$ at 5 minutes, $37.0°C$ at 15 minutes, and $36.8°C$ at 30 minutes. These were well within the range cited as normal by Hill and Shronk (1979) and were well above the means cited as minimal by Phillips (1974). Neonatal temperatures at TBC were found to vary with lengths of the first and second stages of labor, birthweight, month of birth, and time between rupture of the membranes and delivery.

The fact that infants survive quite well held in their mothers' arms comes as no surprise to those of us familiar with the normal conditions that have surrounded childbirth for thousands of years of human evolution and in thousands of settings. The infant is equipped with defenses against excessive heat loss. The vernix caseosa, which covers the body, is primarily composed of fats that provide a degree of insulation and also reduce the rate of evaporation (Adamsons and Towell, 1965). Vasodilation and vasoconstriction are fully functioning processes in the neonate. In addition, the human neonate has unusual amounts of brown fat, adipose tissue that has a high metabolic rate and is especially efficient at warming blood as it flows through areas of concentration (Sinclair, 1978).

Infants can also increase their levels of muscular activity, although there is some question as to whether they can actually shiver. Typically, they flex their bodies in response to decreasing temperature and relax in response to an increase in temperature. These posture changes serve to decrease and increase surface area for conservation and dissipation of heat, respectively.

Finally, the human newborn has available a source of warmth that is almost universal among mammals: a mother. Initial behavioral responses available to the infant that serve to derive warmth and solicitation from the mother include clinging, rooting, grasping, and orienting. The infant is equipped with an impressive repertoire of behaviors that make it attractive to the mother and result in her maintaining proximity to it, thus providing warmth from her body. These will be discussed later in this chapter, but suffice it to say now that infants have at their disposal a wide array of mechanisms for maintaining a body and environmental temperature compatible with survival.

Minimizing weight loss is also a challenge to the neonate, so it is adaptive to minimize caloric output through thermoregulation so that caloric input can be maximized through nursing. During fetal life, most nutrients are in the form of glucose absorbed from the placenta. The glucose directly enters the blood and is transported to the brain, precluding the need for digestive enzymes and other processes associated with digestion. During the last few weeks *in utero,* some of this glucose is stored, so that the full-term infant can survive on these stores for about 24 hours. In order to make the transition to milk consumption, the digestive system must begin functioning, digestive enzymes must be produced, and the infant must be able to suck and swallow.

As with obtaining warmth, the neonate is equipped with behavioral mechanisms that serve to attract the mother and induce her to nurse. At birth, the infant can grasp the mother, orient toward her breast, search for the nipple, and suck once it has latched on. If mother is not there when it is hungry, it cries, inducing her to comfort and feed it. The infant's cry initiates the let-down reflex and elevates breast temperature in the mother, further ensuring that the infant gets what it needs. Once it has been nursed and warmed, the neonate further conserves energy by sleeping for much of the first few weeks of life.

Even in sleep, the infant exhibits behavioral adaptations that enable it to conserve energy: it prefers the prone position which, relative to the supine position, results in lower oxygen consumption (Woodson, 1983). The prone position is also associated with more rapid gastric emptying and improved digestive capabilities (Yu, 1975). Most infants will clearly make known their preference for being prone by trying to move into that position or by intense crying, behaviors that quickly educate their parents to place them in that position.

When things go wrong, the newborn human infant is capable of monitoring and regulating its behavior in an attempt to adapt to stresses. As Woodson (1983) notes, clinical warning signs that are detected by the caretaker or physician are, in many cases, attempts on the part of the infant to adapt to complications. For example, decreased metabolic activity in a jaundiced infant may serve to increase adaptive response to this threat by conserving energy (Prechtl *et al.*, 1973; Woodson, 1983). Premature infants, who spend far more time sleeping than do full-term infants, can also be seen as optimizing their growth and survival potential by conserving energy (Woodson, 1983). Woodson further argues that the clinical expectation of stability in newborn infant behaviors is inappropriate in that it does not take into consideration the neonate's ability to modify its behavior in response to the physiological changes that are normal in the immediate postpartum period.

Birth has been described as a major life crisis event, a time of transition, of abrupt change and reorganization of life's circumstances. With all of the critical events that must take place within minutes of birth, it is no wonder that neonatal mortality is so high in many parts of the world. It is also not surprising that a high degree of ritual is associated with birth in most cultures. Finally, it is no wonder that many people in the United States think that the only safe place for birth is in a hospital where there are highly skilled attendants and sophisticated equipment to intervene should even a single adaptation fail.

THE NEONATAL BRAIN

The neonatal brain undergoes a transition of sorts at the time of birth, although the scale of change is different from that described for immediate adaptation to the extrauterine environment. At birth, the neonatal brain weighs between 300 and 400 g, approximately one-quarter the size it will be in adulthood. Much of fetal and neonatal behavior appears to be regulated by subcortical areas of the brain. At the time of birth, the subcortical parts of the brain (midbrain and hindbrain) are relatively mature, whereas the neocortex is relatively immature. Bronson (1982), reflecting traditional views of infant behavior, notes that since myelinization of sensory pathways into the neocortex begins just before birth, processing in the neocortex is "at best minimal at birth." He further argues that the development of the fetal and neonatal brain parallels human evolutionary history: the more recently evolved parts are less mature at birth and mature more slowly after birth. The transition from subcortical control of behavior to neocortical control begins soon after birth. A great deal of the development of the neocortex from then on is dependent on experience.

Continuing his analogy with human evolutionary history, Bronson argues that most of the behaviors that are observed in newborn infants are processed by phylogenetically older subcortical areas. For example, subcortical components of the visual system can account for the neonate's ability to track moving objects in his visual field, to orient toward peripheral stimuli, and to fix attention briefly on different types of visual stimuli. As evidence, Bronson notes that most of the visual and motor behaviors observed in normal newborns can be elicited in anencephalic infants, those who lack entirely a neocortex and function exclusively at the subcortical level. These infants may survive for several days, until the time the transition to neocortical control normally occurs.

Identification of subcortical motor responses at birth is facilitated by noting the following criteria, according to Bronson (1982): (1) such responses are easily elicited; (2) there is less variation and more stereotypy in the responses; and (3) they can be elicited before term. Good examples of these responses include walking, crawling, and swimming motions that newborn full-term and premature infants exhibit. If one holds up a 1-hour-old infant and lets its feet touch the table, it will straighten out its legs as if to stand. The infant will also move its legs in an alternative walking movement known as "primary walking" (Zelazo *et al.*, 1972). After a few tries at primary walking, movements become more rhythmic, and the infant holds its body straight with its head erect and steady. If placed on its stomach, a newborn infant will attempt to crawl, although it will not make such movements several weeks after birth. Eibl-Eibesfeldt (1975) has an amazing series of photographs that show a premature infant suspended by her hands below a rope, with no assistance. The waning of these behaviors can be attributed, some argue, to the overriding effects of the maturing neocortical processes (McGraw, 1943; Bronson, 1982). Zelazo *et al.* (1972) report, however, that if infants are exercised using walking motions, some of these behaviors can be prolonged indefinitely. In fact, if the infant is "walked" regularly, independent walking develops earlier, suggesting that it may be our child-rearing practices that result in an 11.7 month onset of walking (Bayley, 1970) rather than capabilities inherent in the infant. Zelazo and colleagues suggest that primary walking, in fact, may serve as a stimulus to parents to try to enhance this behavior beyond the waning associated with the transition to neocortical control of behavior. Stratton (1982a) proposes, on the other hand, that walking and crawling movements may have functioned *in utero* to get the fetus into the vertex position, and that to speculate on their function in the neonatal period is fruitless.

As evidence for the former view, Konner (1973) offers data on !Kung infants that suggest that parental treatment and expectations of infants result in onset of walking at an earlier age than expected in Western nations. In fact, some of the physical movements exhibited by neonates, such as placing, walking, crawling, and the Moro reflex, while seen as functionless by neurologists who first described them, are now seen to have function when observed in the context in which they evolved. !Kung infants are carried upright, in a sling, against their mother's skin. Placing, walking, and crawling movements enable the infant to readjust itself at will and may enable it to avoid suffocation, should its face be pressed too hard against its mother's flesh (Konner, 1973).

The period of subcortical control corresponds to Piaget's Stage One of human infant development. This is the stage of reflexive movements and global actions and usually lasts for the first few weeks of life in the human. During this time, a newborn will suck almost anything placed in its mouth and grasp almost anything placed in its hands. Only later will its movements be more refined and will it be more selective in its actions. In a normal human infant, this stage lasts from birth to approximately 1 month. In contrast, the stage lasts less than 2 weeks in macaques, reflecting the greater cerebral maturation evident in monkeys at birth (Parker, 1977).

The period of transition from subcortical to neocortical dominance in behavior processing has implications for Sudden Infant Death Syndrome (SIDS), according to Rovee-Collier and Lipsitt (1982). They note that the greatest risk from SIDS occurs between 2 and 4 months of life, the period during which primary reflex patterns are being replaced by learned behaviors. They characterize this period as one of "neurobehavioral disorganization and disarray" and see it as a critical period for learning certain behaviors. Supports of the subcortical system are being withdrawn from the infant and must be replaced by a learning-dependent neocortex.

Normal neonates respond to breathing obstacles (e.g., the mother's breast) with automatic struggles. Later, however, they must do so using learned responses. Many infants who succumb to SIDS are later determined to have been suffering from slight colds or sniffles before death. Rovee-Collier and Lipsitt suggest that these infants never learned the appropriate response (e.g., breathe through the mouth) and thus do not make the proper adaptation when the nose is occluded. There is, perhaps, in this hypothesis an explanation for why breastfed babies are underrepresented in SIDS statistics. Stratton (1982a) notes that breastfeeding is a challenge for newborn infants, but one that most can meet appropriately. The surmountable challenge prepares them to meet later challenges. Bottlefeeding, on the other hand, is relatively easy and does not provide a challenge to the infants. Bottlefeeding may thus deprive infants of the experiences that prepare them for appropriate responses to later interference with respiration.

Brazelton (1979) argues that, although most neonatal behaviors are under subcortical control, a normal infant is able to modify its responses and regulate its behavior in such a way that can only be explained by a functioning neocortex. For example, a normal infant will react to various stimuli (e.g., auditory, visual, or tactual) with decreasing response levels, eventually habituating or screening out the no longer interesting stimulus. This is adaptive because it reduces unnecessary energy expenditure. The Brazelton Neonatal Behavioral Assessment Scale (NBAS) was designed to test CNS functioning in the newborn as separate from reflex responses, which may be under subcortical control. In addition to 20 reflex measures that are obtained during the exam, there are 26 behavioral responses, all designed to measure infant reactions to stimuli that would be normally encountered in the infant's environment (i.e., a Western Caucasian infant's environment). Although the scale does not explicitly measure neurological functioning, the behaviors that are evaluated are indicative of such.

As an example, one of the behaviors elicited in the NBAS is the infant's response to an auditory stimulus, specifically a bell or rattle being shaken at his ear. If the CNS is intact, the expected reaction is one of a startle with changes in respiration and eye movements on the first trial. After one or two more rings, the normal infant will be able to shut out the stimulus (i.e., habituate to it) and suppress reaction of any kind.

Another item tested is the response to the prick of a pin on the heel. A normal infant will respond by withdrawing the affected heel, becoming alert. An immature or brain-damaged infant will give a total body response to this stimulus and will continue with generalized body movements over a series of trials. This shows an inability to localize the source of pain and demonstrates, in Brazelton's (1973) words, the "all-or-none aspect of an immature organism" (p. 17).

In both examples, higher levels of cortical control are being measured whenever the infant indicates an ability to monitor and alter his response to the stimuli. Other indications of higher cortical control are regulation of state changes (e.g., becoming alert when presented with an initially interesting stimulus or entering a sleep state when the stimulus is no longer interesting) and the ability to be selective in attention to a choice of stimuli. Examples of the latter are the infant's preference for a female over a male voice or for a human over a nonhuman sound.

INFANT STATE

The extent of interaction with people and objects in the newborn infant's world is tied not only to brain development at birth but also to the amount of wakefulness or sleepiness the infant experiences in the first postpartum hours and days. Thus, most studies of infant behavior in the first days of life begin with a concern for infant "state." Peter Wolff (1959) was among the first to explore infant states with his description of six behavior patterns he observed in the first 5 days of life of four infants. Two sleep patterns were observed, termed "regular" and "irregular" sleep. A few spontaneous startles and smooth, even breathing characterize the former, while more body movements and irregular breathing characterize the latter. A third state, "drowsiness," was described as one in which the infant showed a startle response and gross motor activity intermediate between the two sleep states. The final three states he described were "alert inactivity" (wide awake, looking around), "alert activity" (noises, kicking, mouthing), and "crying." Others have adopted these concepts for use in their work, although different terms are frequently encountered. For example, regular sleep is sometimes referred to as "quiet" or "deep" sleep, irregular sleep is called "light", "active," or "REM" sleep (Emde *et al.,* 1975). Alert inactivity is variously referred to as the "quiet, alert state" (Klaus and Kennell, 1976) and "wakefulness" (Emde *et al.,* 1975).

Concern with the variations in terminology and the imprecise methods of assessing infant state led Prechtl and O'Brien (1982) to propose more rigid criteria and terms for studying state changes. The scale they developed depends on presence or absence of four behaviors: eyes open, respirations regular, gross body movements, and vocalization. If a state does not depend on a behavior, that is, if the behavior could be either present or absent, a score of "0" is given (Table 4.1). The results of their criteria are five states, simply numbered. The one removed from their classification is the transitional state, referred to by Wolff and others as "drowsiness." By the new classification, State 1 corresponds to Wolff's "regular sleep," State 2 to "irregular sleep," State 3 to "alert inactivity," State 4 to "alert activity," and State 5 to "crying."

The quiet–alert or wakeful state (State 3, above) is the one in which most learning takes place, as the infant is wide awake, searching with its eyes, fixing eye contact on objects and people, and following voices and faces. It also has strong vocal tone and grasp. This state is usually very short and fleeting in the first several days and weeks after birth. Several studies have reported a period of prolonged wakefulness in the infant during the immediate postpartum period, however, although this period is affected by the amount of medication that the mother received during labor. For example, in a study by Desmond and colleagues (1963), most of the 61 infants entered the quiet–alert state (referred to in this study as "alert exploratory behavior") during the first 10 minutes after birth and spent at least 30 more minutes in this state. Median peak in alerting behavior was reached 1 hour after birth, and none of the infants fell asleep before 65 minutes after birth. Only 17% of the infants whose mothers received no medication during labor failed to follow this pattern, while 40% of those whose mothers had received medication failed to do so. Ten infants demonstrated only fleeting periods of quiet alertness during the first postpartum hours. Nine of these had been subjected to medication during labor.

Theorell *et al.* (1973) found that the timing of cord clamping had an effect on state duration and changes in newborns on the first day of life. As in other studies, these researchers found that infants spent more time awake (States 3,4, and 5) on the first day than they did on the fifth day after birth. Infants whose cords were clamped early (within 10 seconds of birth) spent more time in the quiet–alert state and less time sleeping on the first day than did infants who experienced late cord clamping (more than 3 minutes after birth). The late-clamped infants also had higher blood volumes which the researchers interpret as stressful to the newborn. They suggest that increased sleeping is a response to this stress and propose that, since sleeping reduces opportunities for interaction with the mother, early clamping of the cord enhances development of the mother–infant relationship.

In a randomized clinical trial of 36 mother–infant pairs, the effects of Leboyer and conventional delivery on infant state in the first hour after birth were assessed by Saigal and colleagues (1981). Mothers delivering with the Leboyer method did so in a hospital labor room and held their naked infants until the

TABLE **4.1.** Neonatal Behavioral States[a,b]

State	Eyes open	Respiration regular	Gross movements	Vocalizations
1	× 1	+ 1	× 1	× 1
2	× 1	× 1	0	× 1
3	+ 1	+ 1	× 1	× 1
4	+ 1	× 1	+ 1	× 1
5	0	× 1	+ 1	+ 1

[a]Signs: + 1 = true; × 1 = false; 0 = true or false.
[b]From Prechtl and O'Brien, 1982, with permission of John Wiley and Sons, Inc.

fathers placed them in warm baths for 3–14 minutes, after which the infants were returned to their mothers. Following the conventional method, 18 women delivered in the hospital delivery room and held their infants after they were dried and wrapped in towels. Only four women, two in each group, received epidural anesthetics; none was administered sedatives or tranquilizers. The infants in both groups spent approximately 60% of the first hour in the quiet–alert state and only 10% in the crying state. Although the median times for the two groups differed slightly (Leboyer babies spent 41.5 minutes in the quiet–alert state, while babies delivered by the conventional method spent 35.0 minutes in that state), there were no statistically significant differences between the groups. Unmedicated infants seem primed to spend large chunks of their first hour of life in a state of wakeful alertness, whether or not they have been treated to the Leboyer ritual.

We will see later that this prolonged quiet–alert state in the immediate postpartum period has implications for mother–infant bonding in that it coincides with a period of high arousal in the mother. Both of these periods, however, are, as discussed before, affected by obstetrical medication and perhaps by other procedures used during labor, delivery, and immediately postpartum.

NEONATAL BEHAVIOR

In 1958, John Bowlby introduced into the psychoanalytic literature the concept of species-specific behaviors in human infants. According to him, there are five patterns of behavior that are instinctual in human infants and serve to promote attachment: clinging, crying, smiling, following (with eyes), and sucking. These behaviors elicit caregiving responses from the mother, serve to maintain proximity to her, and ensure survival of the infant. Further, they, and attachment in general, are all part and result of the human "environment of evolutionary adaptedness" (1969), in the context of which all features of a species' morphology, physiology, and behavior, he argues, must be viewed. Without becoming too encumbered with this strict adaptationist approach, I shall review the five infant behaviors and examine ways in which they promote attachment.

Clinging

Clinging is a response found almost universally in nonhuman primates. The Harlows and others have demonstrated that although this behavior is related to the acquisition of food, its primary function seems to be in serving emotional needs. Strepsirhine and monkey infants have an advanced clinging ability at birth and maintain proximity to their mothers with little or no assistance from them. In fact, newborn monkeys have been observed pulling themselves from the birth canal by crawling up toward the mother's breast. Ape infants are less developed at birth and require some assistance from the mother for the first week or two of life. By 2 or 3 months of age, the infants can cling without assistance.

For various reasons, the human infant is unable to support its weight by clinging to the mother until several months after birth. The central nervous and musculoskeletal systems are not developed; the mother lacks body hair to which the infant could cling even if other factors allowed it; and it has lost the ability to grasp with the foot because of the bipedal locomotion that characterizes its species.

Thus, we see a continuum in the primate order: strepsirhine infants can maintain proximity to their mothers with no assistance; apes need assistance for 2 or 3 months; and human infants cannot support their weight at all. For strepsirhines, proximity is infant controlled; for apes, it is bidirectional; and for humans, it is up to the mother to maintain proximity.

Actually, as already mentioned, the human infant clinging response is more readily expressed during the immediate postpartum period than it will be several hours later and for several weeks thereafter. A newborn infant has a grip that would be strong enough to enable it to cling to the mother's body were it not for her hairlessness and its bipedal foot. This strong grasp usually comes as a surprise to parents; I have seen fathers overwhelmed to speechlessness when their fingers were grasped by their newborn infants. There is little question that this response adds a great deal to the attractiveness of the infant to both mother and father. In a sense, it can be seen as a behavior that serves a function other than the one for which it was originally selected.

Crying

Bowlby describes the crying response as one of the ways in which an infant can control his mother's activities. Mothers learn to distinguish the hunger cry from the fright cry and other types of crying, but in almost all instances, any kind of cry will elicit a response, or at least an arousal, in the mother. There is also evidence that a physiological change occurs in the mother upon hearing her infant cry. Lind and his colleagues (1973) report that 54 of 63 mothers they studied demonstrated a significant increase in the amount of blood flow to their breasts. This increased blood flow precedes the let-down or ejection reflex that drives the milk from the mammary ducts to the nipple, thus inducing the mother to nurse her child (Raphael, 1973). Newton (1955) noted that simply hearing any baby cry can cause an immediate release of milk in some women. Thus, the infant cry serves not only to attract the mother to the infant but also induces her to breastfeed.

Although crying is a universal behavior in human infants and usually attracts attention from caregivers, the routine daily crying that we have come to expect may not always have been part of the daily behavior pattern of healthy, normal human infants. As Konner (1972) notes, "on-demand" breastfeeding in the United States means responding immediately to a hunger cry by offering the breast. !Kung women, however, rarely let their infants get so hungry that they cry for food. The infants are constantly in skin-to-skin contact with their mothers who anticipate hunger by reading infant cues such as moving, gurgling, fretting, and changing breathing rhythm. The mother assists the very young infant in nursing; later, the infant will simply find the breast and nurse on its own, obviating the need to cry for attention to hunger needs. In this way, the human infant is much like the nonhuman primate infant who rarely cries except when in acute pain or when separated from its mother.

Other studies have reported that, while rocking movements serve to quiet a crying baby, they are rarely effective below 60 cycles per minute (Bowlby, 1969). At or above that speed, babies stop crying and their heartbeats decline to a normal, relaxed state. Sixty cycles per minute approximates a slow walk in humans. Thus, the response an infant makes to rocking at speeds greater than that is likely a product of millions of years of being carried on mother's hip as she walks in search of food every day. Today's parents often try to reproduce that soothing rhythm by placing the older infant upright in a swing attached to a mechanical arm.

There are at least four good reasons that it would be adaptive for an infant to cry as little as possible and for a parent to keep infant crying at a minimum. Earlier in human evolution, when hominids were more vulnerable to predation than we are today, a crying infant was a clear announcement of the presence of hominids, particularly of the most vulnerable social groups, those of females, infants, and very young children. Infants who rarely cried and mothers who nursed in such a way that the hunger cry was rarely elicited were, therefore, more likely to survive than members of dyads that did not regulate their interaction to reduce hunger and crying episodes.

A second reason that selection may have favored infant and parental behaviors that reduce crying is the profound negative and irritating effect that persistent crying has on adults. In cases of child abuse and infanticide in the United States, very commonly the infant's crying is cited by the perpetrator as a reason for physically abusing or killing the infant (Frodi, 1985). Many mothers report frightening urges to suffocate their infants in response to irritating persistent crying. Crying is particularly annoying when adults and infants are together in one room or, as has been the case throughout our evolutionary history, in close proximity at all times. Infants whose caretakers "let" them cry without intervention may well have been the focus of abuse in the past to the extent that such inattention would be negatively selected in human mothers.

Excessive crying also interferes with parent–infant interaction in a less extreme way. A crying infant is an unusually unattractive being—red face, tightly closed eyes, distorted facial features. Features that are normally attractive become almost repulsive. When prolonged crying finally ceases, the parent is left holding an exhausted, sleeping infant, further decreasing opportunities for interaction.

Third, although most parents can easily distinguish the hunger cry from a cry of pain and respond accordingly, it would have been advantageous in the past for the persistent infant cry to serve as a signal of crisis for which intervention by any older child or adult would be called. In other words, an infant who cries for feeding or any other relatively trivial reasons would perhaps be equivalent to the boy who cried "wolf" when no danger was present. If the infant is known as one who cries "all the time," adults may not take him seriously when a true cry of pain is heard.

Finally, crying is an energetically expensive behavior that may be particularly draining for an infant in the first weeks of life. Crying from hunger further exacerbates the depleted energy stores, and if it has persisted for a long time, the infant may be too exhausted to nurse once it has the opportunity. Any behavior that serves to conserve energy is adaptive for the neonate and for its parent. Thus, if a mother responds to infant hunger and pain in such a way as to minimize crying, she enables the infant and herself to conserve energy and reduce depletion of nutrient reserves.

While newborn crying in the hospital nursery may have been recognized as normal, healthy behavior, recent research has demonstrated that frequent crying has negative physiological impact. Lind *et al.* (1964, cited in Gill *et al.,* 1984) found that crying results in the temporary reestablishment of fetal circulation, meaning that rather than flowing from the heart to the lungs as it does postnatally, blood returns through the foramen ovale between the two atria of the heart and back into systemic circulation. Without having passed through the lungs, the blood carries little oxygen and can create abnormally high systemic pressures. This, in turn, decreases the efficiency of blood oxygen transport and probably adds significant stress to the already stressed newborn infant. Gill and her colleagues (1984) found that infants they observed in a transitional care nursery cried no longer than 40 seconds (mean of 25 seconds) at a time and no more frequently than a mean of every 2 minutes, and they suggest that this may be due to the sheer physical exertion of crying. In other words, newborn infants in hospital nurseries would perhaps cry even more if they were physiologically able.

Smiling

Smiling is a behavior that has received a great deal of attention because it is one of the few human behaviors that most people will accept as universal and perhaps instinctual. The social smile, that is, a smile in direct response to a social stimulus, is supposed to emerge in the fifth week of life. Smiling before that time is variously attributed to gas, reflex, or vagaries of interpretation. Freedman (1974) recorded facial changes associated with gas in newborns and found them to be qualitatively different from the neonatal smile. The former was characterized by writhing, facial reddening, and grimaces, whereas the latter appeared when body and face were relaxed. Freedman also notes that neonatal smiles are more readily elicited by voice than by presentation of a face or other visual stimulus. Smiling, for whatever reason, commonly occurs early in life and has been observed in infants less than 1 hour old. As it will later, this first smile has a powerful effect on most people who observe it, and, although Bowlby calls it "non-functional" (1969:281), it helps to focus the mother's attention on her newborn infant.

Oster (1978) notes that newborn infants have fully functioning muscles for facial expressions, such as smiling, and that this system is developed by 30-weeks gestation. The differences perceived between the smiles of neonates and those of older infants are due to other facial differences and the less developed brain. For example, Oster points out, our perception of facial expressions in neonates is likely affected by other features such as buccal fat pads, lack of teeth and facial hair, and undeveloped cranial bones. Trevarthen (1985) adds that the smiles of older infants are coordinated with vision and hearing, whereas neonatal smiles are not. This ties the development of the so-called "social smile" to cerebral development.

Konner (1979) has suggested that the delayed onset of the social smile is related to decreased gestation length, but that the delay may have been maintained because of its evolutionary significance in societies with high infant mortality. Thus, the strong feelings of attraction that many parents describe in response to the social smile at 3 months may be timed appropriately with the end of a period of fairly high neonatal mortality. A 3-month-old infant has passed a critical period for survival, and parents can then "afford" heavy emotional investment in that child.

Vision

Bowlby suggests that an infant's following with the eyes is an innate releaser of maternal caretaking response. At birth, the human neonate is able to focus clearly on objects approximately 12 inches away (Brazelton *et al.*, 1966). This is roughly the distance from the mother's eyes to her breast when she looks at her infant during breastfeeding. Fantz (1961) demonstrated that newborn infants prefer to look at a human face over any other stimulus. This preference was exhibited in infants less than 10 minutes old (Goren *et al.*, 1975). Stratton (1983) notes that the human face, with its contrasts of light and dark and its movements, is the perfect stimulus for maximal neural firing rate (Haith, 1980), and it is a stimulus that is most likely to be present during the neonatal period. In other words, as Stratton points out, after millions of years of evolution, it is not surprising that the neonatal visual system and the most predicted object in the neonatal environment (mother's face) combine to optimize visual development.

Vision is an extremely important sensory modality for human beings. From the very first moments of life, the human neonate is equipped for visual searching, a process that facilitates further development of that system. Neural activation is necessary for the maintenance of the visual skills present at birth and for the development of new visual skills. Thus, visual stimulation with objects containing patterns of dark and light and contours is adaptive for the development of mature visual skills. It is not surprising that infants in the quiet–alert state spend much of that state searching and attending with their eyes. "The organization of the *information–acquisition* routines are innately given, but the neural tuning for all but the simplest visual patterns . . . is acquired through experience" (Haith, 1980:124 [italics original]). As Haith concludes, why would "nature" have done it any other way?

Rivinus and Katz (1971) propose that, in the primate order, as clinging response at birth diminishes interspecifically, the importance of eye contact increases. In a sense, visual attachment has replaced actual physical attachment, or, as the authors state, "immediate proximal contact behavior is substituted to some extent by more distal contact behavior" (p. 99). Thus, eye contact seems relatively unimportant in mother–infant interaction in the readily clinging strepsirhines and monkeys, is more important in the barely clinging chimpanzee, and is most important in the nonclinging human infant.

Sucking

Stratton (1983) notes "genetic preprogramming of behavior will . . . become established through natural selection only when it allows more effective adaptation to an environmental feature which is important for fitness and which has remained stable over many generations" (p. 303). He further argues that few behaviors meet these criteria more clearly than breastfeeding. Rooting and searching for the nipple are common neonatal responses in mammals, with humans no exception. Soon after birth, human infants turn their heads in response to tactile sensations and tend to direct head movements toward the mother's breast. A tactile stimulus in the area of the mouth elicits sucking. These clearly enhance fitness in neonates for whom an immediate need is nourishment. The availability of nourishment from mother's breast has been a predictable and stable part of the environment of mammalian infants for millenia, so it is no great leap to argue that neonatal rooting, sucking, and orienting, and maternal tendencies to breastfeed, have coevolved in all mammals.

Sucking by the human infant should not be seen, however, as contributing only to physical needs. Wolff (1968) has described two patterns of sucking, one of which he suggests is unique to humans. The first pattern, which he terms *nutritive sucking* is continuous, simultaneous, sucking/swallowing/breathing and is found in all mammals. The second, unique, pattern, termed *nonnutritive sucking,* is characterized by alternating bursts and pauses. As the name implies, this pattern of sucking is associated with a form of behavior that contributes to other than physical development.

Kaye (1977) argues that this behavior prepares the infant for the "taking of turns" that is necessary in communication, and that by responding to the pause, as a mother often does by gently shaking her breast or the infant, she is approximating the dialogue that will characterize later verbal interaction. Baby sucks while mother remains passive; baby pauses and mother becomes active; baby resumes sucking, mother stops movement. Kaye points out that this pattern is similar to that observed in normal adult conversation: person A talks, person B is silent; when person A becomes silent, person B feels an obligation to say something. Nonnutritive sucking also has a calming effect on infants which, in turn, probably enhances mother–infant interaction and increases the time during which learning can take place. Infants who are quieted by a pacifier, thumb, breast, or other object can devote more energy to examining their surroundings than can those who are fretting, crying, or dozing.

Certainly the basis of the various sucking patterns is communication. At least initially, however, the communication is more functional than social. The infant's more immediate need is food, and in order to meet that need, it has to have a way of regulating food intake. Traditionally, we have seen the infant cry as an initiator of the let-down reflex which results in the mother offering her breast. I have argued, however, that crying for food is not routine when mothers and infants are in constant contact. It is not the cry, then, but the burst–pause pattern of sucking that initiates let-down when the infant takes or is first offered the breast. As the milk begins to flow freely, the sucking becomes continuous. Finally, when the infant becomes satiated, it again assumes the burst–pause pattern which effectively communicates its state to a sensitive mother. Thus, as Crook (1979) notes, the two patterns are not simple dichotomies but are part of a continuum, both ends of which relate initially to feeding. Later the burst–pause pattern is used in other forms of communication between mother and infant. The pattern initially used for food acquisition ultimately functions, as well, in perceptual, emotional, and social development.

The human infant has an upper respiratory tract similar to that of other mammals, and unlike that of adult humans; it allows the infant to swallow and breathe at the same time. In infants and most other mammals, the larynx is high in the neck, close to the nasal cavity such that it allows direct passage of air from the nose to the lungs. This separates the nasal breathing pathway from the oral swallowing pathway, so that breathing and swallowing occur independently and simultaneously. It means, however, in Crelin's words, that the infant is an "obligate nose breather" (1973:28). As the infant matures and begins assuming the upright posture of habitual bipedalism, the larynx, tongue, hyoid bone, and pharynx descend in the neck to a position in which the larynx opens into the lower part of the pharynx. By this time, swallowing and breathing must be done separately or choking will result. This may initially seem maladaptive, and indeed many human deaths result from choking each year, but, as Laitman (1984:24) says, it has produced "an anatomical feature of enormous value: a greatly expanded pharyngeal chamber above the vocal cords." This feature, of course, enables humans beyond infancy to produce an almost infinite array of sounds. Unquestionably, language has contributed far more to survival and success of humans than would the ability to swallow and breathe at the same time.

The upper respiratory tract of modern human infants is believed by some to be the best model for that system in adult hominids before 300–400,000 years ago, suggesting that these animals had no greater potential for language than modern human infants and chimpanzees. Laitman (1984), in arguing that the shape of the basicranium (which is often preserved in fossil hominid specimens) relates to the position of the larynx (which is never preserved), suggests that australopithecines had the infant or apelike basicranium/larynx configuration, that *Homo erectus* had a transitional configuration, and that only with *Homo sapiens* does the modern configuration appear. He concludes that australopithecines could not use a vocal language like ours, but they could breathe and swallow at the same time. The larynx had probably descended into the neck in *Homo erectus,* resulting in an increased vocal repertoire, but one not so extensive as that probable with the earliest members of *Homo sapiens.* Obviously, the development of an upper respiratory tract compatible with language could not have occurred until after infancy or breathing would have been incompatible with breastfeeding.

Other Functions of Infant Behaviors

Rivinus and Katz (1971) suggest that, although crying and clinging most likely evolved to maintain proximity to the mother, visual following, smiling, and facial expressions probably contribute more survival value in relation to sensory and cognitive development. They also note another distinction between the two groups of behaviors: crying and clinging are behaviors normally restricted to infancy when maintaining proximity to a caretaker is most important. Visual following and facial expressions, however, persist as interactive mechanisms throughout life, just as need for cognitive stimulation also persists. Thus, one could argue that crying and clinging were behaviors selected in the human infant to attract the mother in the first place, while visual following and smiling were selected to keep her there and interacting. Sucking fulfills another obvious need and, in fact, may be entirely separate from the interactive modes. While nursing their infants, most mothers refrain from interacting with them, verbally or through facial expressions, because these behaviors tend to interrupt nursing. Even eye contact is rare. It is as if, for a while during infancy, the needs of physical growth and cognitive development are met by quite different behaviors.

VARIATION IN NEONATAL BEHAVIOR

Beyond these apparent universal behaviors and capabilities of newborn human infants, there appear to be differences at birth among infants of different cultures and between the genders. These differences are due partially to genetic variation and partially to intrauterine environment (including maternal nutrition and experiences during pregnancy) and labor and delivery practices. The relative weight of each of these effects is unknown.

For example, Brazelton (1977) found that Zinacanteco infants that he examined immediately after birth exhibited freer, more fluid, but less vigorous motor activity than newborn infants he had observed in the United States. Spontaneous startle responses were rare, and the elicited Moro reflex was somewhat subdued in Zinacantecos. These infants were more coordinated in their motor activities. They also remained in the quiet–alert state for longer periods, and no deep or intense crying periods were observed, states that are common in infants in the United States. In accordance with Zinacanteco practice, the newborn infants were ignored in the first few minutes after birth, placed on the hearth with no covering, but they managed to adapt to the colder temperatures with no apparent ill effect. Genetic differences may account for some of the observed differences, but it is equally likely that the birth environment and the lack of medical intervention were partially responsible.

Freedman and Freedman (1979) examined 24 Caucasian and 24 Chinese (Cantonese) newborns in a San Francisco hospital, whose mothers had been carefully matched for parity, age, amount of drugs during birth, income, number of prenatal visits, and gender of the child. They found striking differences between the two groups in results of and reactions to measures on the Cambridge Behavioral and Neurological Assessment Scale. Caucasian babies cried more easily and were harder to control than the Chinese babies. Chinese babies readily adapted their bodies to almost any position in which they were placed, while the Caucasian babies immediately turned their faces to one side when they were placed on their stomachs. When a cloth was placed over the nose, Caucasian babies immediately pushed it away with their hands, while the Chinese babies accepted it and adapted by breathing through their mouths. Chinese babies adapted much more quickly to a light shining in their eyes, while the Caucasian babies continued to blink much longer.

In a second study cited by Freedman and Freedman (1979), researchers examined Navajo infants and found that these infants were even more passive and adapted even more readily than the Chinese babies. In testing for the Moro response, the Navajo babies rarely cried, limb movement was reduced, and they calmed almost immediately. The typical Caucasian reaction to this test is to extend arms and legs in a grasping manner above the chest, cry vigorously, and continue sporadic movements for several seconds.

Australian aborigine infants were also studied by the Freedmans. These infants vigorously fight the cloths placed over the nose and, when placed on their stomachs, can lift their heads up and look around, something a Caucasian infant is unable to do until it is about 1 month old. At birth, when the aborigine infant is lifted by its hands to a sitting position, it is able to support its head, another behavior not exhibited in Caucasian and Chinese infants until several weeks after birth.

Coll and her colleagues (1981) administered the Brazelton Neonatal Behavioral Assessment Scale (NBAS) to 2-day-old infants from three different ethnic groups: Puerto Rican, white, and black. The results indicated that black and white infants habituated to stimuli after fewer trials than required by Puerto Rican infants, that Puerto Rican infants exhibited greater alertness and were able to orient more rapidly to visual and auditory stimuli, and that black infants showed superiority in integrating motor activity and of overall motor tonus. Puerto Rican infants also remained in a quiet–alert state for significantly longer periods and rarely cried. Unlike the other two groups, biomedical parameters (e.g., gestational age, Apgar scores, obstetrical risk factors) accounted for much of the variance on the Brazelton scale seen in Puerto Rican infants. This last finding suggests that the differences in neonatal behavior observed in different sociocultural groups may be due in part to differential effects of obstetric medication and other biomedical variables.

It is also likely that differential selective forces have operated on infants in different parts of the world. For example, African and Australian aborigine infants have been carried for millenia on their mother's hips, often without support of a sling. As an infant monkey who cannot cling to its mother will likely die, so too the infants who were unable to hold their heads up and otherwise support themselves on their mother's hips. If high infant mortality characterized much of our evolutionary history, it is likely that the majority of the motorically weak infants died, whereas the majority of the motorically precocious survived, resulting in a high frequency of strong, alert infants born to tropical peoples. Selection for strong neonates may have relaxed as hominids moved into colder climates of northern Asia and Europe. Rather than being carried on their mother's hips, infants were swaddled or well wrapped for protection from the cold and placed in a sling or back carrier. Motorically weak infants therefore, would not be unfavorably selected.

Gender Differences at Birth

Few would deny that physical differences exist between the genders at birth, but beyond that there is much debate. For example, newborn males have greater muscular strength and are larger and sturdier than newborn girls (Garn, 1958;

Jacklin *et al.*, 1982). Although newborn girls weigh less, on the average, they are more advanced at birth in both skeletal and neurological development (Tanner, 1974).

Females appear to be more receptive to tactile, oral, and perhaps visual stimuli. Bell and Costello (1964) found that female neonates respond more quickly to the removal of a blanket and to a jet of air directed toward them, although Jacklin and colleagues (1982) found no sex differences in tactile sensitivity, as measured by an aesthesiometer. Female neonates also appear to respond more quickly to light (Engel *et al.*, 1968) and are more responsive to sweet tastes, although less willing to work for their food (Nisbett and Gurwitz, 1970).

Hand-to-mouth and hand-to-face contacts are common in newborns, and males and females exhibit the behaviors in equal frequency and duration. The methods of making contact appear to differ, however: females tend to find the hand by searching with the mouth, whereas males more often bring the hand to the mouth (Korner, 1974).

During sleep, males exhibit many more reflex startles than do females, while females excel in reflex smiles and rhythmical mouthing. These differences suggest that the sexes have different ways of discharging neural energy potential: females through the muscles of the mouth and males through total body activation (Korner, 1969).

In my observations of initiation of nursing at TBC, I found that males initiated nursing later than females (Trevathan, 1984). This behavior may be related to observations that females are more "orally receptive" (Freedman, 1974), engage in more "mouth-dominated" actions (Korner, 1973), and exhibit more rhythmic mouthings (Korner, 1969) than newborn boys. Initial active suckling at the breast is not a simple task for any newborn infant. Perhaps females are more "primed" to oral sensations and actions involving the mouth and are thus able to establish nursing earlier.

Labor and Delivery Practices Affecting Neonatal Behavior

Infants of several species exhibit different behaviors according to whether they were delivered vaginally or by cesarean section. These differences can be attributed to at least four factors: (1) Cesarean deliveries usually occur before term, whereas vaginal deliveries usually occur at term; (2) maternal medication is usually greater in cesarean deliveries; (3) the cesarean-delivered infant is not subjected to the uterine contractions and other physical stimuli associated with birth; and (4) related to (3), hormonal experiences vary according to mode and time of delivery. Another likely source of variation, in a different category from the foregoing, is the ability of the mother to interact with her infant.

In general, infants delivered by cesarean section are less active than vaginally delivered infants and tend to sleep more and cry less during the immediate postpartum period. This difference is usually attributed to the effects of maternal medication on the infant. In a comparison of rhesus macaque infants delivered by cesarean section and those delivered vaginally, Meier (1964) found significant differences in activity, number of vocalizations, and number of induced avoidance responses. For all three behaviors, scores were far higher for infants in the vaginal-delivery group. His data and those of similar studies suggested that these differences were independent of the surgical/nonsurgical procedures and independent of gestational age. Meier concludes that the behavioral differences can be accounted for by the differing endocrine experiences of the two groups of infants. During vaginal delivery, hormones are released in the mother and in the fetus that may affect subsequent behavior in an excitatory fashion. These hormones may be responsible for the prolonged quiet–alert state observed in normal, vaginally delivered human infants in the first 2 hours of life.

Probably the obstetric practice that has the most profound effect on neonatal behavior is administration of drugs during labor and delivery. As already noted, obstetrical medications have been shown to affect infant neuromotor functioning, heart rate, and state. Neonatal behavior immediately after birth may not show marked effect from maternal medication, however, a phenomenon that Desmond *et al.* (1966:661) attribute to the "massive, predominantly sympathetic" reaction to delivery that temporarily masks the effect of drugs. Subsequently, once the neonate has reacted to the delivery, depression of respiration, decreased activity, lowered temperature, and poor sucking response may follow. All contribute to morbidity and mortality, this last through lowered weight gain in the days following delivery. Kron and his colleagues (1966), for example, found that in their study of 20 infants, the 10 who were born to mothers who had received obstetrical analgesia (200 mg secobarbital sodium) sucked at significantly lower rates than the 10 whose mothers were unmedicated. As a consequence, the first 10 infants also received less nutrient. Brazelton (1961) also reported greater difficulties in breastfeeding for mothers who had received high doses of medication in labor.

Brackbill and her colleagues (1974) found that amount of medication during labor (specifically meperidine) was directly associated with the amount of time that it took for an infant to habituate to an auditory stimulus. In other words, infants whose mothers had received high doses of meperidine took longer to process auditory information than those whose mothers received low or no doses of the drug. In addition, the longer the time between administration of meperidine and birth, the longer it took the infant to habituate.

These same authors also examined the relationship between drugs administered during labor and performance on the Brazelton Neonatal Behavioral Assessment Scale. Infants whose mothers had received meperidine scored consistently lower on the scale than did those whose mothers had not received the medication (Brackbill *et al.*, 1974). This finding was supported in a more recent study by Hill and Smith (1984). In support of the Desmond *et al.* (1966) claim that drug effects may not be manifested immediately after delivery, Brackbill *et al.* (1974) found no differences in the 1- and 5-minute Apgar scores of infants whose mothers had or had not received medication during labor.

Although obstetrical medication is a major component of parturition today, it is a recently introduced component and one to which there has not been time to develop an adaptation by mothers or infants. In fact, adaptation seems unlikely in our or any other species, and it is precisely the negative sequelae of medication, extending perhaps into years, that have led to a reduction in its use by physicians and midwives today. Parents have probably played the major role in eliminating or restricting the use of medication during labor. In this there is a simple, albeit reductionist, sociobiological explanation. Parent–infant conflict is manifest at the time of delivery to the extent that one party can cause the death of the other. Adult females are perhaps willing to put up with anything short of death or destruction of future childbearing capabilities in order to deliver a healthy offspring. If this can be done with less trauma or pain, however, a female may be quite willing to pursue that option as long as it does not significantly affect her offspring. Thus, until numerous studies demonstrated the dangers to the fetus of obstetrical medication, almost every woman who could, chose a pain-free delivery. Once women became aware of the potential danger to their infants of their selected mode of achieving comfort during labor, their attitudes changed so that, now, many women are trying to achieve drug-free deliveries. A factor that has made this decision more crucial is the delay of childbearing to the third decade and the reduction of family size. A woman in her thirties who plans to have only one or two children thus attempts to avoid any practice that may endanger her few offspring, even if it means a small risk on her part. It appears that the practice of delivering in a hospital resulted in a dramatic decrease in infant and maternal mortality, but that a lower limit was reached because of frequent unnecessary intervention with drugs and instruments. Thus, "natural" childbirth may be the only way of reducing mortality even further and may be an important part of current female reproductive strategy.

Measuring Neonatal Abilities

There is much concern with objectively measuring neonatal behavioral and intellectual capabilities. Most of it has been valuable in that studies have been able to assess risk factors at birth that contribute to low measures on various tests. Primary among these risk factors are hypoxia, obstetrical medication, prematurity, and congenital malformations or diseases. Until the advent of modern medical technology, infants born prematurely usually died, meaning that there was little concern for the effects of premature birth on later development. Infants with congenital problems (e.g., spina bifida, Down's syndrome, PKU, or malformations) also likely died or were killed soon after birth. In fact, any infant who behaved grossly abnormally was likely killed, as is the practice in many cultures today. That leaves us with mild abnormalities, many resulting from hypoxia or other birth stresses, that I would suggest were never noticed in the past before instruments for measuring them were developed. For example, our concern with intellectual achievement has led to a whole class of diagnostic terms such as *slow learner, learning disabled,* and *educably mentally retarded* that may have been less meaningful categories in the past before formal educational institutions.

Our concern for neonatal behavior is also a recent one, a product of dramatically decreased infant mortality. That we have only recently become aware of the capabilities of newborn infants is because depersonification was the more appropriate attitude toward neonates when only 50% were likely to survive. This can be demonstrated in a survey of the attitudes toward neonates in contemporary cultures in which infant mortality remains high.

In many cultures, the infant is ignored during the immediate postpartum period, and all attention is focused on the mother. Where fewer than one-half of all females born reach maturity in a state of health good enough to bear children, it is no wonder that concern is less for the infant, who can be replaced in a year, than for the mother, who will take 20 years to replace. The brief period of neglect that the infant experiences can be seen as a form of selection for the strongest offspring. A newborn who is able to adapt without assistance is more likely to survive in later years than one who requires assistance in establishing respiration and other life functions.

In many cultures, the infant is not recognized as fully human at birth, again reflecting high infant mortality. Ascribing to the infant a name is often the point at which it is recognized as fully human. In a survey of 152 cultures in which the time of naming is specifically stated, only 22 (<15%) named the infant before or on the day of birth. Twenty-six (17%) gave the infant a name 3–4 days after birth, 41 (27%) did so 1 week to 10 days after birth, and the remainder delayed naming to more than 2 weeks after birth. As Newman (1972) points out, if an infant dies before it is named and, thus, before social recognition of its status as human, the body is often disposed of in the same way as a stillbirth or miscarriage. This has obvious economic and social advantages in societies where funerals are expensive and time-consuming. Western cultures are unusual in the practice of naming infants before birth which accords with the suggested association with lowered infant mortality. In fact, another product of lowered infant mortality may well be the controversial belief, held by Roman Catholics and fundamentalist groups in the United States, that human life begins at conception. Like all social movements of the past, the "right-to-life" movement is an outgrowth of a biocultural phenomenon.

At an even further extreme, not only is there concern for neonatal abilities in our culture, recent research also has focused on behavioral characteristics of the fetus. It has been determined, for example, that by the third trimester the fetal taste buds, olfactory system, and visual system are already functioning (Miller, 1984). Even fetal learning has been explored. Studies conducted by De Casper and his colleagues (e.g., DeCasper and Fifer, 1980) have demonstrated that infants recognize sounds to which they were exposed *in utero*. These include the mother's voice, her heartbeat, and the father's voice. Furthermore, not only can neonates discriminate between female voices, they also show preferences for story poems to which they had been exposed frequently *in utero*.

EXTEROGESTATION

In Chapter 1, I suggested that the human infant could be considered an exterogestate fetus for the first few months of life. During this period, human infants share the growth pattern of other primate fetuses, not of other primate infants. For example, ossification of the bones of the phalanges of the human infant at birth is advanced to the same degree as that of 18-week macaque fetuses; these monkeys are born at 24 weeks gestation with the bone development that human infants will not have for several years (Schultz, 1949). Cranial plates in ape infants are fairly well developed at birth, in contrast to the human skull which shows a great deal of molding at birth as the cranial plates slide over one another to allow the head to pass through the pelvic canal. This, in turn, leaves the human infant vulnerable to head damage during the first several months of life.

Later fusion of the cranial sutures is necessary in human infants so that the brain can continue to grow for several years after birth. Other apes must support such powerful jaw and neck muscles that if the cranial plates were so undeveloped at birth that it took several years for closure, the weight of the chewing muscles would pull the skull apart when the infant began eating solid foods. It may be that changes in the diet were necessary for allowing for greater skull flexibility and thus more postbirth brain growth in the hominid line. Once hominids began to use fire to cook food and tools to prepare it, large muscles for chewing food by older infants were no longer necessary. Smaller muscles for mastication meant less downward pressure on the cranial plates, which, in turn, meant that later fusion of these plates was possible.

Chemical development in human infants is also far less developed than in nonhuman primates. Liver enzymes, for example, appear several months after birth (Crelin, 1973). Human infants have gastric enzymes to digest colostrum and milk but do not develop enzymes for other foods for several months. The CNS of human infants is far less developed at birth than that of other haplorhine primates as is reflected in the ability of monkeys and apes to cling to their mothers, supporting their own weight, within hours or days of birth.

Perhaps most importantly, the human infant's brain size at birth is not what would be expected in a survey of the primate order. At birth, it is about 25% of the adult size, measuring approximately 350 cm^3 (21 in^3). By 1 year, it will have more than doubled in size, averaging about 800 cm^3. By age 3, the child's brain will have grown to more than three times its birth size and will be 75% of adult size. In contrast, nonhuman primate infants are born with brains averaging one-half the sizes of adults of their species (e.g., rhesus: 65%; chimpanzee: 41%;

Leutenegger, 1972). If the established trend in the order is for the adult brain to be twice the size of the brain at birth, it again suggests a gestation length of about 18 months for human beings. Actually, if brain weight at birth and adult body weight are plotted against gestation length, both are about twice as large as would be expected for a 9-month gestation period (Sacher and Staffeldt, 1974; Passingham, 1975). Thus, brain growth has accelerated in human evolution both prenatally and postnatally, absolutely and relatively. This is a crucial component of human adaptive strategy, but the usual pattern of completing growth of one-half of the brain before birth was not possible given pelvic structuring associated with bipedalism. Thus, a major shift in relative gestation length occurred, resulting in delaying significant brain growth and associated behavioral development until after gestation. As pointed out in Chapter 1, Martin argues that this shift occurred with *Homo habilis* whose estimated adult brain size was 700 cm^3 (Lewin, 1982). Assuming that pelvic sizes in this species allowed passage of an infant with 350 cm^3, that was the last species that would have fit the expected 1:2 ratio of birth-to-adult brain size. Martin also argues that in order for a pregnant woman to maintain a fetus undergoing accelerated growth of the brain, major changes in metabolic rate and efficiency during pregnancy had to take place. This suggests substantial changes in feeding strategy. Perhaps a component of this change to a high-energy feeding strategy was the increased consumption of animal protein and subsidizing of the pregnant female by group members related to her or to the fetus she was carrying.

I have been arguing that early interruption of *in utero* gestation and associated delayed maturation of several systems occurred because there was no other way to give birth to a fetus undergoing such rapid brain growth. This, in a sense, is negative selection, or selection *against* birth at too late a stage of development. There are advantages to be gained, however, by being born early in the stage of brain development that particularly accrue to an animal as dependent on learning as are hominids. In fact, since so much of our survival depends on learning that takes place during the years of most rapid brain growth, it may have been adaptive to be born at a more undeveloped stage so that brain growth could take place in the presence of environmental stimuli rather than in the relatively unstimulating uterus. The adaptive significance of rapid brain growth in the presence of events of everyday life and the necessity of learning how to deal with them suggests that being born at an early stage of brain development and the associated helplessness of the infant preceded large brains but accompanied bipedalism. In fact, bipedalism may have come about in part as the need arose for the mother to carry a more helpless infant.

If we examine more closely the systems that are developing during the first months of life, the advantage of exterogestation may become more clear. Bronson (1982) has noted that myelinization of the somatosensory, auditory, and visual systems begins at or shortly before birth and continues over the first several years of life. Most importantly, however, myelinization of the visual afferent system occurs rapidly and is completed at age 4 months. Undeniably, vision is the most important means through which primates, including humans, acquire nonlinguistic information about their environment. Furthermore, development of visual acuity is directly dependent on stimulation during the period of rapid growth (see Blakemore and Cooper, 1970), suggesting that proper functioning would not appear in infants exposed only to the visually homogeneous uterus.

The importance of auditory stimulation in infancy cannot be overrated in a species dependent on language. Although neonates do not have the cerebral and anatomical equipment for making language sounds, they do have the ability to perceive sounds and show selective listening preference for linguistic rather than environmental sounds. The language centers of the brain develop in the first 3 years of life as the brain is undergoing its rapid expansion, and these years have been called critical ones for the development of language in the child.

Earlier in the chapter I noted that human neonates are remarkably resistant to negative stimuli (e.g., hypoxia, hypothermia) that have adverse effects on older infants and adults. There is also great flexibility of behavior, and neonates appear to recover more quickly from stresses than they will later. Stratton (1982b) suggests that neonatal immaturity is a protection from "certain kinds of influence which would otherwise provoke adaptations with undesirable long-term consequences" (p. 401). In other words, if infants could be born with greater brain development, after a gestation period of 12–15 months, they would not have the flexibility that enables them to respond to the powerful stresses of parturition and the immediate postpartum period.

Freedman (1974) elaborates on this theme suggesting that altricial development allows for much greater developmental plasticity. In precocial development, events occur somewhat rapidly and close together, such that critical periods are even more critical. A newborn lamb, goat, or gosling has only a short period of time in which to learn to recognize and follow, or imprint upon, its mother. Selection has favored rapid development of various systems with little variation. In altricial species, repeated exposure over longer periods is possible. Furthermore, Freedman argues, slowed development also allows for play and curiosity, behaviors that lead to greater plasticity, learning, and variability.

SUMMARY

In this chapter, I have presented factors in immediate neonatal adaptation that impinge upon infant survival and parent–infant interaction during the first hours and days after birth. Challenges to survival are numerous, and it is no wonder that mortality in the perinatal period has been high throughout most of human history. The physical stresses at birth, great for all primates, are compounded even further in the human because of the relatively large neonatal brain and the relatively narrow female pelvis. Encephalization in hominids has proceeded at the cost of decreased maturity at birth of almost all systems critical for survival. Advantages gained from being born "earlier in the gestation cycle" include greater plasticity and earlier exposure to environmental stimuli important for learning.

No matter how numerous its advantages, however, retardation of growth rates and birth at an earlier stage of gestation could never have occurred had there not been compensating caretaking behaviors on the part of mothers. This is the subject of the next chapter.

5

MOTHER–INFANT INTERACTION IMMEDIATELY AFTER BIRTH

Although the process may not always be perfect, behaviors of mammalian females have been selected to complement the needs and capabilities of their young. Most of the immediate adaptations and needs described in the previous chapter for human infants are those of all mammalian newborn. All infants must, at birth, breathe, warm themselves, find food, and, eventually become attached to, or have the ability to recognize, the provider of those needs. Just as there are similarities in reactions to parturition for most mammals, so too are there similarities in immediate postpartum behaviors. Although the individual behaviors themselves may vary across and within species, there are several types of behavior that are commonly observed and that fulfill fairly specific functions. These include licking or stroking the infants to establish respiration, digestion, and elimination, and to dry them so that maintaining adaptive body heat is possible. Characteristic vocalizations are often noted that function in initiating interaction or nursing and that facilitate recognition. Visual and olfactory communication also enhance recognition. Mothers of most species, although they may not actively assist their infants in establishing nursing, commonly orient their bodies in such a way that the young can find the mammary glands. Finally, mothers and infants have physical or behavioral mechanisms that lead to establishment of some sort of bond between them.

There are, then, two categories of behaviors exhibited in the first hours after birth. One includes those behaviors that directly contribute to neonatal survival, while the second category includes behaviors that enhance mother–infant bonding. The two are not mutually exclusive. For example, licking may serve the immediate need of stimulating respiration, but it also serves to enhance maternal recognition of young and, thus, contributes to bond formation. As I will discuss in Chapter 6, most recent studies of human maternal and infant behaviors have focused exclusively on the role they play in bond formation. Examining the behaviors in an evolutionary perspective forces us to ask a broader question: How have they contributed to survival? But before we can begin to answer this question, we must know something about what mothers and infants do immediately after birth.

There has been extensive research on maternal behaviors in many species of mammals, but very little has been done on the human mother. Peter Stratton (1982a) has pointed out that, over the past two decades, we have amassed great quantities of data on the behavior of newborn human infants, but, although the role of the parents in influencing behavior and development of their newborn infants has received widespread attention, few psychologists and ethologists have paid much attention to what the human mother (or father) was doing in the immediate postpartum period: All research eyes were on the infant.

There are several reasons for this oversight. One can be attributed to the relative ease with which neonates can be observed in hospitals. Until recently, they were usually housed together in newborn nurseries, and getting hospital and parental permission simply to observe their behavior was usually easy. Newborn babies are commonly seen as being not quite human, their awareness of the surrounding environment seems limited, and scientific observation of their behavior appears unobtrusive in the same way that observations of nonhuman animals appear. Mothers, however, are people with rights to privacy, especially during a time as sensitive as labor and delivery. If a behavioral scientist wants to watch immediate postpartum maternal behavior, he or she must surmount obstacles ranging from hospital regulations to parental desire for privacy and modesty.

Another reason that we do not know much about human maternal–infant interaction in the immediate postpartum period is that until recently, at least in many Western countries, mothers and infants did not interact with each other at all during that time, because separation of the two was the norm. This practice has been changing, however, and studies of human maternal behavior at birth have been undertaken in several settings. Now, based on research conducted in several hospital settings and on my own research at TBC, we know more about maternal behaviors at and immediately following birth.

As we have seen, by the time the newborn human infant is 10 minutes old, its body must adapt to an environment completely different from the one it inhabited as an embryo and fetus for the preceding 9 months. Although the first hour of life is probably the single most dangerous one, most infants respond appropriately and survive that period. But, as I have argued previously, the gestation process does not end at birth, but rather it continues for several of the first few months of life outside the uterus, by a process referred to as "exterogestation" (Montagu, 1971). One major difference between uterogestation and exterogestation for human beings is that the primary factors influencing the latter process are psychological and emotional rather than physiological and physical.

During uterogestation, the fetus develops primarily in response to placental functions, hormones, and physiological processes resulting from millions of years of vertebrate and mammalian evolution. After birth, during exterogestation, growth continues as a physical process, but other factors that shape the development of the child are individually determined by mother, father, and other people and environments to which it is exposed.

In the previous chapter, I emphasized the immediate adaptive significance of behaviors such as sucking, clinging, crying, and smiling as proximity-maintaining mechanisms that result in the infant acquiring warmth, nutrients, and protection, all essential to his survival. Regardless of their initial selective advantage, however, these same behaviors also serve to meet a broad range of other, potentially more significant needs. These are the social and emotional needs that make the human infant more than simply a living organism. Even the aforementioned, prolonged, quiet–alert state, while perhaps most important for learning to breathe regularly, has secondary value in its effect on the mother. This prolonged quiet–alert state coincides after birth with a period of high emotional arousal in the mother to provide an optimal time for continuing the bonding process that began *in utero* in what has been called "the closest human relationship" (Newton and Modahl, 1978). Interactions that occur during this period include touching, smiling, kissing, eye contact, and breastfeeding. Some of these interactions are among those that have been called species-specific for human mothers and include preference for left-side holding of the infant, an orderly progression from fingertip touch of the infant's extremities to palmar massaging of the infant's trunk, intense interest in eye-to-eye contact, use of a high-pitched voice when talking to the infant, and initiation of nursing within a few minutes of delivery.

These behaviors complement the ones described in the previous chapter for human infants. They not only enhance survival, but the result is reciprocal interaction, which Klaus and Kennell (1982) say serves to "lock" the mother and infant together: baby initiates an interaction, mother responds, baby continues, mother continues, and so on, as long as it is mutually rewarding to the two. The "dance" terminates when one member of the dyad looks away, falls asleep, or moves away.

Following Klaus and Kennell (1982:71), I have developed a chart listing the mother-to-infant and infant-to-mother interactions (Figure 5.1). Rather than referring simply to human behaviors, as they did, I have structured it to be more generally applicable to most mammalian species. On the right side of the chart, the infant-to-mother side, are behaviors previously described as proximity-maintaining mechanisms, those that enhance survival and, by stimulating further social interaction, help establish the mother–infant bond. These include clinging or following, visual attraction, vocalizations, and suckling. On the left, or mother-to-infant side, are tactile contact, visual, olfactory, and auditory communication, and nursing. All are important in ongoing mother–infant interaction, but they will be discussed here as they are first exhibited on the day of birth.

TACTILE INTERACTION

As mentioned before, in many species, licking the neonate may serve the immediate function of removing fetal membranes or the entire amniotic sac so that the infant can begin to adapt to the outside world. Further licking stimulates breathing and, later, defecation. Montagu (1971) suggests that most mammalian

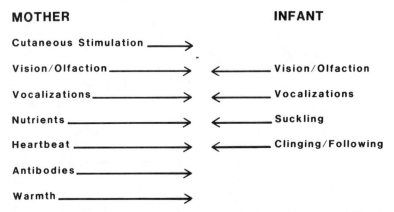

FIGURE 5.1. Mother–infant interactions. After a diagram in "Parent–Infant Bonding" by M. H. Klaus and J. H. Kennell. Modified with permission of C. V. Mosby Company, St. Louis, Missouri. Copyright, 1982.

young would die because of failure of the genitourinary or gastrointestinal systems if they were not licked and notes that the anogenital region is the area most frequently licked and for the longest period of time. Like consumption of the placenta and related birth fluids, licking the neonate may also function for removing odors that would attract predators.

Licking also helps the mother orient the young toward her mammary glands and undoubtedly plays an important role in helping the mother learn the characteristics of her young. In other words, although the behavior was likely selected for its immediate survival functions, it also serves as an initiator of further interaction and as a bonding mechanism.

Sheep, goats, and other mammalian females often lick their neonates in a characteristic pattern, beginning with the head and working back over the entire body to the tail. This may reflect the order of priority of the survival advantages gained: Removing the fluids from the head improves respiration, vision, and escape of heat from a vulnerable part of the body. Her motivation to lick it is so strong that the mother sheep will do all she can to keep him from rising until it is completely licked (Hersher *et al.*, 1963), suggesting that intrinsic signals may override extrinsic ones for this behavior. Most lambs that are not licked within an hour after birth fail to stand and eventually die (Hersher *et al.*, 1963). Under cool or windy conditions, if a lamb or kid is not dried, it may use so much energy simply trying to maintain body temperature that it will be impossible to replace it quickly enough by nursing.

Exceptions to the near universal behavior of postpartum licking include the ocean-dwelling mammals, both those that deliver in the water and those that deliver on land. Elephant seals, for example, make no attempt to clean or lick their neonates, but they do appear to take interest in their smells (Le Bouef *et al.*,

1972). The placentas are not consumed by the mothers. These seals have few predators, so if licking the pup and eating the placenta have antipredator functions, selection need not have favored this behavior. The pups appear to breathe, nurse, and eliminate adequately despite the lack of skin stimulation from licking. The precocial pups flip sand onto their own backs very soon after birth, a practice that probably helps absorb birth fluids and keep them warm.

Another obvious exception to the almost universal mammalian behavior of licking the young is the human species. Instead of licking their young, human mothers make extensive use of their hands in immediate interaction with their infants. Rubbing or massaging the infant is frequently used by mothers or birth attendants as a way of stimulating and maintaining initial respirations. Thus, whatever functions were originally achieved by licking are now fulfilled by the tendency for mothers to use their hands in interacting with their infants in the first few minutes following birth. Lindburg and Hazell (1972) suggest that bathing the infant immediately after birth, a common behavior cross-culturally, has replaced licking as a way of cleaning the infant in our species.

Touch also seems to have a number of other functions. Among those is its suggested role in recognition and attachment. Many mothers have remarked that they did not really believe that they had an infant until they were allowed to hold it. This phenomenon is not restricted to human beings, however. The Harlows demonstrated long ago that tactile and sensory stimulation were more important to young rhesus monkeys than food, and that their mothers gradually lost interest in their young if allowed only to see, but not to touch, them (Harlow, 1958; Harlow *et al.*, 1963).

Stimulation of the skin of the human newborn may also be seen as advantageous when one considers the vernix caseosa, a fatty substance that covers the neonate and served to protect the skin while in the amniotic fluid. Rubbing this substance into the skin of a newborn protects it from drying out in the new environment and may also provide protection from viral and bacterial agents. Furthermore, under conditions where artificial heat is unavailable, this early skin-to-skin stimulation also serves as a means of warming the infant immediately after birth.

In an early study, Rubin (1963:829) noted that "there is a definite progression and an orderly sequence in the nature and amount of contact a mother makes with her child." Most mothers she observed in her hospital study began with fingertip contact over small areas of the infant's body and moved through palmar contact to whole arm contact or encompassing. She further noted that mothers who received a great deal of body contact during labor and delivery were able to use their hands "more effectively" in interacting with their neonates (p. 830).

Klaus *et al.* (1975) reported that, after hospital deliveries in the United States, mothers spent 52% of the first 3 minutes of contact in exploring with their fingertips and 28% in palmar contact of the infant's body. During the last 3 of 9 minutes of contact, a changeover was noted: 26% involved fingertip contact, while palmar contact had increased to 62%. These researchers further suggested that such a pattern, beginning with fingertip contact of infant extremities, moving through palmar contact to fully encompassing, is a species-characteristic behavior for human mothers.

In order to test the hypothesis of a species-characteristic pattern of touch in human mothers immediately postpartum, 66 of the women in TBC sample were observed for the first 10 minutes of contact with their infants (Trevathan, 1981). Touching behaviors were recorded every 10 seconds and subsequently grouped into the seven categories described in Chapter 2 (holding the infant with both hands; holding with one hand; not holding or touching although the infant is with her; holding with one arm, fingertips stroking infant's face; holding with one arm, fingertips stroking infant's extremities; holding with one arm, fingertips stroking infant's trunk; and holding with one arm, palmar massaging of extremities and trunk). The first two categories were recorded only when the mother was doing nothing active with her hands, reflecting a more passive interaction with her infant.

Looking only at percentages of fingertip and palmar contact (Figure 5.2), there was, if anything, a slight decrease in amount of time spent in each of these tactile behavior categories. In the first time interval (3 minutes, 20 seconds), the 41 mothers analyzed spent 18.7% of the time in fingertip contact and 6% of the time in palmar contact of the infants. In the second interval, fingertip contact measured 18.2% and palmar contact measured 3.9%. By the third interval, these had further decreased to 17.8% of the time in fingertip contact and 2.3% in palmar contact. Most of the time was spent in passive holding. For this analysis, only taped observations that began less than 10 minutes after birth were used.

Since there was such a wide variation in the frequencies of each behavior, was any behavior more likely to be preceded or followed by a specific behavior? The frequency of category-to-category sequences based on observations of these 66 women represented a total of 3913 monads (single behaviors) and 3824 dyadic sequences. (Dyads were fewer than monads because the last monad was not followed by any behavior.) The transition matrix (Table 5.1) presents the actual frequencies with which any given behavior was followed by or preceded by any other behavior. [This analytical procedure follows the work of Altmann (1965) on the stochastics of social communication in rhesus macaques.]

In addition to the absolute frequency of each dyadic sequence, Table 5.1 also gives expected frequencies based on the null hypothesis that each maternal behavior is independent of the preceding behavior. (The expected frequencies were derived in the same way that they are for a chi square test.) It is obvious, without further statistical tests, that the observed frequencies deviate significantly from expected frequencies, even when the large N is considered. Thus, the behaviors cannot be assumed to be random occurrences.

By examining the matrix presented in Table 5.2, we can determine which behavior is most likely to follow or precede a given other behavior. The frequencies along the diagonal indicate that persistence in that same behavior is the most likely occurrence, although that may not be the predicted pattern. For example, the mothers were more likely to continue holding with both hands,

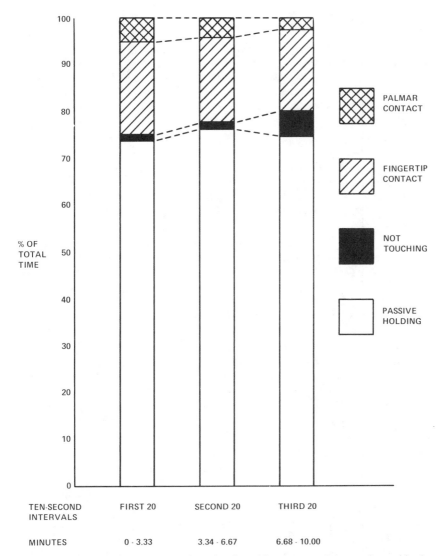

FIGURE 5.2. Maternal touch during the first 10 minutes of interaction with the infant.

even though the expected frequencies suggest that holding with one hand should occur more often in a 10-second segment following holding with both hands. All other behaviors that could have followed holding with both hands occurred one-half or less as often as they should have if behavioral sequences were randomly distributed. The most extreme deviation is noted in column 3. As indicated, not holding the infant, following any other behavior, occurs far less than expected for every category except the persistence of the behavior. The last

TABLE **5.1.** Dyadic Sequences of Maternal Tactile Behavior (in 10-Second Intervals) Based on Observations of 66 Women Over a Period of Ten Minutes[a]

Trial n	Trial $n + 1$							
	Hold both	Hold one	Hold not	Fing. face	Fing. extr.	Fing. trunk	Palmar	Row total
Hold both								
Observed	1003	120	3	57	44	20	.17	1264
Expected	413	517	42	104	87	53	48	
Hold one								
Observed	114	1290	16	44	36	17	19	1536
Expected	502	629	51	126	106	64	58	
Hold not								
Observed	3	12	102	0	0	3	4	124
Expected	40	51	4	10	9	5	5	
Finger face								
Observed	43	49	1	176	21	19	7	316
Expected	103	129	11	26	22	13	12	
Finger extr.								
Observed	35	51	1	17	145	14	9	272
Expected	90	111	9	22	19	11	10	

[a]Each cell presents the number of times any given behavior (n) is followed by a given second behavior ($n + 1$). The second number in each cell is the expected frequency of dyadic sequences based on the null hypothesis that each maternal behavior is independent of the preceding behavior.

154

TABLE 5.2. Transition Matrix for Maternal Tactile Behavior (10-Second Intervals) Based on Observations of 66 Women Over a Period of 10 Minutes[a,b]

Trial n		Trial n + 1							Initial probability
		Hold both	Hold one	Hold not	Fing. face	Fing. extr.	Fing. trunk	Palmar	
Hold both	Observed	1003	120	3	57	44	20	17	
	Frequency	.793	.095	.002	.045	.035	.016	.013	.330
Hold one	Observed	114	1290	16	44	36	17	19	
	Frequency	.074	.840	.010	.029	.023	.011	.012	.402
Hold not	Observed	3	12	102	0	0	3	4	
	Frequency	.024	.097	.823	0	0	.024	.032	.032
Fing. face	Observed	43	49	1	176	21	19	7	
	Frequency	.136	.155	.003	.557	.066	.060	.022	.083
Fing. extr.	Observed	35	51	1	17	145	14	9	
	Frequency	.129	.188	.004	.062	.533	.051	.033	.071
Fing. trunk	Observed	30	22	0	16	9	83	4	
	Frequency	.183	.134	0	.098	.055	.506	.024	.043
Palmar	Observed	22	21	5	4	9	3	84	
	Frequency	.149	.142	.034	.027	.061	.020	.567	.039

[a]Each cell presents the number of times and the frequency that any given behavior (n) is followed by a given second behavior (n + 1). For example, holding with one hand follows holding with both hands almost 10% of the time. A period of not holding the infant is never followed by fingering the face or fingering the extremities. The highest frequencies are found across the diagonal, indicating that persistence in a behavior is the most likely event. The last column, headed by "initial probability" gives the probability that a mother would be in a given state at a given 10-second interval.

[b]Reproduced from Developmental Psychology with permission of John Wiley and Sons, Inc. Copyright 1981.

column, headed by "initial probability," gives the probability that the mother would be in a given state at a given 10-second interval.

So far we have rejected the hypotheses of stochasticity and of invariance. The tactile behaviors appear to be distributed according to some endogenous or exogenous factors that may be different for each mother. A further set of analyses, which examined behavior patterns of (1) Hispanic mothers and Anglo mothers, (2) mothers of boys and mothers of girls, and (3) primiparous and multiparous women, determined that these factors may be contributing to the variability observed.

In general, the Anglo women spent less time not holding their infants and changed state more often than did the Hispanic women. Their more active involvement with their infants is further reflected in Figure 5.3 in which the active states (FF,FE,FT,P) are summed, yielding frequencies of .20 for Hispanic and .385 for Anglo women.

Mothers were more likely not to touch their male infants at all for longer periods of time than were mothers of female infants, although this behavior had a low frequency overall (Figure 5.4). Mothers of males did slightly more active exploring (.24) than did mothers of females (.22).

Finally, tactile movements of primiparous and multiparous women showed significant differences (Figure 5.5). Again, the greatest difference was in the category of not holding: Primiparous mothers spent more time in not touching their infants than did multiparas. The primiparas also showed a slight increase in active exploratory behavior (.26) compared to multiparas (.22).

Another way of viewing these data is to concern ourselves only with the sequences, ignoring the length of time spent in each behavioral state. Thus, only changes of behavior are recorded (Table 5.3). Studies of communication in small groups, where an individual is not expected to talk to himself, have resulted in the development of a formula to derive the expected frequencies of each behavior (Bales et al., 1951):

$$X_{(i,n)} = \frac{S}{i\left(\sum_{j=1}^{n} \frac{1}{j}\right)}$$

Where $X_{(i,n)}$ is the expected number of times that the ith behavior occurred in a selection of n behaviors (in this case, seven), and S is the sum of all behaviors, in this case, 992. The behavior that follows the ith behavior is represented by j. The resulting X^2 for observed differences is significant at the $p < .001$ level.

From the preceding analyses, we may conclude that behaviors vary systematically with gender of the infant, parity, and sociocultural or socioeconomic background of the mother. In sum, they provide no evidence of an invariant pattern of tactile behavior during the first 10 minutes of mother–infant interaction following birth. I would suggest that the behaviors previously observed (Klaus *et al.*, 1970; Rubin, 1963) may actually be the response to the specialized situation of the hospital birth followed by a brief separation of the mother and infant. In fact,

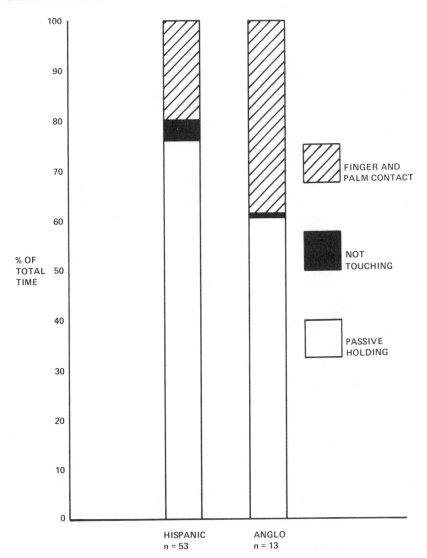

FIGURE 5.3. Maternal touch at first contact with the infant: Anglo and Hispanic women.

in the earlier studies, contact began while the infants were lying in the bed beside their mothers rather than being held by them. In the present study, the infants were always held by their mothers, as they had been from the moment of birth, and most of the maternal tactile behaviors recorded fell into the broad category of "passive holding," a category not used in previous studies.

Based on evidence presented in this study, the more typical pattern of mother–infant interaction may be that of cradling or encompassing the infant for the first few minutes after birth accompanied by palmar massaging for warmth

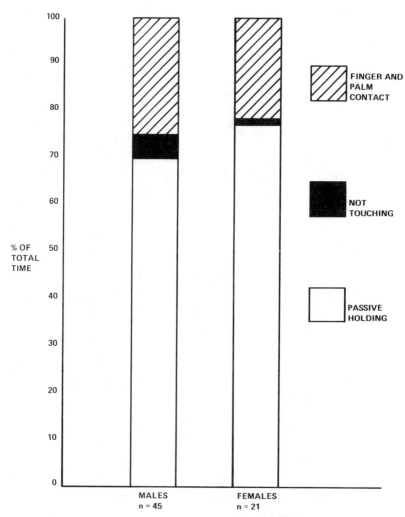

FIGURE 5.4. Maternal touch at first contact with the infant: mothers of boys and
mothers of girls.

and respiration. Finger exploration of face, hands, and extremities then follows
when the mother is not otherwise distracted. In other words, tactile contact with
the infant, including all behaviors described, is a typical response of human
mothers to their newborn infants, but the tactile contact does not necessarily
follow the pattern previously reported.

LEFT-LATERAL PREFERENCE

Another common human behavior that may affect communication in the
tactile, visual, and auditory modes is the tendency for mothers to hold their

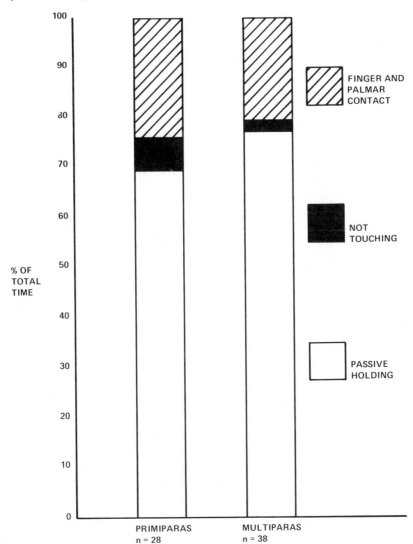

FIGURE 5.5. Maternal touch at first contact with the infant: primiparous and multiparous women.

infants on the left side of their bodies. Salk (1960) found, in a study of 287 women, that 83% of the mothers held their infants on the left side most often during the first 4 days postpartum, and 17% held them on the right. He concluded that left-side preference is established in mothers regardless of handedness since 83.1% ($N = 255$) of the right-handed mothers held their infants on the left side and 78.1% ($N = 32$) of the left-handed mothers held their infants on the left side. He also found that infants exposed to the sound of the human

TABLE **5.3.** Transition Matrix for Changes in Behavioral State Only, Duration Ignored[a–c]

| | Trial $n+1$ | | | | | | | |
	HB	HO	FF	FE	FT	P	HN	Row total
Trial n								
HB	0	123	61	46	22	19	3	274
HO	122	0	44	48	18	18	16	266
FF	44	49	0	24	18	8	1	144
FE	36	55	17	0	18	10	1	137
FT	32	23	14	11	0	3	0	83
P	21	22	4	8	5	0	5	65
HN	4	12	0	0	3	4	0	23
Total	259	284	140	137	84	62	26	992

Rank	Behavior	Observed	Expected
1	HB	274	383
2	HO	266	191
3	FF	144	127
4	FE	137	96
5	FT	83	76
6	P	65	64
7	HN	23	55

[a]Note: $X^2 = 99.54$, $p < .001$.

[b]Note: The first part of this table presents the number of individual tactile behaviors performed by 66 women during a 10-minute observation period. Persistence in a single behavior state over a period of time was counted as a single behavior. Thus, only changes in state were noted for this analysis. In the second half of the table the actual number of times that each behavior occurred is compared with the expected frequency for that behavior, derived by the formula presented on page 156. The resulting X^2 demonstrates a significant departure from randomness.

[c]Reproduced from *Developmental Psychobiology* with permission of John Wiley and Sons, Inc., Copyright, 1981.

heartbeat were thus soothed and gained weight more rapidly than infants not so exposed, suggesting a biological basis for left-side holding of infants.

Weiland and Serber (1970) found that left-side holding of the infant serves to reduce maternal anxiety, a factor most likely related, in turn, to the soothing effect on the infant. Salk's study has been challenged more recently by Detterman (1978) who was unable to replicate his findings that the heartbeat sound had a long-term pacification effect on infants, although he acknowledged that the short-term effects were significant. His findings of no long-term effects have little evolutionary significance if one accepts my argument that excessive crying in human infants is a fairly recent phenomenon.

Others have offered what they term a more parsimonious explanation for left-lateral preference than fetal imprinting on the maternal heartbeat sound (Ginsburg *et al.*, 1979). Turkewitz *et al.* (1968) found that infants more often turn their heads to the right and Miranda (1970) noted that infants prefer to look to the right, suggesting that left-side holding may be a species-specific adaptation to preferences of both mothers and infants. There is evidence that the preferred head-turning direction of the infant actually shapes the maternal placement preference. Ginsburg *et al.* (1979) tested newborn infants less than 48 hours old for head-turning preference upon being placed in a supine position. They later observed maternal lateral placement of these infants and found that most (70%) of the infants who preferred to look to the right were held over their mother's left shoulder while 76% of those who preferred to look to the left were held over their mother's right shoulder. These differences were significant and suggest that neonatal preferences affect their mother's lateral placement. Although no such testing has been done, it is likely that the mothers who respond appropriately to their infant's head-turning preferences have infants who are more satisfied with their position on their mother's body and have more opportunities to interact with and thus learn about their environment.

It is also likely that mothers who respond appropriately to their infant's preferences are more sensitive to their needs. This sensitivity may develop over the first few days of interaction, and it may be enhanced by early contact. In another study, Salk (1970) studied lateral placement in mothers who had been separated from their infants for several days during the neonatal period because of medical complications. He found that, of those who experienced prolonged postpartum separation, 53% held the infants on the left side, and 47% held them on the right. His control sample included 286 women who had only the routine 12–24-hour separation common at the time of his study. In this sample, 77% of the mothers held the infants on the left side, and 23% held them on the right. De Chateau et al., (1978) found that 80–90% of primiparous and multiparous women held their newborn infants to the left of the body midline when there had been no separation from their infants, but that 30–40% of the mothers separated from their infants for the first 24 hours held their infants to the right. They also determined that left-lateral preference was typical of nonpregnant female—but not of male—students, and concluded that left-lateral preference was a genetically determined human female behavior.

In a later study, De Chateau (1983) found that the disparity in lateral preference was also characteristic of fathers, and that couples tended to exhibit the same preferences for holding their infants. College-aged men who had never had children did not exhibit disparity in lateral preference. This again suggests that learning and sensitivity to infant preferences are important in determining lateral-placement behavior.

One way to sort out the role of learning versus innate tendencies for lateral placement is to examine the placement of the infant when it is held by the mother for the first time. This presumably occurs before any learning can take place. Most of the observations reported here were made several days to several weeks after birth, providing plenty of time for parents to coordinate their behaviors with the needs and preferences of their infants. In the present study, an attempt was made to determine side preferences immediately after delivery and for the duration of the first hour after birth for a sample of 100 women (Trevathan, 1982). In 29 cases, the woman giving birth reached between her legs after the delivery of the shoulders and completed the delivery of her own child, bringing it up to her chest. When the father was present, the midwives invited him to complete the delivery of the child after the shoulders had been freed. In these instances, the father usually held the baby aloft above the mother's knees for her to see, although most of the men in these cases seemed so overwhelmed that it was obvious that they were not at all sure of what they were doing. Typically the mother reached up and took the infant from his hands and drew it to her chest, as far as the still-attached umbilical cord would allow. When the birth was difficult or the mother refused to reach down and take her infant, the midwives themselves completed the delivery and placed the infant on the mother's abdomen. The midwives were aware of my interest in lateral preference and attempted not to bias the mother's first reception of her infant.

I recorded the lateral preference of 100 mothers upon first contact immediately postpartum. For the duration of the first hour following delivery, shifts in lateral positioning of the infant were recorded. Six of the original sample were not included in this part of the study because the shifts in position were biased by others interacting with the mother (e.g., the father or a midwife placing the infant on one side or another). For this part of the study, the phrase "most of the time" is defined very simply as more than 31 of the first 60 minutes following birth.

Of the 100 mothers, 71 pulled their infants to their left sides when they first held them, and 29 held them on the right. During the first hour, 75.5% of the mothers held their infants on the left most of the time, and 24.5% held them on the right most of the time ($N = 94$). These results are similar to those obtained by Salk (1960, 1970), and De Chateau *et al.* (1978) (Figure 5.6).

Of the 100 women in this study, only 4 were left-handed (handedness was not obtained for 4 women). In Salk's 1960 sample, 11% were left-handed; De Chateau and colleagues found that 6% of the Swedish mothers in their study were left-handed ($N = 228$). The results of side preference upon first contact with the infant and during most of the first hour are shown according to handedness in Table 5.4. There is no significant association between handedness and lateral preference for the first contact ($X^2 = .105$) or for most of the first hour ($X^2 = .108$). The low number of left-handed mothers in the sample precludes statistical analysis, but two-celled chi square tests of relatedness between handedness and lateral pref-

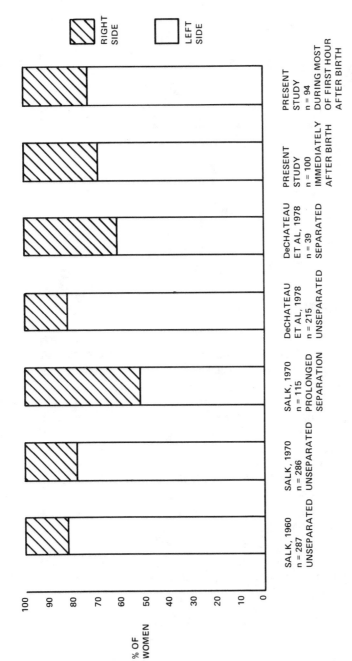

FIGURE 5.6. Summary of studies reporting lateral preference of mothers holding infants.

TABLE **5.4.** Lateral Preference upon First Contact and for Most of the First Hour after Birth[a]

	Lateral preference upon first contact ($N = 96$)	
Subjects	Right	Left
Right-handed mothers	64	28
Left-handed mothers	3	1
	Lateral preference during most of first hour ($N = 90$)	
Right-handed mothers	64	23
Left-handed mothers	3	0

[a]Table reprinted with permission of BIRTH, Blackwell Scientific Publications, Inc., 52 Beacon St., Boston, MA 02108.

erence for right-handed mothers at first contact ($X^2 = 14.08$) and right-handed mothers during most of the first hour ($X^2 = 19.34$) are highly significant ($p<.001$). Not surprisingly, there is also a significant association between side on which the infant was first held and side on which he was mostly held during the first hour. At first contact, 59 women held their infants on the left and for most of the first hour; 11 held right at first contact but held left for most of the first hour; 7 held left at first contact and right for most of the first hour; and 17 held right at first contact and for most of the first hour ($X^2 = 20.99$), $p<.001$).

On postcards sent to the mothers 4 months after birth of the infant, information was requested concerning the side of the body on which the infant was usually carried. Of the 39 responses, 38.5% indicated that they usually carried the infant on the left side, 15.4% usually carried him on the right side, and 46.2% carried the infant about equally on each side. Both of the left-handed mothers who responded carried their infants on their left side. The right-handed mothers were distributed as follows: 13 carried left (36% of the responders), 5 carried right (14%), and 18 carried equally (50%).

During the first hour after birth, there were no significant differences between the side on which the infant was held and maternal interactive behaviors such as patting and rocking, talking to the infant, stroking the face, encompassing the infant, and rubbing and massaging the infant. There were also no statistically significant differences between lateral preference according to parity, socio-cultural/socioeconomic background, marital status, or education. Labor and delivery factors, such as location of the delivery, reaction to labor, length of labor, or administration of oxytocin, did not seem to affect lateral placement of the infant nor did the infant's gender or Apgar scores.

Mothers who held their infants to the left for most of the first hour spent slightly more time looking at their infants *en face* (24.6 minutes) than did mothers who held infants to the right (23.1 minutes), although the differences were not statistically significant ($t = .68$). For those who held left ($N = 48$) during the 10 minutes that a record of tactile behavior was kept, a mean of 15.5 of the 60 units were spent in fingertip exploration of the infant; 10.1 of the units were spent in fingertip exploration of the infant by those who held their infants on the right ($N = 12$). Again, these differences were not statistically significant ($t = 1.45$).

The 51 women who held their infants on the left side for most of the first hour were able to initiate breastfeeding earlier (32.8 minutes after birth) than the 18 who held their infants on the right (45.2 minutes; $t = -2.25$, $p < .05$). Getting the infant to nurse requires much manual dexterity on the part of the mother, which is undoubtedly related to handedness. Probably because left-holding, right-handed mothers have their right hands free to help their infants, there appeared to be an association between handedness and timing of initial breastfeeding, although not necessarily an association between handedness and lateral preference.

The frequency with which the preference for left-side holding seems to be established in human mothers before learning can take place suggests that this behavior may have a biological basis and be a product of past and, perhaps, ongoing adaptations. The genetic assimilation of the maternal behavior of holding the infant on the left side of the body can be explained by demonstrating that it is part of the behavioral repertoire of all mothers, a repertoire that was selected in the course of human evolution because it increased the chances of survival of offspring. Infants who were held on the left perhaps gained weight more rapidly after birth and soothed more readily than those not held on the left. Among early hominid foragers, these two factors contributed substantially to survival of infants. Thus, it can be postulated that women who held their infants to the left produced more surviving offspring than those who did not, and the behavior was selected in the ordinary way.

Huheey (1977) and Bolton (1978) have suggested that right-handedness was itself favorably selected in the course of human evolution because of the tendency of mothers to hold their infants on the left side. That is, right-handed mothers would be more skillful at manipulating objects and, therefore, selectively favored. This approach maintains that handedness and perhaps cerebral lateralization can be explained by the natural tendency of human mothers to hold their infants on the left.

The clinical significance of studies of left-side holding is perhaps less speculative than the evolutionary significance, although the findings are far from conclusive. Bogren (1984) found that 80% of the parents he studied held their infants on the left. Those that did not do so were more likely to have had problems with the pregnancy and were more likely to have had mental symptoms prior to pregnancy, suggesting an inadequacy in those that did not hold their infants on the left side of their bodies. De Chateau and colleagues have suggested that a failure to hold an infant on the left side may be a reflection of maternal insensitivity to her infant's needs (De Chateau *et al.*, 1978), which could, in turn, reflect inherent emotional problems.

Although the present study did not attempt to test for emotional problems or insensitivity, it does suggest that exposure to infants during the first hour enhances the likelihood of manifesting what may be a naturally selected behavior. Thus, the preference for left-lateral placement of the infant appears in human mothers as early as the first few seconds after birth and persists for the first full hour after birth. The preference is independent of handedness, cultural background of the mother, parity, and of other variables associated with pregnancy, labor, and delivery, suggesting further that it is not a learned behavior.

VISUAL COMMUNICATION

For primates, vision is perhaps the most important means of sensory perception. To an even greater extent than most primates, human beings depend on vision for obtaining information about their environment, for communication, and for controlling the behaviors of others with whom they interact. Concern for visual images may begin in the human infant at the moment of birth. Unlike many altricial mammals, whose eyes are closed at birth, human neonates are able to focus binocularly on objects 10–20 in from their faces (Slater and Findlay, 1975), to follow moving objects with their eyes (Brazelton *et al.*, 1966), and to discriminate pattern and form (Fantz, 1961).

Eye contact is one of the few behaviors that is under direct control of the infant, and the eyes appear to be a powerful attraction to the mother. Klaus and his colleagues report that mothers in their study talked about their infants' eyes in 70–80% of the statements made during the first 10 minutes of contact (Klaus and Kennell, 1975). Newman (1975) also observed that the infant's eyes are almost always the first thing remarked upon by its mother. Apprehension and reduced speed of attachment have been observed in mother–infant dyads when one member is blind (Fraiberg, 1974). Others have noted that eye contact is also an important part of the process of father–infant attachment.

It has been suggested that the amount of time that a mother spends in eye contact with her infant, especially in the *en face* position, is associated with the quality of attachment that develops between the two (Robson, 1967). Klaus and Kennell (1976) noted that the mother's interest in her infant's eyes increased during the course of the first 10 minutes of contact. The women in the present study, however, did not exhibit any increase in visual interest in their infants during the first hour, suggesting that this behavior may vary with a number of factors in the mother's background and in the circumstances of labor and delivery (Trevathan, 1983). Table 5.5 lists the absolute time and measures of dispersion for the first hour and for each 10-minute segment in the first hour. The means for

TABLE **5.5.** Amount of Time *En Face* in the First Hour after Birth [a,b]

Time (10-min intervals)	N	Mean/10 min	SD	Range	Percentage of interval
First	69	4.38	1.97	.05– 8.78	43.8
Second	69	3.81	1.96	.00– 8.10	38.1
Third	69	3.79	2.14	.00– 8.80	37.9
Fourth	69	3.83	2.07	.28– 8.82	38.3
Fifth	69	3.51	2.20	.00– 8.08	35.1
Sixth	69	3.85	2.13	.07– 7.87	38.5
Total[c]	97	23.78	8.88	3.83–44.92	39.6

[a]Note: Only total time was recorded for the first 28 subjects; for the remaining women in the study, the time was recorded in each 10-minute segment of the first hour.
[b]Table reprinted with permission, from the *American Journal of Orthopsychiatry*. Copyright 1983 by the American Orthopsychiatric Association, Inc.
[c]Data in mean/hr.

each 10-minute segment vary only slightly, indicating that there is no significant difference in time spent looking at the infant in the six segments ($F = 1.30$, $df = 5,416$). In other words, there is no significant decline or increase in *en face* gazing at the infant during the first hour after birth, as determined by the amount of time spent looking into the infant's face.

When total time looking *en face* was analyzed with other variables, the strongest and most significant association was with sociocultural or socioeconomic background of the mother: Hispanic women spent 22.6 minutes of the first hour *en face;* non-Hispanic women spent 29.9 minutes ($F = 9.96$, $df = 1,90$, $p < .002$). Other variables, including marital status, parity, difficulty of the birth, or duration of the stages of labor had no apparent influence on maternal gazing behavior. Among the Hispanic women, those whose husbands were present at the delivery ($N = 36$) spent slightly more time *en face* than did those whose husbands were not present ($N = 45$), although the differences were not significant (24 minutes for the former group, 21.4 for the latter). Those who described their relationship with their husband as "good" on the prenatal questionnaire spent significantly more time *en face* (23.7 minutes) than did those who said there were problems or that the relationship was "bad" (19.5 minutes), suggesting that a good overall relationship with the father of the child is a contributor to maternal interest in the infant and thus, perhaps, to bonding.

There were also significant differences in *en face* behavior between the women who selected delivery with midwives for philosophical reasons and those who chose TBC care for financial reasons. Those in the former group averaged 27.5 minutes *en face* while those in the latter averaged 21.2 minutes *en face* ($F = 9.48$, $df = 1,17$, $p < .01$). This indicates that women who are motivated for philosophical reasons to choose out-of-hospital birth are perhaps also more motivated to interact with their newborn infants through *en face* gazing.

At least two other factors appeared to influence maternal *en face* behavior in the first hour after birth. An artificial oxytocin is administered intramuscularly postpartum by the midwives if the mother is in danger of losing too much blood. The 16 women who received the ocytocin spent significantly less time looking *en face* at their infants (19.5 minutes) than did the 81 who did not receive an oxytocin (24.6 minutes; $F = 4.55$, $df = 1,95$, $p < .05$). The hormone produces more than the usual cramping, which would draw the mother's attention away from her infant. Because the hormone is administered for excessive bleeding, the apparent association may actually indicate the effects of heavy bleeding on visual behavior rather than the effects of the hormone itself.

The gender of the child did not seem to make much difference in the mother's visual behavior nor did it affect *en face* looking when the child was not of the desired gender. If the desired and actual gender were male (18 cases), however, time *en face* was significantly higher (28.6 minutes) than if the desired and actual gender were female (14 cases, mean 21.2 minutes; $F = 6.5$, $df = 1,30$, $p < .02$). The condition of the infant, as reflected by Apgar scores at 1 and 5 minutes after birth, did not affect amount of time *en face* during the first hour.

Amount of eye contact was not significantly associated with the lateral preference of the mother, but an interesting anecdote suggests that the two factors may be somewhat related. One of the five women who were part of the original sample of 115, but who, for various reasons, were not included in the data analysis, gave birth to twins. She had four boys at home and had many times expressed her strong desire for a girl. Tension was fairly high at the time of birth because of the general difficulty of twin delivery and the hopeful expectancy of all who were present that at least one of the twins would be a girl.

The first infant was born, it was a boy, and the mother smiled briefly and held it on her left side. The first infant was taken by a midwife while the mother delivered the second, 7 minutes later. The child was a girl, and the mother's reaction was obviously one of great pleasure. When she was reunited with both twins the boy was placed on her left and the girl on her right. Although there was no question which child she was most interested in, the mother spent almost the entire hour looking to her left. She knew which child was which, she smiled more at the girl and talked more often to her, but she actually did little more than glance to the right.

In another instance, a woman had shown very little interest in her infant for the first 40 minutes after birth. Her total time looking at her infant, which she held in her right arm, had been less than 5 minutes in that time period. I suggested to one of the midwives that she move the infant to the mother's left to see if that would have an effect on her visual behavior. Almost immediately the mother began giving her full attention to her infant and her total time looking at the infant was more than 20 minutes by the end of the hour. This dyad was not used in the final sample of 110 because of the experimental manipulations, but these two accounts lend support to the proposition that left-side holding enhances interaction.

Eye contact means different things in different cultures. Some believe that the power of the eye can inflict harm; for others, eye contact is made only with intimates; and the steady gaze is almost universally regarded as a threat signal (Argyle, 1978). Although proscriptions about eye contact do not appear to apply to mothers and infants, the results of this study indicate that the total time a mother spends looking *en face* at her infant depends to some extent on her cultural background. Because the Hispanic women in the present study were from a very different socioeconomic background from the Anglo women, however, it is impossible at this point to determine which of the factors, if any, has the most effect on *en face* behavior. As has been noted previously, the two groups of women approached childbirth with different sets of expectations. Among other factors, most of the Anglo women had read a number of the popular books on childbirth, and their awareness of the phenomenon of bonding may have consciously or subconsciously influenced their *en face* behavior. Also, as mentioned previously, the language differences between the Hispanic women and the birth attendants may account for the greater ease with which these women were distracted from focusing on their infants during the first hour. Thus, when advice was given or comments were made by a midwife who was not fluent in their language, more concentration in listening and responding was required of the Spanish-speaking women.

In summary, all of the mothers in the present study spent some time during the first hour after birth looking at their infants *en face*. Although the actual amounts of time were highly variable, the mean for the 97 women was 23.8 minutes, indicating that the eyes and face of the infant are highly attractive to the mother during the first hour postpartum. The mothers who had the highest mean time for *en face* contact were more likely to speak English as a primary language, to have good relationships with their husbands, and to have selected midwifery care for philosophical rather than financial reasons. They were also less likely to have been given an artificial oxytocin for postpartum bleeding and were more likely to have given birth to and desired a male child. Although the behavior itself may be universally exhibited by human mothers, the actual percentage of time spent gazing *en face* at their infants appears to vary with cultural and other factors.

AUDITORY COMMUNICATION

In a number of species, including perhaps our own, there are characteristic vocalizations for both infants and mothers associated with the early postpartum period. Vocalizations between mother and young serve at least three functions: maintaining proximity; facilitating individual recognition; and initiating nursing. Among mammals with precocial offspring, mothers vocalize to locate their young, and infants vocalize to attract their mothers. Walser (1978) reports that in many of the normally silent ungulates, vocal communication is almost constant between mother and young. When calling her young from a distance, a female will use a loud call, but when she is closer to her offspring she uses low frequency vocalizations which Walser describes as soft rumblings or purrs. Infants of many species have characteristic high-frequency, often stacatto-like, cries that they emit when separated from their mothers. There is evidence for many species that individual recognition of these cries develops in the first few days, although other individuals in the group often respond to a distress cry.

Immediately after birth, the female elephant seal turns toward her pup and emits a high-frequency warbling sound. After a few minutes of this, the newborn cries, and the two warble together for several minutes. Such vocal interaction occurs intermittently throughout the 1-month nursing period. The cry is used when the two are separated, suggesting individual recognition of vocalizations. Usually it is up to the precocial pup to get itself to its mother, however. A pup emits a characteristic shrill cry when it is ready to nurse, which results in the mother rolling over on her side to expose her teats. The pup approaches her to initiate nursing, but since it cannot physically gain access to her teat beneath her huge body, the cry has the effect of moving her into position (Le Bouef *et al.,* 1972).

McBride and Kritzler (1951) note that dolphins are vocal from the moment of birth, emitting the high-pitched whistling characteristic of all dolphin communication. They add that "the infant and its mother appear to be in constant vocal communication as shown by the bubbles escaping from their blowholes when whistling is heard" (p. 257). When separated from their mothers, infant dolphins remain in the place of last contact and whistle constantly until they are reunited.

In most primate species, vocalizations between mothers and young in the early postpartum period are not common because the two are rarely separated. There have been, however, a number of descriptions of characteristic "birth cries." Many observers of primate deliveries have reported hearing vocalizations at the time of emergence of the head but before complete delivery of the body (Takeshita, 1961–1962; Brandt and Mitchell, 1971; Kadam and Swayamprabha, 1980; Love, 1978; Graham-Jones and Hill, 1962), a behavior not uncommon in human births. In other cases, a birth cry is heard after expulsion of the entire body. Vocalizations may continue after delivery is completed, but nonhuman primate births are usually described as "surprisingly quiet." I assume the "surprise" is due to the stereotypic expectation that human deliveries are accompanied by loud outbursts from the mother and constant crying of the infant. As I have argued, such is not necessarily the norm in out-of-hospital deliveries, so it may be that, in terms of noise levels, human and nonhuman primate deliveries are not very different. Again, the adaptive significance of quiet births is obvious for all primates.

Takeshita (1961–1962) records a vocalization described as "chi-chi" which was emitted 28 times in rapid succession by a squirrel monkey whose head alone had emerged from the birth canal. A mona monkey infant observed by the same author emitted a birth cry described as "ki" when its entire body emerged. It continued to cry for several minutes afterward. In both cases the infant climbed up its mother's ventrum and found the nipples without assistance. Even when they were not actively suckling, they remained attached to the teat and were quiet.

With the very first cry, the "birth cry," the human mother responds to her infant by stroking and rubbing him, attempting to bring him up to her chest, and making soothing sounds. This cry, qualitatively different from all others he will make, initiates interaction and is the first vocal statement "I exist!" Often the birth cry is not heard for a minute or two after birth as many infants have trouble establishing initial respirations. During this interlude between birth and first cry, mothers are commonly disassociated from the scene, perhaps recovering from the physical exertion of the second stage of labor. Occasionally, in births I observed, the midwives would tell the mothers to vigorously rub their infants to stimulate breathing, but even when they responded they seemed to do so automatically, as if following an outside command for which they had little understanding. A transformation in behavior takes place with that first cry, and, except in rare cases, the mothers are from then on visibly involved with their infants until one or both fall asleep.

There have been a few descriptions of later vocal interactions between mother and infant primates. Goswell and Gartlan (1965), for example, describe various sounds made by a newborn patas monkey including squeals, screams, gecks, and a sound they describe as a "want call." The "gecks" have been described for other primate species as attention-getting and proximity-maintaining mechanisms (Rawlins, 1979).

Nadler (1974:62) describes the development of "coordinated vocalizations" between a mother and infant gorilla on the day of birth. Typically, the infant vocalized and the mother responded with soft "growls." This occurred just after birth and several time during the next 24 hours. The infant's vocalizations were associated with sucking motions, leading Nadler to suggest that the coordination of vocal interaction was a prelude to the establishment of nursing. Eventually, the mother decreased vocalizations and responded to her infant's vocalizations by moving it to a different position on her ventral surface. Thus, although she was not actually assisting it in nursing, the constant repositioning eventually led it to the nipple. The mother in this case was a primipara, and it is possible that she simply did not know how to interpret her infant's vocalizations but that by responding in some manner, particularly by moving it, she was able to help it establish nursing. In general, providing overt assistance in nursing is notably absent in most primate species (see Brandt and Mitchell, 1971; Rawlins, 1979).

One of the characteristics that sets human beings apart from all other animals is the capacity for and dependency on language. Even before birth, the human fetus is exposed to language. It has been demonstrated that from about the twenty-eighth week of pregnancy, a fetus responds actively to sounds. Montagu (1964) reports that fetal heartbeat and movement increase markedly in response to such sounds as washing machines, piano playing, return of a typewriter carriage, concert music, or a sharp, loud noise. Presumably the human voice, at least in the higher pitched or louder ranges, can also be heard by the fetus. Thus, many of the apparent differences among neonates of different cultures may reflect *in utero* rhythms that developed in response to the group's language rhythms in the last few weeks of pregnancy. Perhaps, even before birth, the infant has begun to lay the foundation of his culture's language system which is later reflected in the entrainment process described by Condon and Sander (1974).

Eisenberg *et al.* (1964:264) report that neonate response to noise in the high frequency range is characterized by a greater number of "arousal and orienting-quiet responses." Thus, the neonatal nervous system may be designed to respond more rapidly to the higher frequency of the female voice (Brazelton, 1963). Lang (1972) noted that in home births she attended, the mother picked up the infant immediately after birth, held it in the *en face* position, and spoke to it in a high-pitched voice. Klaus and Kennell (1976) also observed that mothers will talk to other adults present at the birth in a normal voice and will immediately switch to a higher than normally pitched voice, often mid-sentence, when they orient toward their newborn infants. Newman (1975) notes that mothers in her study spoke in a higher than normal tone to their infants. This apparently unconscious raising of her voice may indicate another evolved mechanism that enhances bonding between mother and child. It is not clear, however, whether the orienting response of infants explains the high-pitched voice of mothers or whether the reverse is true.

Voice pitch was ascertained for 68 of the 110 women in my study. Of these, 66 or 92%, spoke in a higher than normally pitched voice, and only 2 spoke in their normal voice (i.e., the pitch did not change when the direction of speech switched from adults to the infant). For the remaining 38 women observed, 34 never spoke to or toward the infant as far as could be judged, and 4 did so but could not be heard well enough directly or from the audiotape to determine whether or not the pitch changed. Speaking to or toward the infant includes all women who were observed to "talk to" their infants, but it also includes some women who did not actually address their infants but elevated the pitch of their voices when looking at the infant while talking to other people.

Since only 2 women did not elevate the pitch of their voices, it was impossible to do any meaningful statistical analyses on these 68 women. Both of those whose pitch did not change were primiparas, both had male infants, both were Hispanic, and both seemed happy during the first hour after birth.

In addition to pitch being important in mother–infant bonding in human beings, verbal interaction itself may be part of that process. As noted before, a reference to the infant's eyes is almost always made by a mother during the first 10 minutes of contact with her newborn infant (Klaus and Kennell, 1982). Newman (1975) observes that this is a mother's way of identifying her infant as an individual and adds two other variables that are part of the first mother-to-infant conversation: (1) relating the infant by analogy to other members of the family or the social group (e.g., "he has his father's nose") and (2) a comment on the infant's presumed inner state, usually hunger (e.g., "do you want to nurse?"). She concludes that these early conversations between mother and child are an important part of acculturation of the newborn into the society in which he is born. Reference to the infant's eyes is, as she describes it, a way of saying "Hello, are you in there?" Referring to the baby by name or describing a resemblance to a family member is a way of identifying the position of the new member in a particular family or society. As Newman notes, the infant is first recognized as an individual (often a big step for a mother who must reconcile the real baby with the idealized baby she has thought about for many months) and then as a member of an organized, larger group.

Daly and Wilson (1982) have discussed the importance of the first postpartum conversations for establishing paternity confidence. Since maternity is always assured at birth, it is important for the mother to enhance the father's confidence in paternity and one way she does so, they suggest, is by demonstrating physical resemblances between the baby and the father. The father, on the other hand, is more likely to exhibit skepticism. Daly and Wilson predict that there will be disproportionate numbers and kinds of comments made by mothers and fathers about the resemblances between the baby and the other parent. The results of their analysis of 68 conversations recorded at birth were that paternal resemblance was stated more often than maternal resemblance, and in almost all cases it was the mother rather than the father who remarked upon that resemblance.

Of the mothers ($N = 107$) in this study, 60% talked actively to their infants during the first hour after birth. In all instances, the mother looked directly into the eyes of the infant when talking to it. There were no significant differences among those who did or did not talk to their infants according to maternal parity, reason for choosing care with midwives, relationship with the child's father, reaction to and duration of labor, degree of difficulty of the delivery, or whether or not fluent speakers of the mother's language were present during delivery.

Talking to the infant during the first hour after birth was significantly associated with mother's sociocultural background ($X^2 = 4.47$, $p<.05$) and with her attitude toward childbirth ($X^2 = 7.71$, $p<.05$). The observed differences between Hispanic and Anglo women may reflect cultural norms about the appropriateness of talking to infants, feelings of comfort the woman had with English-speaking midwives, or a combination of these and other factors.

In almost all instances where the mother was a fluent speaker of both Spanish and English ($N = 7$), she talked to her infant in Spanish and to the midwives in English, freely moving from one language to another. The one exception to this was a woman whose primary language was Spanish and whose husband spoke primarily German. Their common language was English, and she spoke to her infant in that language. During the first hour after this birth, there were phone calls from the father to his parents during which he spoke German and she spoke English, phone calls from the mother to her parents during which she spoke Spanish and he spoke English, and the conversations among themselves (mother, father, and infant) in English.

Introducing the infant to members of the larger social network is often accomplished during the first hour after birth. In the current study, introduction was made directly by visitation or indirectly by a phone call. Slightly more than 71% of the mothers were visited by a friend or relative during the first hour, or they made or received a phone call during that time. In 10 instances, the infant was "asked" to cry into the mouthpiece of the phone as a way of introducing it to the person on the receiving end.

The following transcripts of recordings that began just before birth of the infant provide a little more insight into the drama, excitement, and passion of the first mother–infant interaction:

BIRTH 1: Bilingual Hispanic mother

MIDWIFE:	Push, Karen. The baby's coming out now. Push hard. Good. Coming down. Grab the baby! Grab the whole thing! There you go.
MOTHER:	Oh, my love. Oh, my baby. Oh, I love you.
FATHER:	It's a boy?
MIDWIFE:	Is it really? (laughs) I told you, huh?
MOTHER:	It's a boy?
FATHER:	It's a boy.
MIDWIFE:	One minute Apgar? Let's see . . . a little floppy . . . pink feet . . . (Suctioning with bulb aspirator.)
MOTHER:	What's that?
MIDWIFE:	If he gets that down into his lungs he'll end up with pneumonia.
MOTHER:	(Baby crying) It's alright poor baby, oh, it's alright. Oh my baby, yes, yes. I waited for you so long, now you're here. Oh, my baby, Oh, it's OK, it's OK, I love you. It's OK. (to father) You wanna see it? He's the most beautiful thing (laughs). Never, never, ever seen a baby so beautiful. Oh God, oh baby, I love you. (Baby cries). No, no, no. Oh you do very good, you do very good, good, yes, yes, yes. It's alright. You cry some more? Oh, why you cry? Why you cry, oh yes. shshshshshshsh. No, noooooo.
MIDWIFE:	Give her [mother] some orange juice.
MOTHER:	(To midwife in normal voice pitch) Can I sit up so I can breastfeed the baby? (Baby cries, mother continues to talk, but hard to hear.) Oh, my baby, don't cry, I'm sorry, I love you. Yes, it's alright.
MIDWIFE:	What are you spitting up, fellow?
FATHER:	He's big, huh?

MOTHER: He's the strongest little thing.
MIDWIFE: Got a good grip, huh?
MOTHER: What's the matter?
MIDWIFE: Nothing's the matter, I'm just waiting here for your placenta.
OTHER
MIDWIFE: One more push, Karen.
MOTHER: No, no, no, please, no, no, no. (Then she says the same thing to the baby, in the same rhythm, but much higher-pitched voice). Oh, my baby, oh, my baby. You're so beautiful.

BIRTH 2. Hispanic mother*

MADRE: Mi hijo, mi hijo, mi hijo. ¿Qúe es? ¿Niño?
PARTERA: No sé, mira.
MADRE: Ay es niña. Ay mi bebé. Ya, ya mi hijo. Qué es chiple. Ya mi hijo. Tienes frío. Ya mi hijo, qué tienes. Pobrecito mi hijo está todo chueco.
PARTERA: Gloria, chichi a su bebe.
MADRE: No la quiere. No sé la puedo poner. Tiene hambre.

BIRTH 3. Hispanic mother

MADRE: ¿Qué es?
PARTERA: Niña.
MADRE: Qué mi amor. Mi amor. Niña. Qué mi hijita. Qué mi amor. Ay mi amor. Ay chiquita. Mamita. Mi amor. Chiquita. Ay mi amor. ¿Por qué llora mi amor, por qué? Mi amor.
PARTERA: ¿Tiene un nombre para su bebé?
PADRE: Guadalupe.
PARTERA: ¿Guadalupe qué, nada más?
PADRE: Guadalupe. Es que hoy es día de la virgen de Guadalupe en México.

BIRTH 4. Hispanic mother

MADRE: Qué lindo, es mi hijo, es mío. ¿Qué es? Ay, qué hermoso. Ay, qué hermoso. Mira qué lindo mi hijo. Ay qué hermoso mi hijo. Ay qué lindo.
TIA: Es hombre.
MADRE: ¡Un hombre! tía qué feliz. Ay hasta que salvo, mi hijo, mi hijo. Nadie me lo va a quitar, nadie, nadie. Mi hijo, mi hijo. Qué tonto. Ay qué lindo. ¿Moreno?
TIA: No, no está moreno, está blanco.
MADRE: ¿Blanco? Ya, ya, ya mi hijito. Ya, ya, ya mi papaito. Ya, ya, ya mi papaito. Ya, ya papaito. Ya, ya, chiquitito. Ay, qué

*A translation of the Spanish dialogues is provided in Appendix A.

hermoso. Ay un hombre. Ya, ya, ya chiquito. ¿Por qué llora?
Qué pasó. Ya, ya, ya. Ay qué lindo.

BIRTH 5. Hispanic mother

MADRE: Es niño, ¿verdad? Mi hijo. Es niño. Gracias Dios mío. Mi rey
            lindo. La raźon de mi vida. Mi hijito. Mi vida. Sí mi amor.
            Shshshshshsh Mi cosa linda.
PADRE;   Mira qué uñotas. ¿Te cansaste? Está muy cabezón. ¿Ya está
            chupando?

BIRTH 6. Hispanic mother

MADRE: Gracias mi hija. Ay sí. Está bien. ¿Qué es?
PARTERA: No sé, mira.
MADRE: Gracias Dios mío. Gracias Jesús. En nombre de Cristo Jesús tu
            hijo te doy las gracias y a éstas muchachas. ¿Lo van a bañar mi
            hija or no? ¿Qué es? Qué es?
PARTERA: Mira a tu bebé.
MADRE: No peudo ver. ¿Que es?
PARTERA: Mira a tu bebé, qué es.
MADRE: ¿Hembra o macho?
PARTERA: Mira tú.
MADRE: Macho. Tiene hambre.
PARTERA: Ponga a su bebe en su pecho.
MADRE: No sé cómo darle.
PARTERA: Pero él debe aprender.
MADRE: No sé cómo. Tiene hambre. Mientras denle agua. Mientras
            denle algo pobrecito.
PARTERA: No.
MADRE: ¿Aquí es donde le ponen el nombre a los niños?
PARTERA: ¿El nombre? No ahorita.

ENTRAINMENT

Entrainment is the process by which an infant, or any other normal human
being, moves in rhythm to the spoken word. Using microanalysis of sound films,
Condon and Sander (1974) demonstrated that this interactional synchrony occurs
in neonates as early as 12 hours after birth. The movements of her child in
response to her voice reward the mother and stimulate her to continue talking,
thus prolonging the synchrony as long as the child is in the quiet–alert state.

This entrainment process is one that Papousek and Papousek (1982) suggest
is intuitive because of the simplistic and repetitive nature, which, if under
conscious control, ''would disrupt the dialogue and exhaust the parent in a short
time.'' In these behaviors, they claim, ''are tendencies initiating and supporting

various fundamental integrative processes in the newborn during the early neonatal period'' (p. 384).

Condon and Sander (1974) studied the rhythmic movements of infants using Chinese, English, and discontinuous sounds. The discontinuous sounds did not result in the same degree of correspondence between the infant's movements and the sound as it did in natural speech. The researchers thus suggest that,

> If the infant, from the beginning, moves in precise, shared rhythm with the organization of the speech structure of his culture, then he participates developmentally through complex, sociobiological entrainment processes in millions of repetitions of linguistic forms long before he later uses them in speaking and communicating. By the time he begins to speak, he may have already laid down within himself the form and structure of the language system of his culture (p. 101).

They further suggest that the bonding between mother and child should be regarded as an extension of the cultural milieu in which they participate rather than as an isolated dyadic interaction.

This concept of rhythmic interactions between the mother and infant from the moment of birth is reminiscent of Margaret Mead's description of the cultural rhythm in which the Manus child develops. Immediately after a Manus birth and before the delivery of the placenta, "the nurse holding the baby begins to sing a lullaby in time with the baby's birth wail. As the baby wails and the midwife and her assistant exhort the mother to greater and greater effort, the nurse's voice rises to a crescendo and the new baby becomes part of the rhythm of the world about it" (Mead 1956:345).

Klaus and Kennell (1976) extend this concept of interactive synchrony even further. They note that while *in utero* the fetus must conform to the biorhythms of its mother. For example, there is evidence that the sleep states of the baby *in utero* coincide with the mother's sleep patterns (MacFarlane, 1977). Birth disrupts these synchronous biorhythms, and the mother must help establish new ones. Eventually the mother's interactive state and the infant's quiet–alert state come to co-occur, thus synchronizing their attention and nonattention cycles. Mothers who received no medication during birth are alert and actively interested in their infants for at least an hour after birth, the time in which the infant is also in the quiet–alert–interactive state. Usually the mother wants to nurse within 1½ hours of birth, the infant responds, and both fall into a sound sleep (Klaus and Kennell, 1976; personal observation). Thus, in unmedicated births, synchronous biorhythms may be partially reestablished within an hour after birth.

NURSING

As has been repeatedly emphasized, an important adaptation the infant must make soon after birth is the initiation of nursing, a behavior that is not always easily effected in mammals. Human beings are not the only mammals for whom there is much confusion during the initial nursing period. Rheingold (1963:176) describes initial suckling by dog pups as "fumbling" and uncoordinated. Other terms and phrases recorded during observations of puppies nursing during the first 2 weeks of life included "thrashing about," "mad scramble," "furious," "impatient," and "battle." Unlike many concerned human mothers in Western societies, however, the canine mothers tended to ignore the activity at their nipples; most usually slept right through it.

Finding the teat and nursing are especially challenging for newborn dolphins. The infants are born under water and must swim to the surface to take their first breath on their own. Dolphins are, from the moment of birth, able to keep up with their mothers. Searching for the nipple may begin a few minutes after birth, and nursing is initiated in less than 4 hours (McBride and Kritzler, 1951). The mother provides no direction in first finding the nipple, but she assists nursing by rolling over on her side and moving as little as possible. Suckling need last only a few seconds because the muscles of her abdomen expel the milk into the infant's mouth as soon as it grasps the nipple. During the first 2 weeks, the infant suckles an average of every 26 minutes (McBride and Kritzler, 1951).

Elephant seal pups are precocial and are able to move around, albeit unsteadily, within a few minutes of birth. Other females take active interest in the newborn infant and occasionally aggressive encounters occur. Within an hour of birth, when the mother is lying on her side, the pup locates the nipple and begins suckling, a process that continues for about 1 month. The mother assists in nursing by rolling over on her side, but the infant is always the initiator of a nursing bout, doing so with the characteristic cry described earlier. The dyad rarely moves during the entire month of nursing. Pups nurse approximately two to five times a day with no particular pattern, except that the daily frequency increases as they get older (Le Bouef *et al.,* 1972).

Lambs and kids must usually find the udders on their own, although by licking their infants, the mothers may orient them in the proper direction. Nursing begins within 3 hours of birth and occurs in brief but frequent bursts. Occasionally the mother may assist in nursing by lifting up one of her hindlimbs (Hersher *et al.,* 1963).

Initial suckling attempts by the infant are important for release of oxytocin which enables the mother to recover quickly from the strain of birth. Licking the nipple also serves to increase prolactin concentrations in humans four to six times the normal level (Hwang in Klaus and Kennell, 1976). Prolactin is the hormone that induces milk secretion. Klaus and Kennell (1976) report that prolactin levels increase when the human mother simply touches or holds her baby. Noting that in birds it is the "love hormone," they suggest that the increase in prolactin may further enhance the mother's attachment to her infant.

As soon after human birth as the umbilical cord is cut, it is possible for nursing to begin, although numerous factors affect the timing of initial nursing or "latching on" by neonates. For 954 of the deliveries that took place at TBC between January 1978 and May 1982, I collected data on the time of initial nursing to elicit factors that affected it (Trevathan, 1984). Among the reasons for doing this study was to examine the suggested association between early establishment of nursing and subsequent success and duration of breastfeeding. In several studies, it was demonstrated that nursing within an hour or two after delivery contributed to the establishment of longer and more successful breastfeeding when contrasted with initiating nursing several hours after delivery. For example, in a Brazilian study by Sousa *et al.* (1974), 200 women were divided into two groups, one initiating nursing immediately after delivery, the other initiating 12–14 hours later. At 2 months, 77% of the early-contact mothers were still successfully breastfeeding compared with 27% of the control group.

In another study (Salariya *et al.*, 1978), 111 primiparous women were placed on four different nursing schedules. One group was allowed to nurse 10 minutes after delivery and every 2 hours thereafter; another nursed 10 minutes after delivery, and every 4 hours thereafter. The last two groups began breastfeeding 4–6 hours after delivery, one subsequently nursed every 2 hours, the other every 4 hours. The 2-hourly, early-initiation group nursed significantly longer than any of the other three groups. The 4-hourly, later-initiation group weaned earliest.

Johnson (1976) studied 12 women who planned to breastfeed their infants. Of the 12, 6 were allowed to suckle shortly after birth and 6 had first contact with their infants 16 hours after birth. All of the mothers who suckled on the delivery table were still nursing 2 months later but only 1 of the late-contact mothers was still breastfeeding. Klaus and Kennell (1982) reported longer breastfeeding, fewer infections, and greater mean weight gain for infants whose mothers were allowed to nurse them on the delivery table when compared with those who did not have this contact. Their study was of 38 women, 19 controls and 19 early nursers, in a Guatemalan hospital. In a Swedish study, 58% of early-contact mothers were still breastfeeding at 3 months, while only 26% of the control group continued (De Chateau and Wiberg, 1977). The median lactation period for the early-contact mothers was 2.5 months longer than among the control-group mothers.

Thomson *et al.* (1979) report significant differences in breastfeeding success for 15 women who experienced early contact (15–30 minutes postpartum) with their infants compared to 15 women who first had contact with their infants 12–24 hours postpartum. At 2 months, 60% of the early-contact mothers were successfully breastfeeding, while only 20% of the late-contact group were doing so. They also reported that the early-contact/longer-nursing group showed more positive immediate reactions to their infants; having little or no immediate reaction was related to failure in breastfeeding.

Elander and Lindberg (1984) report differences in breastfeeding success for 30 mother–infant dyads who were separated from each other from 1–6 days in the first week of life when compared with 116 nonseparated dyads. Of the separated mothers, 37% were still nursing at 3 months postpartum, while 72% of the nonseparated group were still nursing. In this particular study, the

TABLE **5.6.** Time of Initial Breastfeeding According to Maternal Parity[a]

Parity	N	Mean time	SD	Range
1	346	46.8	43.2	1–360
2	316	37.7	38.1	1–40
3–5	379	34.6	28.3	1–263
6+	78	28.8	19.4	3–90

[a]From Trevathan, 1984. Copyright Redgrave Publishing Company, Bedford Hills, N.J.

separation resulted from mild illness in the infant (e.g., hyperbilirubinemia, RDS, suspected infection), which likely had confounding effects on the process of breastfeeding. Previous studies (e.g., Tamminen *et al.,* 1983), however, had reported that delayed initiation of breastfeeding because of obstetrical difficulties or infant illness had little effect on the duration of breastfeeding. This suggests that the separation itself played a role in decreasing the success of breastfeeding.

At TBC, women were encouraged to initiate nursing within 1 hour after birth, in part because of the importance of nipple stimulation for oxytocin release. Usually the women made the decision to try to initiate breastfeeding themselves, often responding to rooting movements by the infant. Occasionally they tried nursing at the suggestion of a midwife. The mother trying to initiate nursing and the infant actually "latching on" are two separate actions, however. There were usually several minutes between the initial attempts by the mother and actual suckling by the infant.

Mean time for the initiation of breastfeeding (actual suckling) for the total sample was 27.4 minutes after birth, with a range from 1 to 60 minutes. Slightly more than one-third of the women ($N = 334$) initiated nursing within 20 minutes of birth, 410 began nursing 20–40 minutes after birth, and 210 initiated nursing between 40 and 60 minutes after birth. Anglo women initiated nursing 25 minutes after birth, while Hispanic women began, on the average, 3 minutes later (28 minutes). This difference is not statistically significant.

Primiparas began nursing their infants approximately 3 minutes later than multiparas; nursing initiation times decreased with parity as did within-group variation (Table 5.6). These results suggest that previous experience with birth and infants contributes to initial nursing success. Approximately 80% of the multiparous women had breastfed previous infants.

The length of the first and third stages of labor did not have a significant effect on the time of initial nursing. A long second stage of labor was associated significantly with later initiation of breastfeeding ($F = 14.20$, $p < .001$). This suggests that it takes longer for a woman to recover from a long second stage and, thus, longer to begin focusing on the needs of her infant.

The condition of the newborn infant, as measured by Apgar scores, also had a significant effect on initial nursing. There is an inverse relationship between Apgar scores and time of initial nursing, suggesting that more depressed babies take longer to recover from the delivery and reach a state in which they can begin active suckling. Infants with 1-minute Apgar scores lower than 4 ($N = 24$) began nursing, on the average, 33 minutes after birth. Mean initiation time for those with scores of 4–7 ($N = 236$) was 30 minutes after birth; mean time for those with scores higher than 7 ($N = 694$) was 27 minutes ($F = 7.5$, $p < .001$).

A similar pattern is seen when the 5-minute Apgar scores are examined with respect to nursing initiation: Those with scores lower than 8 ($N = 37$) averaged 35 minutes after birth for first nursing, while those with higher scores initiated, on the average, 27.5 minutes after birth ($F = 9.62$, $p < .01$).

The gender of the infant appeared to have some effect on the timing of initial nursing (Gender and Apgar scores were independent in this sample). Females began nursing 27 minutes after delivery, males 29 minutes after delivery ($F = 4.59$, $p < .05$). In Chapter 4, it was suggested that newborn girls are more "orally receptive" (Freedman, 1974), engage in more "mouth dominated" actions (Korner, 1973), and exhibit more rhythmic mouthings (Korner, 1969) than newborn boys. Initial, active suckling at the breast is not a simple task for any newborn infant. Perhaps, as suggested by these studies, female infants are more "primed" to oral sensations and actions involving the mouth and are thus able to establish nursing earlier.

The primary question of the studies just reviewed was the effects of early initiation of breastfeeding on duration of breastfeeding. Most extended for several months after birth. I was able to follow 743 of the original 954 women through the sixth week postpartum. By this time, 587 (62%) of the women were known to be still breastfeeding their infants, and 156 (16%) were known to have stopped. Even if the 211 (22%) women whom I was unable to follow had all stopped breastfeeding, it is impressive that almost two-thirds of the original sample maintained lactation through the sixth week postpartum. It is likely that many of the 211 who did not return for the 6-week postpartum exam were still nursing, boosting the success rate even higher. Thus, this study confirms the earlier ones that suggested that initiating nursing within an hour or two of birth contributes to greater success in later breastfeeding.

As previously mentioned, when the baby licks its mother's nipple, whether it actually sucks or not, the hormone oxytocin is released into her bloodstream. This hormone helps to contract the uterus, inducing expulsion of the placenta and, once the uterus is empty, further contracts it to stop bleeding. This enables the mother to return to a state of well-being and safety soon after delivery and is thus a significant contribution on the part of the infant to its mother's survival. In the past, before artificial oxytocins were available, early suckling may have made the difference between life and death for some women. Thus, it is likely that early suckling by the infant was selectively favored in human (and mammalian) evolution. Furthermore, if early suckling contributes to longer, more successful nursing, as suggested by this and other studies, there would be another selective advantage to this behavior throughout most of human history when mother's breast was the only source of nourishment for the very young infant.

For the first 3 days, the maternal breast secretes colostrum, and only on the fourth day is the true milk usually available to the baby. Colostrum is composed mostly of serum and white blood corpuscles, and in many cultures (including our own at certain times in our history), it is regarded as a nonfood and even dangerous for the baby, who is not nursed by the mother until the third day. We now know that the colostrum is a rich source of antibodies that provide protection from potentially dangerous gastrointestinal organisms as well as organisms in the environment to which the infant is exposed. Lozoff (1983) has noted that early breastfeeding is not the norm in most non-Western societies, suggesting that this, like other selected behaviors, may have been altered more recently by human cultural practices.

ODOR

There is evidence that the olfactory centers are fairly well-developed in human infants at birth. This fits with Bronson's assessment that the phylogenetically older sections of the brain will mature more rapidly than the more recently evolved parts (Bronson, 1982). Olfaction is the primary mode of interaction with the environment for most mammals, with an exception being higher primates. In fact, for mammals other than primates, it is probably the primary channel of recognition established between mother and infant. Mothers seem to identify their infants through smell and, in many species, lactating females emit a pheromone that enables their infants to recognize them.

Although it is much reduced in primates and especially in humans, olfaction may still play a minor role in promoting attachment and recognition in human mothers and infants. There is, however, no evidence that it emerges on the day of birth. MacFarlane (1977) has demonstrated that 6-day-old breastfed infants show a significant preference for gauze pads from their own mother's breast when given a choice between her pad and that of another nursing woman. This preference was not observed in 2-day-old infants, but by 6 days they seemed to recognize their own mother's scent, suggesting that learning from repeated exposure was involved in the process.

There is also evidence that mothers can learn to distinguish their own infants from others by odor alone. Porter and his colleagues (1983) tested 20 mothers after an average of 23 hours of exposure to their infants after birth. Of these, 16 were able to distinguish clothing worn by their own infants from similar clothing worn by another infant of the same age. In a second experiment, they tested 17 women who had an average of only 2½ hours of contact with their infants following cesarean delivery. Of these women, 13 were able to identify correctly by smell the clothing worn by their own infants. The mechanisms involved are uncertain, but these authors suggest several possible explanations. One is that there is a phenotypic similarity between relatives that enables a mother to recognize her infant as smelling somewhat like herself. Rapid learning could also be involved and is the most likely mechanism for odor identification in ungulates, who are able to recognize their infants after only a few minutes exposure to them. Finally, mothers could impart an odor to their infants, after even a few minutes interaction, that enables recognition after a period of separation.

Regardless of the mechanism responsible, the evidence that mothers can recognize their infants by odor adds to our understanding of the mother–infant bonding process. Porter and his colleagues (1983) point out that although visual and auditory cues may be more important in later mother–infant interaction, olfactory cues may be a more important channel of recognition in the first few hours postpartum. The physical appearance of a neonate changes fairly rapidly over the first week of life, and recognition of individual cries may develop more slowly. Thus, olfaction may have been "an ideal channel for mothers to use in identifying their infants," particularly in the past (Porter *et al.*, 1983:153).

Nicholson (1984:625) proposes what he calls the "semiochemical–addiction bonding hypothesis" which suggests a primary role for olfaction in human–human bonding. He notes that infants in the first year of life and females at the end of pregnancy and during lactation excrete unusually high levels of sebum. In addition, the vernix caseosa has a high component of sebum. He also argues that kissing itself enhances bonding because of the high number of sebaceous glands in the scalp and facial region. Thus, the chemicals associated with this sebum secretion, he argues, make the infant attractive to the mother, make the mother attractive to the male at a particularly vulnerable time (i.e., after giving birth), and perhaps enable the infant to more readily recognize its mother's odor.

ETHOGRAMS OF MATERNAL BEHAVIOR IMMEDIATELY AFTER BIRTH

Many of the behaviors observed postpartum in mammals can be incorporated into an ethogram for a given species. This is not to imply that a rigid, invariant pattern is observed in any mammalian species. Those who have made extensive observations of maternal behavior in species such as rats, rabbits, dogs, and cats conclude that the patterned behaviors that they have observed are largely under neurohormonal control but depend heavily on experience, learning, and socialization. In other words, it may be that hormones provide the appropriate initial stimulus, but how the mother proceeds in reaction to that stimulus depends, to some extent, on her own experiences in life, the number, state, and perhaps "personality" of her offspring, and other environmental stimuli.

The laboratory rat, for example, tears the fetal membrane from each pup after delivery, vigorously licks the infant all over, increasing concentration on the anogenital region which stimulates the pup to urinate and defecate. After all have been born, the mother continues to lick the pups, characteristically retrieves each pup that strays, repairs the nest if necessary, and finally settles down to allow the pups to nurse. All of this seems to be part of the total delivery pattern for the rat (Rosenblatt and Lehrman, 1963).

Parturition behavior in the domestic cat was also described in Chapter 3. Schneirla *et al.* (1963) suggest that physiological changes in the female set off a pattern of behavior that begins with focusing the cat's attention on her own body. As each kitten is born, her attention shifts to the neonate, and she licks each one until it is dry. The birth fluids and placenta are consumed. Once parturition has been completed, the cat begins to focus attention on her kittens and spends approximately the next 12 hours resting with them. Nursing begins anytime from during parturition to 2 hours postpartum. The mother assumes a posture, encircling the kittens, which provides them with warmth, protection, and access to nutrients, all of immediate survival value. The altricial neonate orients itself toward the mother's ventrum, probably through tactual and olfactory cues, and slowly propels itself toward the nipple, moving its head back and forth, rooting, until the nipple is found.

Schneirla *et al.* (1963) had predicted that maternal behavior would be different in reaction to the first born compared to the last-born kitten. This prediction seemed logical because of changes in novelty of the stimulus, in the environment of the birth location, and in the number of other kittens in need of attention. In general, however, they found no significant differences in behaviors in succeeding kitten births, suggesting her reaction was more closely tied to internal than to external stimuli. They caution that this does not imply rigidity in the patterning of behavior. Licking, for example, is an invariant behavior, but it is not always done immediately after birth of a kitten. Other things may distract the mother for a few minutes.

Many other species, as diverse as sheep, goats, and primates, follow similar patterns, as has been pointed out in Chapter 3. No matter where one is in the world, it is easy to predict parturition and immediate postpartum behavior in domestic cats, sheep, and other species. In Chapter 3, I proposed an ethogram for human parturition that describes the female's reactions to labor and delivery. This ethogram can be continued for the first hour postpartum because there are behaviors used in interacting with the newborn infant that are common enough to be described as characteristic.

After the end of the second stage of labor, a woman usually appears exhausted but elated, although occasionally indifference, disgust, or despair is noted. The infant is placed on its mother's abdomen, the cord still attached and pulsating. Rubbing of the infant by the mother may begin immediately, and she often makes high-pitched vocalizations directed toward the infant. Birth attendants are involved in assessing the newborn and assisting it to establish respirations, if necessary. They also attend the mother, watching especially for postpartum bleeding.

The cord is cut when it stops pulsating, usually about 2 minutes after delivery. Once the cord is cut, the infant can be drawn up toward the mother's breasts, typically on the left side of her body, and she will often attempt to establish breastfeeding, although rarely does the infant suckle at the initial placement on the breast. Commonly, the mother and infant expend effort at making eye contact with each other. Touching, rubbing, and stroking continue. Almost invariably, the mother smiles at her infant, and many women talk actively to their infants during the first hour after birth. When the infant cries, common responses include patting, rocking, rubbing, and shushing sounds.

Usually within ½ hour of birth, the mother experiences contractions of the third stage, which result in separation of the placenta from the uterine wall and expulsion. Once delivered, the placenta is examined for completeness and set aside. Slight postpartum bleeding is normal. If the father or other family members are present, they express great interest in the infant and often try to take it from the mother for a few minutes. Interaction between the mother and infant continues for up to 1 hour after birth while each are in a prolonged "quiet–alert" state, but by the end of that time, most mothers and infants have fallen asleep.

Species-Specific Behavior?

In proposing an ethogram, I am suggesting that the behaviors described are exhibited by virtually all human females delivering under normal circumstances. Of course, there is a great deal of cross-cultural and temporal variation in the definition of "normal" as it is applied to childbirth. In order to make it broadly applicable, I define "normal" delivery as one that fits the following criteria: (1) no medications used; (2) vertex presentation of a single, healthy infant; and (3) assistance from at least one other person. Although I acknowledge that the practice is far from widespread, I add a fourth criterion, that the mother and infant be in contact with each other for the first hour or so after birth, otherwise, the concept of characteristic interaction patterns is meaningless.

Can it be argued that the behaviors I have described for human mothers are species specific as some have proposed? To meet this definition, according to Jolly (1985:189–190), a behavior must exhibit the following characteristics:

1. Be widespread or universal throughout the species
2. Be stereotyped in pattern on the motor side
3. Be responsive to highly simplified models, containing only a few cues of the total normal situation on the perceptual side

For example, to meet criterion 3, the pattern must emerge with just the sight of the infant in the absence of directional orders from others, such as "take your baby," or "rub your baby." On the other hand, the behavior is most likely learned, according to Jolly, if it exhibits:

1. Variability among individuals of a species

2. Variability in motor pattern
3. Variability in types and possible multiplicity or complexity of perceptual cues

It has already been noted that, although certain maternal tactile behaviors occur more frequently than others, there is no evidence of a patterned sequence from fingertip contact of infant extremities to full palmar massaging of the trunk, as had been suggested in previous studies. The fact that the sequence of seven tactile behaviors (holding with one or both hands, fingertip stroking of the face, extremities or trunk, palmar contact, or not holding at all) varied significantly with the sex of the child, maternal parity, and sociocultural or socioeconomic background also suggests that the pattern of tactile contact is not species specific. I observed similar tactile responses in an adoptive mother who received her infant 3 minutes after birth, suggesting that parturition and its associated hormonal changes are not necessary to explain the behavior. My conclusion is that tactile contact of the infant, including encompassing and finger exploration of the face, is a typical response of human mothers to their newborn infants, but that the tactile contact does not follow a strict, species-specific pattern.

Although it was not exhibited by all of the mothers in the study, there is evidence of a statistically significant preference for holding the infant on the left side of the body. It has been demonstrated in previous studies that left-side holding exposes the infant to the maternal heartbeat sound and serves to soothe it, in addition to contributing to greater weight gain early in infancy (Salk, 1960). It has also been postulated that left-side holding serves to reduce maternal anxiety (Weiland and Serber, 1970). Furthermore, infants more often turn their heads to the right (Turkewitz *et al.*, 1976) and prefer to look to the right (Miranda, 1970), so left-side holding may be a species-specific adaptation to preferences of both mothers and infants.

It is apparent that eye contact between mother and infant is important in enhancing recognition and in forming attachment between the two. All mothers in this study spent some time during the first hour after birth in eye contact with their infants, but the actual amounts of time were variable. Although the behavior itself may appear in all human mothers, the percentage of time in eye contact with the infants appears to vary with cultural and other factors.

Can we conclude that speaking to the infant in a high-pitched voice is a species-specific behavior of all human mothers? It seems to be common for all adults, and even for older children, to elevate their voices when talking to infants, small children, or small animals. Thus, it could be a universal response to any small, cuddly object. Since infants orient more readily to a sound in the high-pitched range, it is a behavior that would be favored in all people talking to infants.

The orienting response of the infant could also explain how the high-pitched voice could be selected for in mothers in the course of human evolution. Thus, an alternative approach would be to suggest that it is a species-specific response in women but is a learned response in others. More observations of different dyads in a variety of cultural circumstances would be necessary before conclusions of species specificity are warranted.

Although the evidence gathered in this study of 110 women does not support the hypothesis of species-specific behaviors following the strictest of definitions, it does support the conclusion that left-side holding, tactile explorations, eye-to-eye contact, and talking to the infant in a high-pitched voice are common responses to newborns and are within the behavioral repertoire of all women. Which responses are exhibited and how closely they fit the model of species-specific behaviors depends to some extent on the background of the mother and the birth environment.

Any behavior that is so widely distributed in a species can perhaps be assumed to have current or past adaptive significance and thus be a product of natural selection. Given the wide range of human experience, it can be assumed further that any behavior found universally in that species likely has a biological basis. The onset of maternal behavior in most animals seems to be dependent on a number of variables including hormonal state, parturition, and exposure to newborn infants. Hormonal state and parturition can generally be considered physiological universals, and birth results in an offspring; thus to postulate a stereotyped immediate reaction to a newborn is not an illogical extension of three variables that are part of the experience of all parturient women.

To argue that many of the behaviors associated with parturition are products of past selective forces is not to deny the vast changes, mostly human-produced, that have taken place in that environment over the last two million years. We know that one of humankind's most distinctive characteristics is the variability in environments occupied by members of our species, variability that is, again, natural and human-produced. How then, can we argue for species-characteristic behaviors that are supposedly adapted to a "human" environment? How can we expect to see behavioral similarities in !Kung women, who deliver almost alone, and in Western women, who deliver in hospitals with great varieties of medical and technological aids? What is even remotely similar in those women and their environments that would suggest behavioral universals?

Certainly, we can argue that similar hormonal, physiological, and physical experiences are part of parturition for all human females. Bowlby (1969) and others have argued that one predictable feature of the human environment of evolutionary adaptedness that is found in all contemporary cultures is the mother–infant relationship. Although the components of a "family" are highly variable in our and other species, the core of the mother and infant is practically invariant, for obvious reasons. Thus, although male–female relationships have varied through time and across cultures, resulting in few universal behaviors, many mother–infant behaviors should remain as they have been for millions of years. Primary among these, again with obvious adaptive significance, are proximity-maintaining behaviors. A universal goal of infants of all mammalian species is being near mother, the source of food, warmth, and protection. Likewise, although her life is not in immediate danger if she behaves otherwise, a universal goal of mothers is to provide food, warmth, and protection to the infant who represents her genetic investment. The infant goal is very immediate, whereas the maternal goal is ultimate, but the result, because of natural selection, is a convergence of mother and infant behaviors in maintaining proximity. Just as in the pursuit of any goal, however, there are alternative ways of maintaining a mother–infant relationship, and there are few behaviors that approach those termed *fixed-action patterns* by ethologists. In fact, while a few of the very basic interactive behaviors may be "instinctive," most proximity-maintaining behaviors are undoubtedly learned and are, thus, environmentally labile.

In assessing the "causes" of behavior, we must look at various levels. Typically, in the ethological and sociobiological literature, one encounters categories of causation including "proximate," "ontogenetic," "ultimate," and "phylogenetic." Within each of these, however, there are various "subcauses." For example, consider the various answers to the following question: "Why does a mother react to her crying, hungry infant by picking him up and breastfeeding him?"

1. Survival of the infant, and thus her genetic investment, is dependent on her responding that way; natural selection has shaped the response (*ultimate o̵ phylogenetic*).
2. In the culture or family in which she grew up, mothers respond to crying infants that way (*ontogenetic*).
3. The cry causes secretion of oxytocin, which, in turn, initiates the let-down reflex, which induces the mother to nurse (*proximate*).
4. She has strong emotional feelings for this infant and suffers when he cries like this (*ontogenetic*).
5. The cry irritates her and those present, so she reacts this way to stop the annoying stimulus (*proximate*).

Perhaps all of these can explain why a mother acts in a certain way. They are, in Bowlby's words, the "factors that activate a particular behavioral system" (1969:126). The function of the series of behaviors is separate and one most clearly related to "cause" 1 listed above: survival of the organism. Bowlby saw cause and function as two separate factors, whereas today we are able to see them as two parts of a continuum from proximate to ultimate causation. Bowlby also saw distinctions in behaviors that were of consequence to the individual and those that were of consequence to the population, a distinction that is now blurred by the same perceived continuum. If sociobiological theory has done nothing else, it has enabled us to see human individual, cultural, and species behaviors as parts of a whole rather than as three rigidly separated classes. Our success of a species is due, in large measure, to our ability to use idiosyncratic and population-shaped (learned) behaviors to reach the same goals as those accomplished by species-specific behaviors in many other animals. This does not mean, however, that the more flexible behaviors are any less the product of natural selection than the more invariant behaviors.

SUMMARY

In this chapter, evidence has been presented that mothers of different cultural backgrounds behave in predictable ways when they meet their newborn infants immediately after birth. Some of the behaviors observed are believed to contribute directly to survival, while others appear to play an important role in individual recognition and bond formation. The next chapter reviews numerous studies that have been done of the significance of the first hour after birth for bond formation. In most, the behaviors observed at birth have not been found to be associated, in any particular way, with later expressions or measures of attachment. The conclusions of these studies have often been that the interactions in the early hours postpartum have little effect on the later relationship, and that, therefore, being together in that time period is not important for bonding. Again, I suggest that we can gain a different understanding of the process of early bond formation if we ask broader questions and if we place it in an evolutionary context.

6

MOTHER–INFANT BONDING
AT BIRTH

"Bonding" has become somewhat of a catchword, commonly used by parents talking about their children and prospective parents talking about the anticipated birth of their child. The latter may hope that there is "an opportunity for bonding"; the former may note that they feel "more bonded" to one child than to another. Like any other term that once had very specific meaning, the use of the word in common parlance has resulted in a great deal of controversy. To the parents, bonding may mean something as broad and undefinable as "falling in love." To an ethologist, the term may be equated with "imprinting."

There are various ways of defining bonding, but all describe the relationship between two individuals. Synonyms include love, attraction, fidelity, attachment, and affection. The term *bond* can be used to describe the relationship between lovers, spouses, parent and child, siblings, and even humans and pets. A common assumption, however, is that all of these bonds between humans ultimately can be traced to the very first one, that of mother and infant. A typical argument is that this first bond lays the foundation for all subsequent bonds, and, further, the nature of this first bond will affect future bonds. In other words, if the mother–infant bond "fails," future bonds are in jeopardy.

Various theories have been offered to explain the origin of the mother–infant bond. Freud suggested that attachment of child to mother was related to the hunger drive of the infant. Others agreed that nursing was the occasion on which an infant learned to "like to be with others" (Dollard and Miller, 1950, cited in Bowlby, 1969). Later, the Harlows and their colleagues at the University of Wisconsin primate center demonstrated that the need for food could not explain fully the origins of the mother–infant bond, at least in rhesus monkeys. Rhesus infants who were given a choice of a wire mother with milk or a cloth mother without milk, always chose to cling to the cloth mother, indicating that food was only a secondary factor in the attachment process; the primary influence was something else (Harlow and Harlow, 1965).

John Bowlby's ideas on attachment are sometimes referred to as the "ethological attachment theory" (Waters and Deane, 1982) because basic to his theory is that the mother–infant bond is rooted in naturally selected species-specific behaviors (Bowlby, 1969). Bonding between mothers and infants, he argues, is an environmentally stable system, a system expressed in each species as a part and product of the "environment of adaptedness." Like other ethologists, Bowlby argues that species have unique behavioral repertoires just as they have unique morphological characteristics. Arguing for the adaptive significance of behavioral patterns is simply a logical extension of arguments concerning the adaptive significance of morphological or physiological patterns. Thus, as internal gestation contributes to survival by affording greater protection to the fetus, so maternal behaviors at birth (leading ultimately to a strong mother–infant bond) contribute to survival by affording greater protection to the newborn infant. For a given individual, the proximate outcomes may be warmth, nutrition, and concealment; the ultimate outcome may be greater rate of survival of the genes of members whose behaviors carry them successfully through the postpartum period.

The adaptive significance of caretaking behavior as it contributes to infant survival is obvious. Bowlby (1969) argues that attachment behaviors that are observed today are products of our evolutionary past, of a time period when attachment was necessary for protection from predators. In the early course of human evolution, a strong mother–infant bond in the presence of dangers from predation meant the difference between life and death for the infant. Presumably, during a lengthy period in the evolution of our species, the dangers of predation, hairlessness, and an ineffectual clinging response in the infant coincided long enough for strong selective pressures to favor the emergence of proximity-maintaining behaviors on the part of mother and infant. The main force appearing in the first few hours after birth simply may have been to imprint upon the mother the image of her infant so strongly that she did not forget, even for a moment, that she had an infant when escape or rapid movement became necessary. All sensory channels may be involved in imprinting on the mother the visual, tactile, auditory, and olfactory image of her newborn infant. We know from evidence on hospital births, where separation and anesthesia are the norm, that women occasionally forget that they have given birth (Arms, 1975).

Contemporary evolutionary theory incorporates the concept of *inclusive fitness*. Thus, a behavior is more likely to become "fixed" in a species if it contributes not only to the survival of the individual who first manifests it but also to the survival and subsequent reproductive success of all of that individual's kin. Attachment, for example, as it accompanies helplessness in human infants, can be regarded as disadvantageous to the parent. It means greater investment of time and energy, slower reproductive rate, and if nursing continues for 2 or 3 years for each infant, smaller numbers of offspring. The advantages for the offspring and thus for the parental genetic investment, however, can be calculated in terms of larger brain size and expanded social education which in turn facilitate the development of sociosexual and caretaking activities for each succeeding generation. The sum outweighs the disadvantages for a single generation. Human reproductive strategy can be seen as opting for quality over quantity in that emphasis is placed on maximizing survival of offspring rather than maximizing numbers. Bonding and any maternal behavior that facilitates it fits well within this model.

MOTHER–INFANT BONDING IN NONHUMAN MAMMALS

An examination of the literature on mother–infant bonding in mammals suggests several issues that can be addressed. These include the following questions: (1) How strong or specific is the mother–infant bond? (2) What factors influence bond formation or failure? (3) Is there a critical, sensitive, or optimal period for bond formation in the first few hours postpartum? (4) What are the consequences of failure to form a bond or of maternal deprivation in general? and (5) Can any of the first four questions be asked or answered for human mothers and infants?

The direction of the bond must also be considered: Who bonds with whom? Much of the original work on attachment was done on bird species with precocial young; the process was described as "imprinting." According to the early thinking, chicks, ducklings, goslings, and other precocial young are primed to follow the first moving object to which they are exposed during a critical or sensitive period soon after hatching. Typically, of course, this first moving object is the mother, and selection favored rapid learning of her identity so that her young would follow her, remaining in her protective custody while being led to food and water. For the most part, this bonding process is unidirectional: The young assume most of the responsibility for maintaining proximity to the appropriate care provider. If the following response is evoked by an inappropriate figure, (i.e., if the bird "imprints" on an object or animal other than the mother), the chances of survival are greatly diminished. Even if the young should survive infancy without parental care, there is evidence, for a number of species, that normal sexual behavior fails to develop in young that imprint on other than adults of their own species. Thus, selection for attachment within a fairly defined period of time has been strong in a number of avian species with precocial young.

With mammals, the process becomes more complicated, and there is no evidence that attachment in the two classes has similar phylogenetic roots. Thus, caution has been advised in attempting to describe the phenomenon in mammals, using examples and terminology derived from bird studies.

Strength and Specificity of the Mother–Infant Bond

The strength and specificity of the mother–infant bond in mammals is closely associated with a number of factors in the behavioral ecology of the species. These factors include the degree of altriciality or precociality of the offspring, the degree of sociality of the species, and whether or not the species is predator or prey. These factors are themselves closely interconnected, so it is difficult to treat them separately. Gubernick (1981), for example, argues that one of the best predictors of degree of mother–infant bonding found in a species is the social structure, that is whether adult members are typically solitary, pair-bonded, or live in multiadult social groups. He suggests that species that are normally solitary will not form strong filial attachments whereas gregarious species will.

All of the foregoing factors can be subsumed under one general principle: What is the likelihood that a mix-up of offspring could occur under natural circumstances? Natural selection should consistently favor caretakers who invest in offspring closely related to them. Thus, mechanisms for recognizing one's own offspring will evolve when it is likely that unrelated young will be in close proximity to related young. A strong and specific bond will be characteristic in this case. Furthermore, the speed of bond formation should be associated also with the likelihood of a mix-up. For example, if females deliver in isolation but rejoin a social group several hours later, the bond may develop gradually over that time period. If a female typically delivers in the midst of other females and young, fairly rapid bond formation would be favored.

In mammals, the specificity and direction of the bond are associated somewhat with the degree of altriciality or precociality of the young, a factor more closely related to the ecology than to the taxonomy of the species. Typically, species whose young fall at the altricial end of the continuum give birth to large litters of unfurred, relatively immobile young whose eyes are not opened and who are usually cached in burrows or nests. Most of the burden of maintaining parent–infant interaction falls upon the mothers of altricial young. On the precocial end of the continuum are young that are born fully furred and able to follow or cling to their mothers soon after birth and, thus, can play an equal or predominant role in maintaining the mother–infant bond. Mothers of precocial young usually give birth to only one or two offspring at a time. Within an order and even a family, one finds example species for both states: altricial rabbits and precocial hares in the family Leporidae, order Lagomorpha; altricial Norway rats and precocial spiny mice in the family Muridae, order Rodentia; altricial dogs and precocial spotted hyenas in the order Carnivora.

Altriciality and precociality are related, to some extent, to the species' place on the continuum of predator to prey. Predators, who are usually capable of protecting themselves and whose young are rarely preyed upon, can "afford" to have helpless, defenseless, sightless young. Animals who are prey of other species and depend on flight for avoidance "need" young that are fairly well-developed and can keep up with the mother and/or the herd soon after birth. Almost all species of the order Carnivora have altricial young, whereas almost all ungulate species have precocial young. Correspondingly, in predator species, the mother–infant bond is often not specific, whereas in prey species, a strong and specific mother–infant bond is typical.

There are numerous exceptions to this generalization, but, in some cases, the exceptions actually support the rule. For example, lions and hyenas, among whom maternal–infant bonds are strong, are often cited as exceptions to the expectation that selection favors weaker parent–infant bonds in predator species (see Gubernick, 1981). In these species, however, cannibalism by unrelated conspecifics is reportedly high (Wilson, 1975). It should also be noted that both of the species have a form of social organization in which several females with young may be in proximity resulting in a higher likelihood of contact with alien young. As was suggested previously, a strong bond is favored under circumstances in which a mix-up of offspring is likely to occur.

Schaller reports that communal nursing is common among lions. This is not surprising, since female lions in a pride are closely related to each other. Apparently a mixed strategy has been adopted: when effects are long-term and general, selective attention to own offspring may not be favored over communal feeding of own and related young. When effects are immediate and critical, however, selection would favor selective attention to own young, as in the case of threatened infanticide by an adult male. In solitary carnivorous species, a strong bond with individual young would not be under much selective pressure. For a solitary mother, the young following her are usually, by definition, her own. Occasionally, chance encounters do occur, and mothers have been observed leaving the encounter site with alien young, indicating that neither mother nor infant recognize each other as individuals (Schaller, 1972).

In general, mothers of altricial young appear to bond to the nest site, and it is fairly easy to foist adoption on the species: "An infant in my nest must be my own offspring." Cats have mothered rats, rats have mothered mice, and dogs have mothered cats. Females of altricial young, who characteristically deliver in nests far removed and even defended from conspecifics, would not have been subjected to selection for a strong and specific bond.

Marsupials deliver what are perhaps the most altricial of all mammalian young and thus provide good examples of bonding between mothers and helpless young. Among most marsupials, young can be substituted in the pouch as long as it is done during the period of permanent occupation. Bonding to a specific offspring seems to begin with the first ventures from the pouch. This fits with the expectation that a strong bond would not be selected favorably unless or until it is likely that a mix-up of young would occur. In the red kangaroo, for example, excursions from the pouch first occur at about 190 days after "birth," and the young are usually allowed to return to the pouch at will until about 45 days later. Pouch gestation in this species is apparently complete at 235 days. When red kangaroo young become separated from their mothers, they give a special call to which all mothers vocally respond. The mother whose young is missing searches actively, examining all available young until her own is located (Ewer, 1968). In some sense this is similar to the phenomenon noted in humans, wherein the cry of a hungry infant elicits a response (i.e., let-down) in most nearby lactating mothers, but usually it is only the infant's own mother who attempts to feed him.

Red kangaroo mothers apparently learn the characteristics, including vocal sounds, of their own infants and respond to them as individuals. Learning of individual characteristics has been demonstrated even when the young are of a species different from the mother. In one experiment (cited in Ewer, 1968), a wallaby infant was substituted in the pouch for an infant red kangaroo. Typically, the mother makes the decision of when the infant reaches the "point of no return'' to the pouch. In this substitution experiment, she responded to the stage of development of the young and allowed him to return to the pouch until 267 days postbirth, which is the pouch gestation period of wallabies. As mentioned earlier, the red kangaroo usually rejects return attempts by her young at 235 days.

In other altricial species, recognition of individual young develops through time. This is consistent with the idea that individual recognition is related to the likelihood of mixing up the young of two or more mothers. As long as the infants are immobile and remain in the nest, there is little likelihood that substitution of young will take place. Once they begin moving on their own and leaving the nest for brief periods, a mix-up of young is more likely. It is then that mothers of altricial young begin to show recognition of their own offspring.

To some extent, however, recognition of individual young is evoked according to the location of the infant at a given time, indicating that recognition is not very specific in all cases. Ewer (1968) notes, for example, that a female giant rat will retrieve nonconspecific young when they are detected outside of the nest, but once they have been placed inside the nest, the ''alien'' signal is elicited and she attacks. A housecat will approach the rear-end of an alien kitten and lick it as she does her own young, but when the kitten turns around, it is apparently recognized as alien and the mother hisses and swats at it. As Ewer says, ''clearly for the cat, one end said 'youngster-to-be-cleaned' while the other end bore the message 'stranger to be driven away''' (1968:257). Again this is somewhat similar to the effects of the hungry infant cry on a human mother. The cry and her subsequent let-down mean to her ''hungry infant, get ready to nurse,'' regardless of the social inappriateness of this response today.

Observations of naturalistic behavior of pinnepeds indicate fairly specific mother–infant bonds, which accords well with the synchronized breeding and whelping of most of the communal species. Alaskan fur seals, for example, refuse to allow any pup but their own to nurse. Bartholomew (1959) reports that the mother smells but does not groom or lick her pup after birth, but she will retrieve and carry it when necessary. She allows no other females near her pup in the first few hours after birth. Pups are generally left alone on shore, mothers returning from sea to nurse not more than 1 day in 7. Hungry pups will, at this time, attempt to nurse any female, although she rebuffs all except her own.

Most elephant seals observed by Le Bouef and his colleagues (1972) nursed only their own pups and refused all nursing attempts by alien pups. Adoptive nursing and occasional nursing of an alien pup were not uncommon. Of those mothers observed, 11 of 50 nursed their own and an alien pup, at least occasionally; 8 nursed or adopted other young after their own pups died. Providing enough milk for more than one pup is apparently difficult for this species, and in cases where females tried to nurse more than one at a time, both pups usually died. In a case where both survived, they were much smaller than normal at weaning and may not have survived their first year.

One obvious advantage of a fairly strong bond in this species, and perhaps in most others, is the allocation of food to one young at a time. Indiscriminant nursing reduces survival of own, as well as alien, young and would obviously be a negatively selected behavior, as observed in cases when weaker bonds prevailed. Thus, a strong mother–infant bond can be seen as a method of allocating scarce resources and a way of ensuring that all young, especially one's own, get adequate nourishment. Le Bouef *et al.* (1972) note, however, that most elephant seal pups try to nurse females other than their mothers, adding to their own nutrient stores when and if the females respond. Obvious advantages accrue to the pup who successfully nurses another female in that it increases its fitness, perhaps at the expense of a competitor. This is not done without risk, however: The observers documented 40 cases, in one season, of pups being bitten by alien females when they attempted to nurse. Several of these resulted in death of the pups.

Even if a pup succeeded in "scavenging" food from alien mothers, a lone infant elephant seal is highly vulnerable to being bitten by adults other than its mother and being trampled to death by charging bulls, who move through the harem in search of breeding conquests, oblivious to the existence of the tiny pups. The Le Bouef *et al.* (1972) data indicate that preweaning mortality for pups separated from their mothers approaches 70%, and even those who survive do so with smaller fat stores than mothered pups and likely have higher mortality once at sea. In the long run, it is apparent that the best strategy for mother and young elephant seals is the one most commonly observed: mothers bonded to and nursing only their own young.

In primates, the likelihood of a mix-up of young is variable among species, but the mother–infant bond appears to be generally strong and specific. The young are somewhat precocial and thus play a major role in maintaining proximity to their mothers. As was noted in Chapter 3, many primate neonates are able to assist themselves in emergence from the birth canal by crawling up their mother's abdomen. Since infants take such active roles in their own deliveries and mothers also use their hands in assisting delivery, it is highly unlikely that a mix-up of infants would occur under natural circumstances. Furthermore, although most primates are gregarious, it would be most unusual for two parturient females to deliver simultaneously in close proximity. Thus, unlike ungulates and pinnipeds, there has not been selective pressure in this order for rapidly forming mother–infant bonds. Primate mothers and infants can thus take time to learn about one another. But because interest in infants by other group members is high in many social species, it is important that the bond develop somewhat early and that it ultimately be specific.

Adoption. In most cases, there is little selective pressure for females to adopt alien young. There are, however, certain conditions under which adoption is advantageous, especially if one's own offspring dies. For most mammals, there is a relationship between the birth interval and the length of lactation. For example, in most primate species, lactation inhibits ovulation and thus prolongs the interbirth interval. If the infant dies and lactation ceases, then the female may resume cycling again, enabling her to conceive after a reduced interval. Thus, in most cases, adoption and nursing of alien young would be disadvantageous for a slowly reproducing species. If the infant is closely related to the adopting mother, however, her inclusive fitness could be increased, depending on the time of adoption, the degree of relatedness between the two, and the time that might be necessary to recover from the previous pregnancy. In other words, it may be to her advantage to delay pregnancy for a few months, and nursing an alien young may be the only way that can be effected.

Another clear example of an advantage gained through adoption of alien young is provided by the elephant seal. In this species, there may be strong selective pressure to adopt an alien pup if one's own pup dies: All females observed by Le Bouef *et al.* (1972) who did *not* nurse pups also were not seen copulating. Apparently, nursing in this species stimulates postpartum estrus so that, unless a female adopts an alien young after hers dies or disappears, she will have at least two unsuccessful breeding seasons. This selective pressure would be increased even further if the infant she adopts is genetically related to her in any way, a likely event in harem-dwelling species.

Finally, in species in which learning plays a major role in the caretaking of infants and inexperience results in high infant mortality, adoption of an alien young after death of her own provides a female with the opportunity to "practice" raising an offspring. Although this may prolong the time before she can conceive again, this enables her to gain greater experience in caretaking, which may result in increased survival rate of her subsequent offspring. Adoption of young by nulliparous females or those who have lost their own infants is common in a number of primate species. The value of "practice mothering" is usually cited as a selective premium for adoption. A mother may also gain from allowing infant sharing: should she herself be killed, the chances are better that her offspring will be adopted by another female.

Proximate Factors Affecting Mother–Infant Bonding

Proximate factors influencing bonding of mother to young include parturition, hormones, and exposure to the infants. Parturition itself undoubtedly plays a role in directing a female's attention to her young. Most mammalian females focus on their anogenital region as parturition approaches, increasing their attention and licking when contractions begin. With delivery of the young, licking continues, of self, placenta, and infant. Although licking of the young is necessary for proper functioning of respiration, digestion, and elimination, it may also be an important initiator of bond formation, especially in those species in which olfactory cues play a major role.

In an experiment of cross-fostering in rats, Denenberg *et al.* (1963) found that fostering was far more successful if effected before a newborn pup had been cleaned by its natural mother. This again implicates the significance of licking the young and perhaps ingesting hormones associated with the birth fluids in the establishment of the mother–infant relationship.

Hormonal changes at the end of pregnancy and during parturition and early nursing have also been implicated in bond formation. Research on rats, mice, and rabbits has been useful in teasing apart the effects of hormones and environment (i.e., exposure to young) on mothering behavior. To demonstrate endocrine regulation of the onset of maternal behaviors, a series of experimental manipulations on these animals (e.g., hysterectomy, premature delivery by cesarean section, injection of hormones, and exposure to young) have been performed. The results indicate that maternal behavior can be experimentally induced in nonpregnant, nonlactating females of several species with hormone injections and blood transfusions from parturient females. Determining the role of specific hormones has been difficult, however, and many studies have had conflicting results.

Prolactin was one of the first to be explored because, in birds, it is the hormone that stimulates broodiness, incubation of eggs, and feeding of the young (Zarrow *et al.*, 1971). Results of experimental administration of prolactin in mammals have been inconclusive, however. After a series of recent experiments with rats, Bridges *et al.* (1985) have suggested that a problem with earlier studies of prolactin was related to the timing of administration of the hormone. They conclude that prolactin plays a role in inducing maternal behavior in the rat when it is combined with the gonadal steroids, estradiol and progesterone, and when it is applied during a time equivalent to the period of gestation, rather than restricted to the period just before parturition. Earlier studies may have failed to elucidate the role of prolactin because they relied on acute administration during a short time, a situation quite unlike that experienced by the normal female rat during pregnancy and parturition. These studies further point out the fallacy of treating birth as an incident isolated from pregnancy and the extended postpartum period.

Additional support for hormonal roles in postpartum maternal behavior comes from studies of rats delivered by cesarean section before term (and thus before hormonal changes at the end of pregnancy): in most cases, the rats are not responsive to their pups until the time at which normal delivery would have occurred (Moltz and Leon, 1972). Hysterectomies at various points during pregnancy also have an effect on maternal behavior in rats. This procedure results in rapid drops in the level of progesterone and rises in estrogen, mimicking the changes at parturition; the latency to retrieve young was also reduced in these females.

Recent experiments point to the importance of oxytocin in the development of maternal behavior. Virgin rats, injected with oxytocin directly into the brain, were placed in cages with newborn pups. Of the rats, 42% began to show maternal behaviors toward the pups within 20 minutes of the injections (Pedersen and Prange, 1979). Later studies showed that similar maternal behavior could be evoked in ovariectomized rats treated with estrogen when oxytocin, arginine vasopressin, and $PGF_{2\alpha}$ were injected directly into the brain in separate experiments (Pedersen *et al.*, 1982). Behaviors varied with dosage, and latency of onset was longer with arginine vasopressin than for the other two hormones.

Studies of other rodents, such as hamsters, gerbils, and mice, have revealed similar relationships between hormones and exposure to young. Most have as their conclusion that the onset of maternal behavior is governed by hormonal changes at the end of pregnancy but that these behaviors are maintained only by stimulation from the young (see Rosenblatt and Siegel, 1981). In other words, endocrine actions prepare the maternal system "to a point that renders it acutely responsive to the sight, sound, and odor of young" (Moltz and Leon, 1972:20). If pups are removed at parturition, mothering behavior in rats declines rapidly in 4 days (Rosenblatt and Lehrman, 1963). On the other hand, postpartum removal of ovaries, adrenal glands, or the pituitary gland does not appear to alter mothering behavior, except as it affects nursing.

In an early study of hormonal influence on maternal behavior in primates, Tinklepaugh and Hartman (1930) reported that a pregnant rhesus macaque, 3 weeks from her due date, showed no interest in the newborn infant of her cage mate. Her interest in another newborn and its placenta was markedly high 3 days from her due date, suggesting that hormonal changes had an effect on her behavior. Among squirrel monkeys, only females in their last 2 weeks of pregnancy responded fully and consistently to young infants (Rosenblum, 1972). Cross and Harlow (1963) reported a study in which rhesus females who had shown no interest in viewing infants during the last 2 weeks of their first pregnancy exhibited a dramatic increase in interest following delivery.

For many primate species, however, hormonal effects of parturition are not at all crucial for the emergence of maternal behavior or interest in neonates. Langurs and other colobines are noted for their unusually high interest in newborn infants and their tolerance for infant-sharing. Fifteen minutes after a birth witnessed by McKenna (1974) at the San Diego Zoo, a mother Hanuman langur (*Presbytis entellus*) allowed a 3-year-old juvenile female to hold her neonate for 3 minutes. Wooldridge (1971) reports infant-sharing 7 hours after birth in *Colobus guerza*. Although similar behaviors have been observed in many other species, there is no evidence of hormonal changes associated with this interest in neonates.

Interest in infants is also high among marmosets, particularly among adult males who have been observed taking and licking a neonate within minutes after birth. In a test of blood prolactin levels in male marmosets (*Callithrix jacchus*) that carried offspring more than 60% of the time, Dixson and George (1982) found five times higher levels than in males that did not carry infants, indicating endocrine changes associated with paternal care. The researchers suggest that it is actual physical contact with young that stimulates these changes, since levels in individual males were highest when they had most recently been carrying young. It is likely, although not yet demonstrated, that there are further behavioral consequences of elevated prolactin levels in these males. Here again is evidence that extrinsic factors interact with intrinsic factors to produce caretaking behaviors and interest in neonates.

Sensitive or Critical Periods for Bonding

Jay Rosenblatt has paid special attention to the period that he refers to as the "transition" from hormonal control of onset to infant-determined maintenance of maternal behavior in rats (Rosenblatt, 1975; Rosenblatt and Siegel, 1981). Several hours of contact with pups are usually required for the firm establishment of maternal behavior. He argues that the time when this transition is taking place is especially important, perhaps critical, in the continuation of a successful mother–infant relationship. In other words, it is a critical period for bonding in rats and perhaps in several other species.

This critical period for bonding has been especially well studied in goats. In an early study, Klopfer (1971) noted that the period may be as brief as the first 5 minutes after birth. When the newborn kid is removed immediately after birth, most mothers refuse to reaccept their own or any other kid when the separation lasts an hour or more. Dams who are allowed just 5 minutes of contact reaccept their own kid, even after 3 hours of separation. An additional conclusion from the early studies on bonding in goats was that the bond not only formed within a short time period, it was also highly specific, in that mothers with brief exposures to their neonates refused to accept any but their own. Later studies, however, revealed that dams with brief exposure to young would later reaccept any kid, their own or an alien one, as long as it had not been "marked" by another mother (Gubernick, 1980). This accords well with the probable circumstances under which the mother–infant bond in goats evolved. Even for those giving birth with other parturient and newly delivered females close by, the initial contact with the neonate, including licking and consumption of the placenta and membranes, would be sufficient for marking or "labeling" to take place so that a mix-up of young would be unlikely. Individual recognition of young beyond this, therefore, could develop more slowly.

Experiments with ewes have demonstrated that the sensitive period for attachment to and acceptance of lambs is less than 12 hours after birth, but that this period can be extended if parturition is induced with estrogens (Poindron *et al.*, 1979). Thus, as with rats, the onset of maternal behavior is likely under hormonal control, and the authors suggest that the fading of the sensitive period is associated with the transition from intrinsic to extrinsic regulation of maternal behavior. If the lambs are not present at the time of transition, there is no stimulus to maintain maternal responsiveness to young, and attachment fails to develop. Separation of ewes and lambs 2–4 days after parturition has little effect on maternal behavior because, apparently, attachment deriving from contact with the young during the transition period has been established.

As already suggested, extremely rapid bond formation, such as has been described for goats and sheep, is "unnecessary" unless there is a good chance that the young will be mixed with others in the first few minutes or hours after birth. This is not the situation for most species and certainly not the case for higher primates and human beings who live in groups too small for synchronous deliveries to be common and who have a level of awareness that would preclude great confusion over individual identity during the postpartum period. Thus, it is untenable to argue for a rapidly forming bond in most mammalian species including our own. This does not mean, as has been discussed, that the first postpartum hours are not important for the development of the mother–young relationship in all species.

Consequences of Bond Failure or Maternal Deprivation

Maternal deprivation has long-term social and emotional consequences for infants of most mammalian species, and the short-term negative effects of hypothermia and exposure to predation are obvious. There are also physiological consequences of separation that have more immediate effects and may have implications for the practice of separating human mothers and infants for even brief periods immediately postpartum. Kuhn *et al.* (1978) have demonstrated that if rats are removed from their mothers, they show a significant decline (50%) in the production of ornithine decarboxylase (ODC), an enzyme important for growth of the brain and other rapidly developing organs. This decline occurs despite the fact that pups are kept warm and well fed. Further experiments indicated that the decline in ODC activity is related directly to decreased production of growth hormone (GH), although maternal deprivation has no apparent effect on production of other anterior pituitary hormones. In other words, deprivation has a fairly specific effect on GH, rather than an overall suppressive effect on all hormones of the anterior pituitary, and its effect is different from that of stress in general. Kuhn *et al.* conclude that maternal deprivation has a specific neuroendocrine response, including a decrease in GH production which, in turn, results in a decrease in ODC activity. Noting that human failure-to-thrive infants also have impaired secretion of GH, they suggest that similar mechanisms may operate in human infants who are separated from their mothers. They also note that the effects of GH and ODC suppression in rats are quickly reversed if the pups are reunited with their mothers, suggesting few long-term effects of temporary separation. If short-term deprivation impairs growth of the brain and other vital organs in the critical postpartum days, the effects may be irreversible.

BONDING IN HUMAN MOTHERS AND INFANTS

I have addressed the issue of bond strength and specificity, the factors influencing mother–infant bonding, and the optimal timing for bond formation in selected mammalian species. It now remains to determine whether or not any of the principles derived from animal studies can be applied to human beings or can enhance our understanding of human mother–infant bonding.

The first issue of concern is bond specificity and strength. Primate models suggest that the mother–infant bond in most species is bidirectional from the moment of birth. Infants of most species are precocial enough that they can maintain proximity to their mothers by clinging to them and by suckling whenever they want. On her part, the mother helps the infant cling in the early postpartum period and does not provide any obstacles to access to her nipples. Individual recognition probably begins with licking and visual inspection of the infant immediately after birth, but there is no evidence that a highly specific bond develops rapidly in a short period of time, as some have suggested it does in sheep and goats. Infant-sharing is tolerated in several species very soon after birth, but infants and mothers appear to have little uncertainty about who belongs to whom, so it is likely that a fairly strong and specific bond is developed within a few hours of delivery. I am unaware of any experimental research that could define that period more precisely.

Does this tell us anything about human mothers and infants? One major difference is the relative altriciality of the human infant, rendering the task of maintaining proximity entirely up to the mother. As noted earlier, the infant is not without mechanisms for attracting her, but, should she forget it or decide to abandon it, there is little that the infant can do other than cry intensely.

As with other species, the physical and hormonal experience of parturition serves to focus a woman's attention on her body and her newborn infant. Although she does not lick it, she visually and tactually inspects her neonate after birth, learning individual characteristics. The learning process thus begins at birth, but it is highly unlikely that it is completed within a few hours of birth. Because human females rarely deliver synchronously under natural circumstances, there is no need for rapid bond formation. I would suggest, however, that by the second or third day after birth, a mother who has been in constant contact with her infant could distinguish it from all others of equal age. This strong and specific bond must ultimately form so that the mother is motivated to provide the high level of care needed by the helpless infant. Such attachment and motivation can develop in an adoptive mother as well, so neither the experience of parturition nor close biological relatedness is necessary for a strong mother–infant bond in human beings.

Hormonal Effects in Human Mother–Infant Bonding

Researchers are hesitant to implicate hormones as effectors of human maternal behavior. It is, to me, untenable to claim that they play no role whatsoever and that all maternal behavior immediately postpartum is under conscious control. Unfortunately, little more can be said about the role of specific hormones in maternal behavior. It is difficult enough to draw conclusions about the hormones affecting rat maternal behavior, suggesting that it would be impossible to tease apart the effects on humans. An example of the difficulties is the evidence that human maternal behavior seems somewhat altered by elective cesarean delivery, but it is not known what factors predominate in effecting this difference: the surgery itself, heavy medication, hormones, or the enforced separation of mother and infant that usually follows operative delivery.

Recent research has stimulated new thinking on the role of endogenous opiates in reducing pain sensitivity and enhancing a sense of well-being in humans. It has also been suggested that these natural opiates contribute to maternal–infant bonding because of their unusually high levels in mothers and infants during and immediately after delivery (Odent, 1984). β-Endorphins have been isolated from amniotic fluid at term and during labor. Maternal plasma levels of β-endorphins rise at delivery, and they are at high levels in infants during the first few days postpartum (Goland *et al.*, 1981; Moss *et al.*, 1982). Kimball (1979) has reviewed studies of the effects of β-endorphins and suggests that the following be considered:

1. They are associated with the release of prolactin and thus may play a role in mediating nursing behavior.
2. They have been shown to suppress hostility, anxiety, and irritability, and to increase affectionate behavior.
3. Their effects are far stronger than those of morphine but produce similar dependency behavior and addictive response.
4. Production increases during difficult and prolonged delivery.
5. Levels at the time of elective cesarean deliveries are much lower than those at vaginal deliveries.
6. High levels in fetuses at term are associated with high levels of corticosteroids, prolactin, and lung surfactants, which are, in turn, associated with low incidence of respiratory distress syndrome (RDS) and hyaline membrane disease.

This research has prompted Kimball to ask, "What purpose in biologic evolution and selective survival is served by a natural hormone that produces lactation, affectional behavior, and addictive dependency?" (1979:127).

As with any other study of the effects of hormones on human behavior a study on the effects of β-endorphins will be impossible to conduct in a way that would yield conclusive results. That will not stop speculation, however. What we appear to have discovered is a mechanism that reduces negative input and enhances positive feelings about an event that could potentially be (and often is) an entirely negative reinforcement for reproductive behavior. In fact, one argument for the evolution of "concealed ovulation" in hominid females is that it was a by-product of women consciously trying to avoid conception because of their fear of the pain of childbirth (Burley, 1979). Those that were successful at determining when they were ovulating avoided intercourse at that time and had fewer offspring. Those who could not detect their ovulation had more offspring and eventually, assuming this to be a genetically based trait, most females of the species were unable to detect their own ovulatory periods. I would argue, however, that childbirth is not always regarded as a painful and overall negative experience. Certainly, many women have described a feeling of euphoria during unmedicated childbirth, and I have known several women who say they would give birth several times a year if such were possible and if they did not have to care for that many children. These positive feelings may result, in part, from the natural opiates released during delivery and nursing.

Thus, I think there are answers to Kimball's question, although they are not yet well grounded in scientific research. It seems clear that any endogenous hormone that produces a sense of well-being and affectionate behavior at the time of delivery would have selective advantage in any species, no less our own. Such a positive state leads a mother to engage in interactions with her infant and eventually nursing begins. This, in itself, is a reward and a positive reinforcer of maternal behavior. The reward of milk induces the infant to continue suckling; the pleasure a woman receives from nursing induces her to continue nursing her infant. The initiation of interaction may be under hormonal control, but its continuation is the result of classical conditioning and learning.

Whittlestone (1978) argues that the pleasurable sensations that many women derive from nursing reinforce the mother–infant bond and further increase levels of oxytocin and prolactin which he calls ''maternal solicitude'' hormones. Other pleasurable reinforcers that I and others have suggested are tactile sensations, eye-to-eye contact, heartbeat sounds, and verbal interaction. Brody (1981) has argued that the simple pleasures of the postpartum period are sufficient in themselves to explain the motivation on the part of most mothers and infants to continue interacting for the mutually rewarding benefits.

The transition from internal to external stimulation of maternal behavior may thus occur very early in humans, perhaps minutes after delivery. But that does not deny the role of hormones in initiating that response. On the other hand, one cannot argue for a dependency on hormones for the development of maternal behavior in humans. Thousands of cesarean-delivered, bottle-feeding, and/or adoptive mothers offer proof of the ability of maternal solicitude to develop in the absence of hormonal precursors.

There are factors, however, that can inhibit normal hormone production and perhaps can affect maternal behavior in a negative way. Primary among these are fear and anxiety, which, during labor, inhibit contractions and intensify the feelings of pain perceived by the woman (Kimball, 1979; Connolly *et al.,* 1978). Anxiety also inhibits the production of prolactin and oxytocin, thus interfering with lactation and preventing a mother and child from experiencing the pleasurable sensations of nursing. As has been mentioned, one cause of anxiety is lack of emotional support during labor and delivery, further reinforcing the significance of birth attendants. Another cause of anxiety in a parturient female is lack of contact with her neonate, suggesting that contact during the neonatal period may be important for mother–infant bonding. The importance of this period is the subject of the next section of this chapter.

Timing of Bond Formation in Human Beings

The first hour after birth has been called, variously, a critical period, a sensitive period, and a relatively unimportant period in the human mother–infant bonding process. There is evidence that all three are appropriate, depending on what factors are of concern.

The term *critical period* has been used by ethologists and psychologists to describe specific periods that are necessary for learning crucial behaviors. Others have suggested that the term is best reserved for describing developmental or maturational changes that are physical or physiological, rather than behavioral. For example, during gestation, there is a brief period of time during which various limbs and organs are being developed. Certain drugs and viruses are known to interfere with these processes, and if their development is disrupted during a critical period, the limbs or organs may never develop normally. A specific example is rubella: if a woman is exposed to this virus during the first 16 weeks of pregnancy, it is likely that her child will have defects of vision, hearing, and the heart. After that critical period, the virus has little or no effect on the developing fetus.

Another example of a critical period is the ninth week of gestation when sex differentiation occurs. Exposure to androgen from the gonads of a male fetus triggers development of testes and other primary sex characteristics of males. If exposure does not occur during this critical period, the fetus will develop phenotypically as a female even though it is genotypically a male. On the other hand, a genotypic female will develop into a phenotypic male if exposed to androgens during this critical period for sex differentiation.

Ethologists and psychologists, beginning with James and Spalding in the nineteenth century, have used the term *critical period* when referring to the time during which baby chicks imprint on their mother or a substitute (Kimble and Garmezy, 1968). Lorenz, in his work with geese and ducks, noted that the critical period for imprinting in these species is from hatching to 36 hours. It now seems preferable to use the term *sensitive period* for this time because it refers to a behavioral process that is largely influenced by learning in the presence of certain environmental stimuli (Hinde, 1974). It also should be noted, however, that certain physical processes develop during this period that are necessary for imprinting to occur: in birds, the development of locomotion, vision, hearing, and the overall CNS must be such that following is elicited and possible. In that sense, the timing of the maturation of certain systems that enable imprinting can be seen as occurring in a critical period.

The use of the term *critical period* implies a degree of rigidity in the development of a system that is usually reserved for physical of physiological changes in human ontogeny. Rarely is it appropriately used in describing behavioral systems in that the term implies a dependence on biological programming that most people find untenable for human beings. The term further implies death or malformation in the event of failure. Despite these restrictions, I shall later argue that the hour immediately after birth fits the definition of a critical period during most of human evolution (although not necessarily critical for attachment), and only recently has it become relatively unimportant.

Postpartum Separation of Human Mother and Infant

Recent reviews of statistics concerning child abuse and developmental disorders in the United States has prompted the suggestion that separation of human mother and infant for long periods after birth can result in mothering disorders similar to those described previously for other mammals. For example, an unusually high percentage of battered and failure-to-thrive children have been prematures, who were separated from their mothers for several weeks following birth, suggesting that poor or abusive caretaking may be the result of extensive postpartum separation (Elmer and Gregg, 1967; Klein and Stern, 1971; Barnett *et al.*, 1970; Sameroff and Chandler, 1975). Fanaroff *et al.* (1972) report that, although only 7–8% of live births in the United States are premature each year, a range from 25 to 41% of battered infants were premtaures.

In contrast, Egeland and Vaughn (1981) have suggested that the higher incidence of child abuse and neglect among infants who were prematures may be due to factors other than separation. For example, premature delivery is inversely related to the amount of prenatal care, and it may be that aspects of the personality or individual circumstances of the woman lead her to avoid prenatal care and also lead her to provide less-than-adequate or even abusive care to her infant. These may include nonacceptance of the pregnancy, lack of familial support, poverty, and isolation. Another reason Egeland and Vaughn propose for the association between prematurity and child abuse is the greater difficulty in caretaking presented by the premature infant. In other words, separation may be part of the problem affecting failure of bond formation, but there are clearly other factors involved.

Others have suggested that even short-term separation may lead to mothering disorders. Until this century, separation of mothers and infants after birth was not common. In fact, women typically gave birth at home (and still do in most of the world), and separation, even if desired, was possible only for women who could afford wet nurses and nannies.

The movement of birth from home to hospital took place gradually until, by 1961, 97% of all U.S. births took place in hospitals (Devitt, 1977). There are several reasons behind the transition: physician and consumer pressure, high maternal and infant mortality rates, decline in number of practicing midwives, and increased use of drugs and technological innovations in birth (e.g., forceps, pain relief medication, operative delivery). With the transition, childbirth became a medical procedure and was seen more as an illness rather than a normal physiological process. As if to reinforce this idea and the push for births to take place in hospitals, there was a significant decline in maternal and infant mortality: In 1935, when 37% of all births took place in hospitals, maternal mortality rate was 58.2 per 10,000 and neonatal mortality rate was 32.4 per 1000. By 1961, the former figure had dropped to 3.7, the latter to 18.4 (Devitt, 1977). It should be noted, however, that health and nutrition of all women improved during those years, as did the percentage who sought prenatal care. The number of families living in poverty also decreased. Many have concluded that the drop in mortality is due primarily to improvements in socioeconomic status, and that healthy women with normal pregnancies have not benefited significantly from the movement of birth from home to hospital (Devitt, 1977).

Even in the hospital, it was not normal for mothers and infants to be separated until concern for disease, particularly maternal sepsis, reached such proportions that strict isolation procedures began to be followed. Infants were kept in large nurseries where it was easier for staff members to monitor them. Visitation was discouraged or not allowed, and mothers were confined to their wards for the long period of recovery. In fact, in many cases the very reason the woman was in the hospital for delivery was that she was in ill health and could not care for her newborn, necessitating nursery care (McBryde, 1951).

In the late 1930s, concern for infection caused a reversal of previous trends in some areas. Epidemics of infectious diarrhea were common in hospital nurseries, and mortality was high. At Duke University Hospital in Durham, North Carolina, the medical staff decided to adopt a universal policy of rooming-in and to abolish the nursery, in hopes of avoiding a serious epidemic. More than 2000 mother–infant pairs (all white, since blacks were sent home within a day of delivery!) experienced rooming-in between 1947 and 1950. During this 3-year period, the percentage of mothers breastfeeding rose from 35 to 58.5. There was also a 90% decrease of telephone calls from mothers during the first week after discharge, suggesting an increased confidence in ability to care for the infant (McBryde, 1951).

Although the initial reasons behind the rooming-in policy were medical, the psychological and emotional consequences soon became paramount. McBryde argues the advantages of close contact for a self-regulating schedule for breastfeeding, emotional contentment of the infant, heightened paternal interest and involvement, and maternal satisfaction. Citing Maloney (1949), he notes that "the early closeness of the parent–child relationship, as it is initiated in rooming-in, may be the first step in forming the proper close family relationship." He further notes that, by rooming in with its mother, an infant "gets as good care as a puppy and a kitten, who thrive nutritionally and psychologically better than many human offspring" (1951:626).

The Proposed Maternal Sensitive Period

Klaus, Kennell, and colleagues (1975, 1976, 1982) have called the early hours after birth the "maternal sensitive period" in which the mother is most sensitive to her infant, and bonding takes place most readily. Studies conducted by these researchers at Case Western Reserve University Hospital have been used to support their proposal. In one study (Klaus *et al.*, 1972), 28 primiparous mothers of normal, full-term infants were divided into two groups evenly matched for education, socioeconomic status, and gender of the child. Of these, 14 were placed in the "extended-contact" group: they were allowed to hold their infants for 1 full hour within 2 hours of delivery and were given 15 extra hours of contact in the first 3 days of the infant's life. The second group experienced the routine postdelivery pattern followed by the hospital: a brief glimpse of the infant at birth, brief contact at 6–8 hours, and, after that, 20- to 30-minute feedings every 4 hours.

At 1 month, when the mothers brought their infants in for a physical examination with a pediatrician, their behavior was observed by people who did not know the experimental groups to which the mothers belonged. The extended-contact mothers spent significantly more time standing beside the doctor, anxiously watching what he did, while the control group had significantly more mothers who remained seated and detached during the examination. The extended-contact mothers were also more likely to soothe the infant when it cried during the examination, and the control group was more likely to ignore the infant when it cried. At a second examination at 1 year (Kennell *et al.*, 1974), the extended-contact mothers still spent more time assisting the physician and soothing the infants when they cried. At 2 years, the mothers in the extended-contact group used a richer vocabulary when talking with their infants (Ringler *et al.*, 1975), and at 5 years, the children of these mothers were found to have significantly higher scores on IQ and language tests (Ringler *et al.*, 1976).

In a similar study by these same researchers, 19 Guatemalan mothers were given their infants in the delivery room during the episiotomy repair, then left alone with them for 45 minutes. A second group of 19 was separated from their infants, according to the hospital routine. The mean weight gain of the infants 35 days later was significantly greater in the extended-contact group. In another Guatemalan study, mothers in the extended-contact group spent significantly more time fondling, kissing, looking *en face,* gazing at, and encompassing their infants when observed 12 hours after birth (Klaus and Kennell, 1976).

These studies by Klaus, Kennell, and their colleagues prompted numerous similar studies, changes in hospital routines, and a fair amount of criticism of their work. Some studies reached similar conclusions. In Sweden, De Chateau (1976) conducted a study that allowed an experimental group of mothers an extra hour of skin-to-skin contact with their infants immediately after birth. At 36 hours, these mothers showed more holding, encompassing, and looking *en face* than did mothers who experienced routine separation from their infants during the first hour. Their infants cried less and smiled more than did the infants of the routine-care mothers.

Kontos (1978) produced similar results in her study of 48 mother–infant dyads, 12 of whom were given 1 extra hour of contact beginning 30–45 minutes after birth. These groups were observed at 1 month and 3 months postpartum; the differences persisted.

Anisfeld and Lipper (1983) reported that women who had had uninterrupted contact with their infants during the first hour postpartum exhibited significantly more affectionate behaviors toward their infants 2 days after birth when compared to women who had been separated for several hours after birth. Their study was of 59 women, 29 of whom were treated by early-contact procedures, and the remainder were separated from their infants. The researchers further found that the effects of early contact were notably greater for women who had low levels of social support, suggesting a therapeutic role for offering opportunities for early interaction.

Peterson and Mehl (1978) found, in a study of 46 families, that the most significant predictor of maternal attachment was the amount of separation during the first 72 hours postpartum. Indicators of attachment selected by these researchers included how soon after delivery the mother felt the child belonged to her, her confidence in caring for the child, how much time she willingly spent with the infant, how long it took her to respond to infant cries, her overall feelings about her child, her behavior toward her child during an interview, and statements made by others about her behavior. Variables that were associated with high maternal attachment scores were little or no separation from the infant, a positive birth experience, long labor, and a positive attitude toward childbirth.

Responding to the suggestion that separation of mother and infant immediately postpartum may interfere with the bonding process, hospitals and physicians all over the United States began altering their practices of routine separation of mother and infant. Even the normally conservative American Medical Association adopted a statement supporting bonding as their official policy in 1978. Advocates of alternatives in childbirth saw the bonding research as support for their views that birth should take place at home, or at least in a homelike atmosphere, where mother, father, and child are in more or less constant contact. Kennell and Klaus became heroes among those looking for less medical intervention and more humanization in birth.

Criticism

Soon after publication of studies of the bonding phenomenon, criticism of the studies began to come from various sources. Many note that the studies lacked the procedural and methodological controls that are expected in normal scientific procedure (see Svejda *et al.,* 1980; Lamb, 1982; Siegel, 1982; Thomson and Kramer, 1984). Studies have been difficult to replicate, and when attempts were made, results across studies have been inconsistent. For example, in one study, control and experimental mothers might be found to differ in frequency of fondling their infants but not in frequency of smiling at them. Another study might obtain opposite results: smiling differed between the two groups but fondling did not. Typically, dozens of measures have been used with only a few showing significant differences between groups.

Defining bonding or attachment behavior has proved extremely difficult, and again, there has been much variability in definition across samples (see Herbert *et al.*, 1982). One study used "mother leaning on elbow" as a measure of difference between the control and extended contact groups (De Chateau and Wiberg, 1977). As Svejda and colleagues (1980) point out, it is unclear how this particular behavior relates to attachment, although Winberg and De Chateau (1982) defend the idea that her position affects a mother's ability to interact with her infant, particularly in the *en face* position. Other examples of measures that seem peripheral to bonding include the mother's eagerness to return to work, degree of paternal involvement in infant care, timing of toilet training, and mother's reactions during a pediatric exam.

This last is particularly interesting to me in that I attempted to use it as a measure of attachment in my study of mostly Hispanic women. Following Klaus and colleagues (1972), the mothers were scored on the basis of their interaction with the infants during an examination of the infant 5 days after birth. Specifically observed and recorded were their reactions when the infants' heels were pricked for collection of blood for the PKU test. This procedure almost always elicited intense crying from the infants. A mother was given a score of zero if she remained seated and detached during the exam, a score of 1 if she seemed somewhat concerned, and a score of 2 if she seemed extremely concerned and anxious. When the infant cried during the PKU test, her reaction was scored as zero, if she ignored the infant, 1 if she soothed but seemed unconcerned, and 2 if she soothed and seemed anxious.

The results indicated that none of the women seemed detached and uninterested during the PKU test, and only one woman completely ignored her infant while it was crying. On the one hand, I might conclude that all of these women were "well-bonded" and that that was due, in part, to the fact that they had had uninterrupted contact with their infants. When comparing Anglo and Hispanic women, however, the latter consistently scored higher. Is this because the Hispanic women were "more bonded" to their infants, or did those women show more concern because the procedure was not explained thoroughly enough by the midwife who was not fluent in Spanish? I concluded that the "PKU score" was not actually measuring attachment to the infant but familiarity or unfamiliarity with the situation.

Feminists have objected to a number of the measures that have been used to define attachment, suggesting that bonding theory was being used to keep women in their places (Arney, 1980). Again, there is an example from the early Case Western studies. At an interview at 1 month, the 28 mothers in the control and extended-contact groups were asked if they had been out since the baby had been born, and, if so, how did it feel? If the mother answered that she had been out and if felt good, she earned no points. If she had gone out but thought about the baby, 1 point. Going out and worrying about the baby earned her 2 points;

and finally, not going out at all earned her 3, the highest number of points. The message is: mothers are better if they stay at home (Arney, 1980).

I also tried that question on the women in my study 2 weeks after delivery. The question turned out to be more of an indicator of cultural variation in acceptable forms of behavior rather than a measure of attachment. The Hispanic women, if they went out, always took their infants with them. They seemed unfamiliar with the concept of leaving the infant in the care of anyone else or with the concept of getting away from the infant for a while.

In summary, it appears that most of the early studies of the maternal sensitive period have been flawed for various methodological reasons and have produced inconclusive results. So far, it has not been demonstrated to most people's satisfaction that events during the first hour after birth have long-term benefits to the mother or infant. Most of us who were born between 1935 and 1975 in the United States can attest to our health and that of our mothers, despite the fact that we were separated from each other for several hours or even days after birth.*

Like Michael Lamb of the University of Utah, one of the most outspoken critics of the recent bonding research (1982, 1983), I would be careful to acknowledge the commendable social value of the works in humanizing the birth process for American families. I would not go so far as to say that the first hour after birth is *not* a sensitive period, however, nor would I agree with Lamb's statement that parenting behavior is among the most unlikely behaviors to be stereotyped in a species so highly dependent on learning as our own (Lamb, 1983). He is most certainly correct for most of parenting behavior, but I would argue that maternal behavior, at least in the first hour after birth, is one of the *most* likely behaviors to be biologically based, and thus stereotyped, in our and any other species. I proposed this latter at the end of the last chapter and would like to address further the "sensitive period" issue here.

AN EVOLUTIONARY PERSPECTIVE ON THE FIRST HOUR AFTER BIRTH

I believe that the first our after birth *is* a sensitive period for human mother-to-infant bonding, but that its importance has varied throughout human evolution and is still highly variable among popultions today. In the ensuing pages it will be argued that it was actually a critical period for survival and bonding of mothers and infants for much of hominid evolution. With the increase in neonatal mortality during the last 10,000 years, however, it became adaptive to separate mothers and infants in the first hour after birth and to delay bond

---

*It is intriguing that this is the age group that has experienced spiralling divorce rates, increased incidence of child abuse, and greater extent of familial alienation than that seen in previous generations, and the temptation to associate these problems with U.S. birth practices is hard to resist.

formation, an idea I will discuss in Chapter 7. Finally, I will argue that, because mortality has been greatly reduced in some contemporary populations, and because far fewer offspring are produced in the lifetimes of many contemporary women and parental investment per child has increased, the sensitive first hour after birth has again become a component of female reproductive and parenting strategy. In other words, the sensitive period exists as it always has, but whether or not it is essential for attachment or survival varies through time and space.

Why am I convinced of its existence when there is so much evidence against its long-term significance? Consider the intense physical and emotional experience of giving birth and the hormonal actions that accompany the process. The mother has been aware of the existence of this child for several months. She has felt its movements and may have even talked to it. The newborn infant is finally present in living, breathing form, and, like a wrapped package that is explored upon opening, the mother is especially interested in finding out about it. To continue the wrapped package analogy, we all know the excitement of unwrapping gifts and the sense of discovery felt upon opening a gift box. We also know the disappointment felt when someone else opens a package intended for us. The value and meaning of the gift itself, in the long run, may not have anything to do with whether or not we actually opened it, but there is added pleasure in doing so. So it is with the newborn infant. The later, long-term relations between parent and child may have nothing to do with whether or not the father was present at the birth or whether or not the mother and infant were together for the first hour getting-acquainted period. They missed out, however, on a special period of excitement that *in itself* is valuable and meaningful.

But, there is much more to it than that. It is also an important time for physical adaptation and adjustment of both mother and infant. Touching and massaging the infant stimulates breathing, provides warmth, and serves to rub the fatty vernix caseosa into the skin, which may prevent dehydration. If she holds it over her heart, on the left side of her body, the mother may be quieting the infant with the rhythmic beat that was an important part of its intrauterine environment. Holding it on the left may also facilitate eye contact, in that most infants prefer to turn their heads and look to the right. While she looks at the infant, she may talk to it, elevating the pitch of her voice. The neonatal auditory system is especially receptive to voices in the higher pitched range, and a female voice usually serves to quiet newborn infants.

The infant may lick, nuzzle, or even suckle the mother's breast in the immediate postpartum period. Nipple contact stimulates release of oxytocin into her bloodstream, which results in uterine contractions, expulsion of the placenta, and inhibition of postpartum bleeding. The colostrum that the infant ingests provides immunological protection and is its only natural source of Vitamin K, a substance essential for normal clotting of blood, necessary, for example, for preventing hemorrhage at the site of the umbilical cord. In addition, this early suckling may enhance later breastfeeding success.

Today, at least in technologically advanced nations, if massage does not stimulate breathing, there are instruments that can do so. Commercial creams and oils can replace the vernix that moistens the infant's skin and helps prevent dehydration. If mother's arms do not keep the infant warm, radiant heaters will. There are musical toys and wind-up rockers to soothe it, if it does not hear its mother's heartbeat. If her eyes and her voice do not stimulate the development of its visual and auditory systems, mobiles, toys, stuffed animals, and television will.

Exogenous oxytocin is available to encourage expulsion of the placenta and inhibit postpartum bleeding, so it is no longer necessary that the infant lick its mother's breast to stimulate release of endogenous oxytocin. If the breastfeeding cycle is not initiated early and later fails to be established, artificial substitutes are readily available. Vitamin K shots are routinely given in hospital births today to aid clotting of blood, so it is not necessary that the infant receive that with the colostrum in early nursing. Antibiotics and intensive medical care can take care of most infections the infant gets as a result of lack of immunological protection from the colostrum.

But what about the mothers and infants of past centuries and millennia? For these people, the biological and behavioral mechanisms that are manifested immediately postpartum were the products of millions of years of selection to ensure survival of mothers and infants during the most vulnerable periods in any lifetime. It was not just desirable, it was *critical* that hominid mothers of the distant past be with their infants after birth. For them, it was not simply a sensitive or optimal period for bonding, it was a period critical for survival. Following Bowlby, I argue that these behaviors are all part and result of the human "environment of evolutionary adaptedness" and reflect adaptations that contributed to survival of mothers and infants in the early stages of hominid evolution, perhaps up to the Neolithic. With that stage, the entire human mother–infant relationship may have changed, as will be discussed in the next chapter.

The results of most of the bonding studies lead us to conclude that, in today's technological world, there is scant evidence that contact between mothers and infants during the immediate postpartum period is necessary for survival or for optimal bond formation. Although mothers from a variety of backgrounds exhibit similar behaviors when interacting with their infants during this period, there is little basis on which we can argue current selective pressures to maintain these behaviors. Perhaps we can only say that they are relicts from our past that have no significant function in today's world.

It is now impossible to find human populations living under circumstances even remotely similar to those under which behaviors or even morphologies unique to hominids evolved. We are able to create environments in which individuals survive and reproduce who would have never been able to do so under natural circumstances. In fact, we can demonstrate that, as with other domesticated species, we have favored morphological and behavioral characteristics that would be useless or even maladaptive were we suddenly confronted with our own past "environment of evolutionary adaptedness."

Examples supporting this can be drawn from every population and at every life stage, but nowhere is it more clearly illustrated than with the neonatal period. Today, no matter what takes place during this time, our infants survive and develop social skill that are acceptable, for the most part, within the culture in which they were acquired. Biological mothers are not necessary for this process, nor even is an adult female. Fathers can substitute easily, as can older siblings. But few of these substitutes would have been adequate 10,000 years ago. At that time, the only infants who survived were those whose bond with their mothers began at birth and continued to an age at which food, protection, and nurturance could be derived from other sources. As with other species, natural selection thus favored mechanisms, hormonal or otherwise, which ensured that each mother–infant dyad had optimal opportunity to initiate that bonding process, even while the infant was *in utero*.

7

AN EVOLUTIONARY PERSPECTIVE ON HUMAN BIRTH AND BONDING: CONCLUSIONS

Because competing selective forces operate on a given population, character complex, or trait, all evolutionary change can be seen as occurring with compromise. The compromises themselves result from a weighing of costs and benefits of reproductive success. For example, the long, brightly colored tail of the peacock makes him more attractive to females of his species, but an upper limit is reached when selection for long tail feathers results in young males succumbing to predators before they are able to mate for the first time. Selection will gradually eliminate the longest and brightest while still enhancing the reproductive success of the "long, bright" at the expense of the "short, dull." Tail-feather length and color will then stabilize at the optimum. As Maynard Smith (1972) and others have pointed out, the optimal strategy for enhancing reproductive success also will depend on what it is that others of the species are doing. In other words, conspecifics are as important in determining optimal reproductive strategy as are predators, food-limiting, and other environmental factors.

As I suggested in the first chapter, human reproductive strategy is a result of a long series of compromises, of weighing the costs and benefits of each new adaptation. Table 7.1 represents a compilation of these compromises with, whenever possible, estimates of the approximate time of occurrence of each. The first compromise on the list is that of sexual reproduction, which entails the costs of meiosis, recombination, and mate-finding. The compromise pays off in cases where new variability allows a population to respond to environmental change or to expand into an uninhabited niche. Thus, as long as there is fluctuation in the microenvironments inhabited by a given species, sexual reproduction will be favored.

The next step was that of internal gestation and viviparity, which resulted in more care for offspring but reduced the quantity that could be produced each generation. The cost was a decrease in absolute numbers produced, but the benefit was an increase in relative numbers of those that survived to reproduce. Similar costs and benefits are associated with lactation.

The success of the primates has often been attributed to their ancestors moving into an arboreal niche (see Le Gros Clark, 1959). The benefits gained, however,

TABLE **7.1.** Evolution of the Human Female Reproductive Strategy

Event	Costs	Benefits
Sex (1 billion years ago)	Reduced number of offspring through meiosis, recombination; increased time and energy finding a mate; parent–offspring conflict	Increased variability; greater likelihood of survival in unpredictable environment; elimination of unfavorable alleles
Viviparity (Mammalia: 220 million years ago)	Time and energy for internal fertilization and gestation; reduced number produced	Protection of zygote so that greater percentage survives
Lactation (Mammalia)	Energy for production of milk	Provisioning young so that more survive to independence
Arboreality (Primates: 65 million years ago)	Decreased numbers of young	Quality of care for single young
Hemochorial placenta (Haplorhini: ca. 40 million years ago)	Decreased variability between generations; higher rate of abortion due to incompatible pregnancies	More efficient delivery of oxygen to developing brain
Bipedalism (Hominidae: 5–10 million years ago)	Constraints on brain size; more difficult parturition; infant unable to cling with feet	Hands free to manipulate environment; energy-efficient in nonarboreal environment
Encephalization (*Homo:* 2 million years ago)	Greater difficulties at birth	Higher intelligence
Secondary altriciality (*Homo:* 2 million years ago)	Greater demands on mother	Exposure to environmental stimuli while brain is developing
Birth attendants (ca. 35,000 years ago)	Risks of infection to mother and infant; overmanipulative interference	Lowered mortality for mother and infant; emotional support for mother
Early interaction and nursing	Bond to infant who may die or be killed	Enhance survival; stronger bond; enhance breastfeeding success
Birth in hospital (20th Century)	Lack of emotional support for mothers; dangers of medication and technological intervention; interrupted contact between mother and infant	Increased survival of mother and infant
Birth at home (renewed, 1970s)	Greater mortality and morbidity(?); more time and energy for preparation	More emotional support for mother; constant contact among mother, father, and infant

were not without expense, in that the numbers of offspring produced were limited by the ability to care for young in the uneven substrate of the trees. In general, arboreal mammals have fewer young per litter than terrestrial mammals, indicating that one of the costs of living in the trees is a reduction in numbers of offspring. Presumably, the cost is balanced by the increased quality of care that can be provided a single infant.

Evolution of a hemochorial placenta in haplorhine primates was another conservative step, in that phenotypic variability between generations was reduced, but the quality of care provided the usually singleton fetus was increased. Thus, the benefits of greater phenotypic variability between generations, which had been cited as the major advantage of sexual reproduction, became less advantageous when weighed against the gains deriving from intensified investment during gestation, especially that contributing to brain growth.

Before going any further in the analysis of evolutionary compromises, I should point out that the process is not a simple zig-zag, with complete adjustment or adaptation taking place. Rather, the process of evolution is a mosaic of behavioral, morphological, and physiological changes. The secret to success is the ability to respond behaviorally to a morphological or environmental change, but occasionally there is a lag time during which accommodation or adaptation takes place. It is during this lag time that natural selection operates, eliminating those individuals that fail to develop appropriate behavioral responses or that take longer to do so than other members of the population. For example, in hominid evolution, secondary altriciality of the neonate, resulting from the interaction of selection for bipedalism and increased brain size, could not occur without appropriate behavioral responses on the part of the mother. For a time, there was likely a mismatch between the needs of the infants and the responses of the mothers, providing a fertile field for selection.

Several mammalian species provide examples of the mismatch between infant needs and parental caretaking responses. Some of these have been described previously by Ewer (1968). Richards (1969) notes, for example, that the female golden hamster exhibits more maternal behavior toward pups of 6–10 days of age than to newborn pups. Gestation period in this species is 16 days, rather than the 20–25 days typical of other small rodents. He suggests that the shortened gestation period is of recent evolution and that the maternal response has not yet made the adjustment. In other words, the mothers are still responding to pups of the ancestral stage of development.

In a species of spiny mouse (*Acomys cahirensis*) of the family Muridae, just the opposite pattern prevails. *Acomys* young are born precocial (rare in Rodentia), and it has been suggested that the length of gestation has recently increased in this species (Dieterlen, 1962, cited in Ewer, 1968). Pregnant females have an apparently strong desire to care for young several days before birth, and they will groom and suckle any available young. In fact, if other young are not available, preparturient spiny mice have been observed grooming adults in ways appropriate only for pups. They have also been known to cut the cord, lick, and eat the placenta of young not their own. Eventually, it is presumed, selection will favor an evening out of these behaviors so that the maternal responses are appropriate for the "premature" golden hamster and the "postmature" spiny mouse.

Another example of what can be termed a "mismatch" in behaviors is related to changes not in gestation length but in social behavior. Grey seal (*Halichoerus grypus*) females originally gave birth alone or in very small groups. Because the chances of a mix-up in young were low, there was no selective pressure to ensure the rapid formation of a strong mother–infant bond. Recently, however, the grey seals have begun to deliver their young in large, crowded rookeries. Because the mothers do not bond to a specific young, or vice versa, nursing is done promiscuously. Not surprisingly, only the stronger and seaward-located young are nursed, and mortality among pups is high. Presumably, under these circumstances, selection will favor the development of a stronger mother–infant bond, so that mothers nurse only young recognized as their own, as is the case with most other seal species (Smith, 1968, cited in Ewer, 1968).

A final example of a mismatch in maternal and neonatal behaviors may be found in the delayed onset of the social smile in humans. How is it that this powerful elicitor of maternal interaction develops only at 3–4 months of age in all normal infants in all sociocultural settings? It would seem that selection would favor its appearance soon after birth, when the human infant is most vulnerable and perhaps least attractive to its caretakers. Konner (1979) suggests that, among other reasons, the delayed onset of the social smile can be seen as an artifact of shortened gestation in our species. Thus, the infant begins smiling at the time of ancestral birth, 12 months after conception. Perhaps this is another example of a mismatch of maternal and infant behaviors: the mother is "ready" for that smile soon after birth, while the infant is not "ready" to produce it until 3 months later.

I have pointed out these mismatches because I think they have been important in the evolution of the human female reproductive strategy. As Hrdy and Williams (1983) have noted, most of the literature on reproductive strategies in sexually reproducing animals suggests that selection has operated only on males, because, the argument runs, females are usually the limiting resource, and they can reproduce, no matter how dull, ugly, dim-witted, unsexy, or passive they are. The only way that selection operates on females, it is implied, is on the physical and physiological abilities to conceive, bear, and care for offspring. Thus, to paraphrase an admirer of coast redwoods, "if you've seen one female, you've seen them all." Of course, this is not the case, and I would argue that with each major step in the evolution of the human female reproductive strategy, there were periods of incomplete adaptation or "mismatches," wherein only those females who could respond appropriately were able to increase their fitness. In other words, selection has acted with vigor on hominid females and has done so at a minimum of five major points in human evolution.

READJUSTMENTS IN BIRTH AND THE MOTHER–INFANT
BOND THROUGHOUT HUMAN EVOLUTION

As was pointed out in Chapters 1 and 3, difficult parturition is part of the evolutionary history of all higher primates, due primarily to the large size of the neonate relative to maternal body (and pelvis) size. Human parturition has been affected by three additional factors: anatomical adaptation for habitual bipedalism, increased brain size and elaboration, and secondary altriciality of the newborn infant. The third is, to some extent, a result of the first two factors, but all three interact in a way that increases interdependency of mothers and neonates and leads to a dependency on others during parturition.

During the past five million years, there have been at least five major transitions in human biology and culture that have resulted in changes in parturition and the mother–infant relationship: (1) the origin of bipedalism and associated greater difficulties in parturition; (2) secondary altriciality of the neonate associated with encephalization in the genus *Homo;* (3) the behavioral adaptation of obligate midwifery with further encephalization; (4) postpartum separation and decreased contact between mother and infant following agriculture and sedentism; and (5) technological effects on birth and infant care in the industrial age. Each of these transitions placed different demands on females giving birth to and caring for dependent young.

In the following pages, I shall propose possible scenarios describing these transitions. The first two were developed extensively in Chapter 1, so I shall simply provide a summary here. The last three transitions are less concerned with the physical and physiological aspects of birth but more with the emotional aspects of birth and associated changes in the mother–infant bond. As scenarios, these descriptions have not yet achieved the status of models against which can be designed tests using data from primate and human ethology, demography, and human sociocultural studies. I hope that, eventually, the proposed scenarios can be elaborated into models and that parts of the models can be elaborated, in turn, into testable hypotheses.

First Transition: The Pongid–Hominid Divergence

The first transition of concern occurred with the origin of the pongid and hominid clades. Brain expansion is characteristic of evolution in both clades, and the process probably began with their origin. In the pongid line, locomotor adaptation for brachiation and increased body size resulted in easier parturition than that presumed for their ancestors. Selective pressures operating on hominids to rearrange the pelvis for bipedalism resulted in a smaller birth canal which, coupled with even slight cranial expansion, resulted in greater difficulties in parturition than seen in most primates today.

One of the difficulties encountered by hominids was a change in orientation of the fetal emergence pattern, as reviewed in Chapter 1. Two patterns have been proposed. One proposal is that the australopithecine fetal head entered the pelvic basin in a transverse position and rotated to an anteroposterior position to exit, as it does in normal human birth today (Berge *et al.*, 1984). Another proposal is that the head entered in the transverse position and, because of the extremely narrow transverse dimensions of both the inlet and outlet, remained in that position for emergence (Tague and Lovejoy, 1985). Regardless of which pattern was actually followed, the series of rotations or twisting of the neck that would have been necessary for the shoulders to emerge would place additional stress on the fetal neck and spine and may have led to higher mortality. Only with increased attention and assistance on the part of the mother could infants be delivered without injury.

As has been pointed out previously, nonhuman primates typically use their hands in assisting delivery of their infants. Exceptions include the squirrel monkeys, who have been noted not only to have the closest cephalopelvic fit in the order (excepting humans) but also may have the highest neonatal mortality. Apparently mortality can be reduced if manual assistance by primate mothers is offered.

It has been suggested that the earliest hominids may have retained enough features of arboreality that they returned to the trees for sleeping, safety, and feeding (Lewin, 1983). Stern and Susman (1983) suggest that females of the species *Australopithecus afarensis* were, like female orangutans and gorillas, more arboreal than males. If this argument should be supported by further analysis of locomotor adaptations in this species, I would suggest that females of *A. afarensis*, like female orangutans, often returned to the trees to give birth. Their smaller size made them more vulnerable and thus more likely to seek safety in the trees. If they had skillful use of their hands during delivery, the safest place for birth would have been in the trees.

Once delivered, the australopithecine mother and infant would have had other problems not encountered by the other primates. To appreciate these difficulties, it will be useful to look at the familiar model for early hominids, the common chimpanzee. Chimpanzee females typically give birth to infants whose developmental maturity falls somewhere between that of monkeys and that of modern human infants. The young are born covered with hair, their eyes are open, and although they are not strong enough to cling to their mothers without some assistance from them, they are able to do so within several days. For approximately the first 4 months of life, the infant clings to the ventral surface of its mother, riding under her belly when she moves quadrupedally. Often for the first several weeks of life and whenever the infant has trouble clinging, the mother will provide support with one hand. She also aids the infant in finding the nipple and assists in nursing for the first several months of its life.

If prehominid females followed a similar pattern, they were faced with fairly strong selective pressures on behavior approximately five million years ago when the transition to bipedalism and increased mobility accompanied the appearance of a new group of primates, the hominids. Undoubtedly for a while, most mothers continued to behave during parturition and toward their neonates in ways similar to those hypothesized for their ancestors. Because of their bipedal foot, infants had even more difficulty clinging to their mothers. But, despite the fact that it made clinging virtually impossible, bipedalism was advantageous for carrying infants, because the hands were not necessary for locomotion.

In summary, the major challenges to parturition faced by the first hominids were those imposed by the evolution of bipedalism. This made the birth process even more difficult than for most primates and required greater skills on the part of the mother in assisting the delivery of the infant and in caring for it in the first days of its life. These initial challenges were obviously met successfully by some female hominids, whose descendents survived to meet the greater challenges that bipedalism imposed on hominid evolution in placing limits on the size of the neonatal brain.

Second Transition: Encephalization in the Genus *Homo*

As mentioned previously, brain size probably expanded slightly during the first two or three million years in the evolution of the hominid (and pongid) clade. By approximately two million years ago, however, it had reached the maximum size that could be born to a mammalian lineage that followed the typical pattern of completing half of brain growth *in utero*. It was at this point, with the origin of the genus *Homo,* that a shift in the usual growth pattern occurred so that more than half the growth of the brain took place after birth. Essentially, the way that members of the genus *Homo* met the problem of producing young too large for successful delivery was not to increase the size of the birth canal but to expand the lower limits on encephalization at birth by producing young "prematurely" when the fetus had not yet reached normal neonatal size. As a result, neonatal brain and motor development are far lower at birth than any other closely related primate neonate. This, in turn, required increased maternal attention at birth and a different pattern of caretaking during the several weeks and months thereafter.

The usual caretaking pattern exhibited by mothers of altricial young is to leave them behind in a nest or burrow as the adults forage. The significance of what has been called "secondary altriciality" in the human infant is that it implies an ancestral pattern of delivering more precocial infants. A characteristic that evolved in our ancestors, who delivered precocial young, is a milk content appropriate for infants who are in more or less constant contact with their mothers and can nurse whenever they want. This places upon hominids yet another phylogenetic constraint: not only does the milk composition fit the needs of an infant for whom the breast is always available, but the protein and fat content is so low that the breast *must* always be available for proper growth and development of the infant.

Thus, early *Homo* mothers could not leave their altricial infants behind in a nest while they foraged during the day. No longer could infants cling at all to their mothers, and yet the composition of milk remained such that infants had to be in continuous contact with their mothers (Lozoff *et al.* 1977, Blurton Jones, 1972). Selection favored those mothers who devised ways to keep their infants with them and yet were able to continue to exploit food resources efficiently. Eventually, hominid females developed the sling for carrying their young, enabling them to gather food with both hands in order to meet their own needs and the needs of those dependent on them (Tanner and Zihlman, 1976). As maternal nurturing behavior became more finely tuned to the needs of the infant during and after birth, infant mortality decreased and social bonds became even more tightly cemented because of the longer, more intensive period of dependency in the young.

The newly evolved nurturing pattern included keeping the infant in more or less constant contact, nursing on demand, maintaining high mobility during the day, and sleeping in small groups at night. Nursing on demand had several effects, one of which was to keep infants quiet during the day and night. Crying infants attract predators, and, especially at night when diurnal hominids were most vulnerable, it was important to keep infant crying at a minimum. In addition, nursing on demand likely kept early hominid females from ovulating during at least a 2-year period following birth, resulting in a 3–4-year birth interval.

In summary, the decrease in relative gestation length that was a byproduct of selection for bipedal locomotion at the origin of the hominid clade and for encephalization in the genus *Homo* resulted in greater altriciality of the neonate. This, in turn, placed greater demands on females in delivering and caring for more helpless infants. The ability to provide optimal care for her young depended on the skills of the female herself and on the amount of assistance she could receive from others in her social group. Ultimately, selection favored some degree of investment in young by adult males (Lovejoy, 1981) and provisioning of juveniles by adults (Lancaster and Lancaster, 1983). Thus, these characteristics of human social organization may owe their origin, in part, to secondary altriciality of the hominid infant (Fisher, 1982).

Third Transition: Further Encephalization and Obligate Midwifery

As encephalization proceeded even further in the hominid lineage, selection favored even smaller relative brain size in the neonate. Encephalization also may have meant increased awareness of the dangers of birth. *Homo* mothers of the Middle Paleolithic not only encountered greater difficulties in delivering very altricial infants, but they were perhaps more aware than any of their fellow or ancestral primate females of the vulnerable position of themselves and their infants during birth. Up until that time, hominid females probably sought privacy when delivering, as do most primates today. All others things being equal, it is likely advantageous to deliver alone because of the greater vulnerability to infection for the mother and infant and increased chances of injury resulting from too eager attention of others at birth. In hominids, however, all other things are not equal. I would argue that with the increase in encephalization at this time, there was a third behavioral transition, a point at which assistance at childbirth made a difference in mortality of *Homo* mothers and infants. Again not only was parturition more difficult, the genus became encumbered with a unique need of obligate midwifery.

Certainly the primary contribution made by birth attendants in the past and today was that of emotional support to the parturient woman. I would suggest, however, that there are a number of points at which manipulative assistance may have been important in reducing mortality. To appreciate this, it perhaps will be useful to review briefly parturition in nonhuman haplorhine primates. In most monkey and ape deliveries described in the literature, the infant emerges in a vertex position with the occiput against the mother's sacrum and the face toward that of its mother. After the head emerges, she may then pull it up toward her along the normal flexion of its body. If the occiput emerges with the face away from the mother, she will likely pull the infant backward, risking injuring it in the process. For an animal that typically delivers on an uneven substrate (e.g., in the trees), the use of the hands in assisting delivery is critical.

Human infants rarely emerge with the face toward the pubis. This type of presentation is referred to as "persistent posterior" and is associated with increased likelihood of perineal lacerations, prolonged delivery, arrest at the perineum, and more extensive molding of the cranial plates. Presumably a change in normal orientation of the fetus has thus occurred with the evolution of the female pelvis associated with bipedalism and encephalization. This change has affected the entire emergence pattern of the fetus and, thus, the mother's response to that emergence. If she uses her hands to assist delivery, she pulls the infant against the normal flexion of its body, again with the risk of injury, particularly to the nerves of the neck. This kind of injury can be prevented if another person intervenes to help guide the neonatal head as the shoulders emerge. Certainly women can and have given birth unassisted for millinea, but with some assistance from other adults, mortality is reduced. Eventually, as selection favored further assistance during birth, the behavior became a part of normal parturition in hominids. With the genus *Homo,* the costs of increased chance of infection were far outweighed by the benefits of assistance and emotional support in accomplishing a successful delivery of a healthy infant. As with sexual reproduction, viviparity, and so on, the practice of being attended at birth was not added to the reproductive strategy of hominids without competing selection pressures.

For a while, there was a variety of procedures followed: some females continued to labor and deliver alone, some had a minor amount of emotional support and assistance, and a few had the help of older adults experienced at giving birth themselves or assisting at numerous deliveries. If the last group experienced a mortality reduction of only one in 1000 births, the behavior would have enough selective advantage to reach very high frequencies in less than a million years.

The altruistic behavior of midwifery need not have a genetic basis, however. A male who assists his mate in parturition or a mother who assists her daughter will have more surviving offspring to whom to pass this behavior, either through learning or a genetically based tendency. Either way, the percentage of those adopting or inheriting the behavior will increase through time because of greater survival rate of mothers and young.

As the hominid brain increased from 700 to 1200 cm^3, selection continued to favor a gestation period that was shorter than would be expected for that adult brain size. This was itself a process that took a long time to develop successfully. There are a number of points at which failure was likely. Some fetuses gestated too long and were thus too large at delivery to pass intact through the birth canal or did so causing great trauma and perhaps death to their mothers. Some may have been born when the passage through the canal was successful, but their physiological development was not advanced enough to enable survival outside of the uterus. Even those who were born without trauma and made a successful transition to the extrauterine environment may not have survived if their mothers lacked the skills or motivation to provide extra care for the more helpless infant. Again, even with assistance at birth, mortality was likely high, not only until selection shaped the coincidence of infants small enough for safe deliveries yet developed enough to breathe on their own, but also until mothers were capable of responding to and satisfying infant needs. To some extent, this second transition, taking place over the course of a million years, was an elaboration of adaptation to the first with the important addition of assistance and support at birth.

As hominid populations spread into colder regions of the world, climate may have also affected their behavior at birth. Winter and night temperatures during much of the year in temperate regions preclude a woman from moving far away from the campfires to deliver her infant. Rather, she is more likely to move to a corner of the shelter (cave, tent, brush hut) and to deliver with other females close by. Because of their proximity and natural interest in and curiosity about birth and neonates, these nearby women probably occasionally offered assistance. Simply picking up the neonate out of curiosity and rubbing or massaging it in some cases would have enhanced respiration enough that mortality was reduced. Eventually selection would favor development of a tradition of providing assistance at birth.

Even if the woman left the shelter to give birth, she would be more likely to be accompanied by an assistant. A parturient woman encumbered with heavy clothing would find it difficult to deliver her infant unassisted. Again, even if one or two sought assistance while most others tried it alone, the survival differential would be enough to account for eventual incorporation of the practice in group tradition.

A final selective advantage to having others present at birth may be found in the anecdotal evidence that people who witness a birth become bonded to the infant (see Klaus and Kennell, 1982). Thus, in areas or times of high maternal mortality, other women are present to bond to the infant and will perhaps be more inclined to care for it if the mother dies. If attendants are relatives of the mother or infant, as is often the case in contemporary cultures, their own genes are represented in the infant.

The transition from the Middle to the Upper Paleolithic was marked by major morphological, physiological, behavioral, and sociocultural changes. Eric Trinkaus (1984) proposes that Middle Paleolithic Neandertal populations were characterized by large birth canals, large-brained neonates, a 12-month gestation period, and somewhat simple technology. In contrast, he argues, Upper Paleolithic humans gave birth after a 9-month gestation and had notably more elaborate cultural traditions. In other words, according to Trinkaus, the reduction in the length of gestation from 12 to 9 months was a punctuational event in the transition to anatomically modern human beings.

His argument for a reduction in gestation is based primarily on the unusual pelvic morphology of Neandertals, particularly the distinguishing characteristic of a thin, elongated pubic bone relative to modern humans. Neandertals of both sexes have much greater distance from the hip to the pubic symphysis than early modern and contemporary human beings, according to Trinkaus. These differences are seen by Wolpoff (1980) as adaptations to delivering large infants with large brains. Trinkaus argues that early moderns do not show evidence of being any smaller, less stocky, or smaller brained than Neandertals, and yet their pubic morphology does not reflect adaptations to delivering relatively large neonates. This suggests that other factors are involved, and Trinkaus argues that Neandertal pubes are larger because they gave birth to neonates with a cranial volume 15–25% greater than that of modern human neonates. This, he concludes, was the result of a gestation period of 11–12 months. In other words, the differences in pelvic morphology of Neandertals and early moderns are due to differences in gestation length: almost 1 year for Neandertals, the more familiar 9 months for early modern populations.

The selective advantages Trinkaus cites for the decreased gestation period include reduction in birth spacing, decreased energetic costs to the mother of pregnancy (although I would suggest that the energetic costs of a lengthened lactation period may be even greater than the savings of 3 fewer months of gestation), and enhanced neurological development of the child, due to exposure to earlier extrauterine stimuli. Trinkaus argues that these advantages could only be realized when cultural evolution had reached the stage that more vulnerable infants could be supported, a stage reached in the Upper Paleolithic.

Karen Rosenberg (1986) has countered Trinkaus' argument on morphological grounds, arguing that elongated pubes are found in australopithecines and in some anatomically modern humans as well, suggesting that this feature is more closely associated with maternal:fetal body size than with gestation length. Female pelvic dimensions are thus longer in any population in which mothers and neonates are large. Rosenberg further argues that large pelvic inlets in Neandertals are within the range predicted for modern humans of Neandertal body weight, suggesting that Neandertal infants at birth were as similar in proportion to their mothers as modern infants. She thus concludes that those infants were at a similar stage of development and dependence as newborn infants today (Rosenberg, 1986).

There are also counterarguments on physiological, behavioral, and sociocultural grounds. I have argued that delayed brain development and reduction in relative gestation length took place over a minimum of a million years, as constant readjustments took place in neonatal developmental state and maternal ability to care for a less precocial infant. When one considers the number of changes that had to take place in gestational physiology, neonatal physiology, and maternal behavior, gradualism is, to me, a much more parsimonious way of explaining shortened gestation than punctuationalism. Probably the most dramatic readjustment that had to take place in decreasing gestation length was in the fetal and neonatal respiratory systems; none of the technological skills possessed by Upper Paleolithic hominids could have saved the lives of neonates with the kinds of respiratory problems encountered in prematurely born infants today. A dramatic decrease in gestation length has far more life-threatening consequences than reduced ability to cling, to thermoregulate, and to seek nourishment.

The cultural transition that marked the Upper Paleolithic reflects an elaboration of subsistence skills and sociocultural complexity that undoubtedly resulted in improved infant care and decreased infant mortality, as Trinkaus suggests. Increased efficiency in food extraction certainly resulted in improved nutrition during gestation and lactation. Trinkaus cites evidence of expanded sociocultural complexity and suggests that there may have been more time and motivation for providing care to pregnant and parturient women and to mothers and infants during the postpartum period. Perhaps people became more skilled at simple obstetrical assistance, but even more critical would have been the availability of care-providers for the mother and infant after birth. If home bases were more stable and technology for defending them were improved, it is likely that women were able to remain "at home" for a few days or weeks after giving birth, enabling them to return more rapidly to good physical condition and to establish successful nursing. Relatives and other group members had the technological capability of providing for them during that time, as Trinkaus has suggested.

Human population during most of the Pleistocene grew only slightly (some suggest rates as low as .001 to .003% per year; see Cohen, 1980), remaining in equilibrium, just as does any natural animal population tied to fluctuations in resources (Lee and DeVore 1968). This equilibrium was maintained by biological mechanisms (e.g., the interaction of resource limitations, nutritional needs, and lactation demands) and by cultural mechanisms (e.g., infanticide, especially when practiced preferentially upon female infants, and taboos against sexual intercourse). Furthermore, difficulties in delivery, including slight cephalopelvic disproportion, asphyxia resulting from delayed second stage, and maternal sepsis, contributed not insignificantly to maintaining human populations just above replacement level, a level compatible with resource availability under foraging conditions. Thus, giving birth alone or with unskilled attendants can be seen as part of the total adaptive strategy for maintaining a foraging way of life under somewhat harsh circumstances.

As many have argued, physiological, ecological, and cultural mechanisms acted to keep human populations in balance with the ecological niche of hunting and gathering. The ceiling was raised significantly with the occupation of a different niche, that is, that of a controller and producer of resources, the next transition to be discussed. It has been argued that any long-term increase in resources or migration to an area of greater abundance also resulted in an increase in population (Cohen, 1980), and I would argue that the same effect derived from increased vigilance by others at childbirth.

Many authors (see Cohen, 1980) have noted that life expectancy for females in prehistoric populations is 2–4 years less than that of males. The difference is due primarily to the hazards of childbearing. Again, any behavior that serves to reduce those hazards increases life expectancy for females and contributes to population expansion. Consider that successful intervention in a difficult first delivery of a young primipara potentially could result in a short-term increase of perhaps six people: the young mother not only survives, but her firstborn and perhaps as many as five subsequent offspring also will live to reproduce themselves. One need not invoke mathematical formulae to see the long-term significance of a single midwife helping a single mother and infant through labor, delivery, and the postpartum period.

Many have argued that population increase preceded and perhaps caused the transition to agriculture in the Middle East and other parts of the world (see Binford, 1968; Flannery, 1973; Boserup, 1965). An abundance of wild foods is usually cited as the major reason for this increase, but I suggest that the behavior of seeking and providing assistance at childbirth also entered the population growth equation by reducing maternal and neonatal mortality such that increases occurred.

The Fourth Transition: The Neolithic

It is reasonable to assume that by the time of transition to domestication of plants and animals and increased sedentism, midwifery had been fairly well established as a tradition if not a profession. There is today a wide range of variation in the ways in which midwifery skills are practiced in various cultures of the world. Some techniques probably enhance survival of mother and infants, whereas others likely contribute to increased mortality. This variation has been reviewed extensively in the anthropological literature, so I have chosen not to focus on midwifery from a cross-cultural perspective. The major transition in the Neolithic that is of concern to this treatise was a change in the relationship between mother and child. This was directly related to sedentism and dietary changes.

In a foraging society, a woman contributes substantially to the collection of food for the group. She is highly mobile, carries her infant with her at all times, and typically gives birth every fourth year. Thus, an infant experiences about 4 years of intense contact and interaction with its mother, father, and other relatives. Konner (1976:220) notes that the infant is indulged during this period and spends its entire childhood in a "dense social context." He further notes that the close attachment between mother and infant is made possible, in part, because of this social context in which the mother is provided extensive physical and emotional support.

In contrast, mothers in many agricultural communities may be isolated from other group members by the nature of individual family dwellings and by economic division of labor. In many cases, women work in the fields and carry their infants with them, but often they will set the infants aside in a cradle or on a cradleboard as they conduct garden or household chores, picking them up occasionally for nursing. In this context, the signal for nursing is often a cry of hunger—resulting in nursing "on demand." Infants older than 2 years may be cared for primarily by older siblings. Because a woman does not have to carry her infant with her at all times, it is no longer necessary that there be a long birth interval. Actually, much the opposite prevails: in agricultural communities, children are usually an economic asset, thus there is incentive to have as many healthy offspring as possible. Increased consumption of carbohydrate-rich foods, decreased mobility, and nursing at infrequent intervals all interact to make this possible, enabling women to conceive within 10–15 months of the last birth. Weaning earlier is made possible by the availability of appropriate infant foods in the form of cereal grains and, in some places, milk from domesticated animals. Ultimately the birth interval is reduced to approximately 2 years, resulting in population increase.

This was not accomplished without an increase in infant mortality, however, primarily due to infectious diseases and malnutrition associated with weaning and periodic food shortages. This increased infant mortality provides a clue to the solution of another conundrum one encounters in examining ethnographic reports of contemporary cultures of low technology. In examining birth practices in cultures making up the Human Relations Area Files (HRAF), one is first struck with the fact that, commonly, mothers and infants are not together during the period that has been previously described as the "maternal sensitive period," that is, the first hour after birth. I consulted the HRAF literature on childbirth in 174 cultures. Rarely is it explicitly stated that the mother and infant are or are not together for the first hour after birth, but detail is usually provided on things that take place during that hour such as bathing the infant, rubbing it with special substances, and dressing or swaddling the infant. Often these attentions to the infant do not begin until the placenta is delivered. Since this process usually takes about 15 minutes, I have inferred that, based on other events described for the immediate postpartum period, contact between mother and infant is interrupted at birth and that reunion often does not occur until at least 30 minutes have passed. This seemed to be true for 76 of the cultures I surveyed in the HRAF. For 47 of them, interruption of contact between mother and infant appears minimal, and for 51 there were no descriptions of events in the first hour after birth. Thus, of the cultures on which information was available, I infer that for 62%, separation of mother and infant occurred for up to 30 minutes postpartum.

On the one hand, it might be argued that this in itself is proof that a maternal sensitive period does not exist. On the other hand, however, one might wonder that if this period is so good for bonding, why are women in most societies deprived of their best opportunity to form attachment to their infants? Again, as with sexual reproduction, viviparity, and so forth, we have a compromise between competing strategies. Consideration of the apparent contradiction between biologically mediated behaviors to ensure the health of the mother and infant and cultural practices that prevent these interactions has led Lynn Udick and me (Udick and McCallum, 1978; Trevathan and Udick, 1981) to propose that if it is likely that a newborn infant will not survive the early hours of its life, it may be best to delay formation of the bond between mother and child until a critical period has passed.

Data on perinatal mortality do not note the hour of death, but it is likely that the first hour is the most dangerous, and that, once the infant has passed that hour, its chances for survival increase considerably. Since most women have their infants with them almost constantly after the cleansing and other rituals of the first hour, bonding likely takes place readily, and the chances of survival are greater.

In many non-Western cultures with high infant mortality, few females ever reach childbearing age in a state of health that enables them to conceive and carry a fetus to term. In these groups, survival of the mother is of far greater concern than survival of the child. After all, if the newborn dies, the woman can have another child within a year, but if the mother herself dies, it will take many years to replace her. Thus, in many groups, attention is focused primarily on the mother for the first hour or so after birth as the attendants make efforts to bring her back to a state of health as quickly as possible. Often the newborn infant is ignored during this period of repair, and only when they are sure that the mother is stable do the attendants turn their attention to the infant. The mother then receives her child for the first time after she has been cared for and is more likely to give her full attention to her infant. This early period of inattention also selects for stronger infants who are more likely to survive subsequent dangers.

Inherent in this is the idea that it is detrimental to the mother's emotional health to form a strong bond with an infant who dies shortly after birth. Although there is evidence to the contrary (cf., Klaus and Kennell, 1976) it seems that a woman who had not held and nursed her child may have an easier time adjusting to its death than a woman who receives her neonate immediately after birth. Since ovulation can be affected by emotional stress, a woman who bonds to a child who subsequently dies may have trouble conceiving again. Thus, under conditions of high neonatal mortality, it may be adaptive not to bond to an infant until it is relatively safe beyond the first hour.

Delaying bond formation is no more clearly adaptive than in situations where infanticide may occur. Tonkinson (1978:64) notes that if a Mardudjara aborigine neonate is to be killed, it must happen before the mother sees the child's face or hears it cry. Otherwise, according to the aborigine women, she will "become so overwhelmed by compassion that she will not allow its death." Thomas (1958) notes a similar practice among !Kung women who try to kill their infants before the first breath and before "the time her love for the baby wells up in her so that the act would be impossible forever after. She must think of the child she has already and act quickly, before she hears her infant's voice, before the baby moves or waves its feet; she must not look at it for long or hold it. . . . "(p. 163). Without knowledge of research on the maternal sensitive period these women are recognizing the importance of the first postpartum interactions for mother–infant bonding.

Infant and maternal mortality have been high throughout recent human history, and today, only a few Western nations have been successful at reducing those rates. Only recently have reliable artificial means of birth control been developed. Today, mothers in Western cultures with low infant mortality can emotionally "afford" to bond to their infants immediately after birth. Our low perinatal death rate gives us the luxury of taking advantage of the optimal period for bonding in the first hour after birth. In groups where perinatal mortality rates remain high, bonding between mother and infant during the first hour may not be adaptive.

The Fifth Transition: Industrialization

It has been proposed that interactive behaviors immediately after birth that initially contributed to survival became less adaptive or even maladaptive when neonatal mortality increased. At the time of delivery, survival of the mother assumed primary focus until medical technology enabled both mother and infant to receive constant attention in the early hours and days following birth. For the last 50 years or so, most women in Western nations have approached pregnancy and delivery with the expectation of a positive outcome (i.e., a healthy, normal child). This is in contrast to people of developing nations and cultures where, as was noted in Chapter 4, people do not even recognize the infant as human and bestow upon it a name until it has lived a certain number of days or weeks. In other words, the expectation is as often that a neonate will die as that it will live.

Human mothers and infants still have within their behavioral repertoires the tendencies to interact with each other in ways that serve two functions previously reviewed: (1) to reduce infant and maternal mortality; and (2) to enhance mother–infant bonding. From the time of the Neolithic, they were perhaps separated for the early postpartum hours to avoid maternal emotional investment in an infant who was likely to die or be killed. Thus, the benefits of interaction for the first function were outweighed by the possible negative consequences of the second function should the infant not survive. Today, technological intervention has replaced with greater success the natural behaviors that once contributed to survival. Mortality at all life stages has been reduced significantly, while the birth rate in most of the world has remained high, resulting in the all-too-familiar population avalanche (Dubos, 1965) in which we are now caught.

Technological advances have also meant, as has been noted, that biological mothers are no longer necessary for the health and development of normal children. Thus, the entire mother–infant relationship has undergone substantial changes in the past century. Modern contraceptive techniques, economic conditions, and the movement of significant numbers of women into the work force have resulted in a decrease in the number of infants born to many women in their lifetimes. Thus, most women make conscious decisions about childbearing, choosing to avoid it altogether, to have 2.2 children, or to use no birth control and "let nature take its course."

Prenatal care has replaced taboo and ritual as the most likely way of ensuring delivery of healthy, normal infants. Further insurance has been gained by the almost universal practice in many developed nations of having birth take place in a hospital monitored by highly skilled medical personnel and modern machines. Obstetrical medication enables women to avoid the painful stimuli of labor and delivery to the extent that many remark that they have never really experienced childbirth. In the interests of survival, infants are usually removed to a nursery for monitoring in the critical postpartum hours, while mothers return to their rooms in an entirely different part of the hospital. Several hours or days later, the two are reunited or introduced to each other for the first time, and the mother must *learn* to interact with and care for her newborn infant.

Today, a Western mother typically bottle-feeds her infant and puts it to sleep in an infant bed, usually in its own room, away from its parents. The infant is fed approximately every 4 hours, and any crying between feeds is ignored, unless there is suspicion of illness or other "true" crisis. Mobiles are hung above the bed to provide entertainment and enhance intellectual development, and when the infant is out of bed it can be placed in an infant seat, swing, or rocker that winds up to simulate the movement of adult walking. Certainly, there are frequent periods of fairly intense interaction between parents and infants, but the extent of interaction is far less than that experienced by human infants for millinea.

And yet these infants grow up to be perfectly normal, healthy adults, as predicted by those who argue that the greatest key to success of our species is our behavioral flexibility, especially during infancy and childhood. But I would argue that there are limits to this flexibility and to the degree of alienation that women can achieve from parturition and from their infants. Robert LeVine

(1977), in writing about child rearing as cultural adaptation, discusses Bowlby's proposal that mother–infant attachment is a product of past selective pressures and that:

> [A]s descendants of the survivors of those environmental conditions, contemporary humans are innately programmed for attachment, and child-rearing practices everywhere must be accommodated to this universal tendency. In this respect, then, child-rearing practices reflect the environmental pressures that acted on our hominid ancestors, and they can vary culturally only within limits established in the distant evolutionary past without inflicting developmental damage on the child (p. 16).

Today, we are perhaps experiencing a sixth transition in mother–infant relationships as some parents have begun to question the degree to which modern birth practices "inflict developmental damage" on their infants and emotional damage on themselves. In Chapter 4, I noted that, with awareness of the dangers of obstetrical medication, many women are seeking to forego drugs during pregnancy and delivery as much as possible. Without drugs, however, the intense need that a parturient woman has for emotional support during labor and delivery must be met by some other means. Few medical people are able to provide this for the numerous women who deliver in hospitals daily. As a result of this unmet need, many women are seeking alternatives to birth in hospitals and with physicians, returning to the midwife with whom women have labored for thousands, perhaps millions of years.

These "new" ways of giving birth are themselves products of our greatly reduced infant mortality and our expectation that we will give birth to a healthy child, no matter what. LeVine (1977) notes that there are three universal goals to parenting: (1) physical survival and health of the child; (2) socialization of the child so that he or she can be economically independent in adulthood; and (3) acquisition by the child of behaviors that maximize other cultural values such as morality, prestige, intellectual achievement, religious piety, self-realization, or creativity. In cultures where infant mortality is high, parents emphasize goal No. 1 to the near exclusion of the other two goals, at least in early infancy. In societies, such as our own, where infant mortality is realtively low, No. 1 is taken completely for granted, No. 2 somewhat for granted, and, thus, most of parental investment goes into fulfilling goal No. 3. Home birth and midwifery are part of the seeking to fulfill this final goal. Since they assume that a healthy child will be born, some parents seek to have the birth take place in an atmosphere that is deemed best for the baby's and their emotional and spiritual health.

Neolocality has reached such an extreme that when a woman approaches term there may be no one residing nearby to assist her at delivery or in the postpartum period, except her husband. This, coupled with active control of reproduction and renewed interest in the emotional aspects of birth, has resulted in increased participation by fathers in birth and child care. Even when birth takes place in hospitals, husbands often accompany their wives in labor and delivery. In home births, fathers are often incorporated in the delivery process in almost ritual roles: "catching" their infants once the shoulders have emerged or cutting the umbilical cord.

Arguments that "breast is best" and group-support organizations such as La Leche League have resulted in an increase in the percentage of breastfeeding mothers in Western nations. "Natural mothering" advocates have encouraged feeding on demand and keeping infants and mothers together almost constantly for the first several months of life. Front and back baby carriers have replaced both the sling of ancient times and the baby carriage and stroller of more recent times. It has even become more common to hear of the "family bed" again, a sleeping arrangement that further decreases the amount of time mothers and infants are separated (Thevenin, 1976). All of these behaviors, which seem revolutionary and even ill-advised by Western standards, have been, and still are in most of the world, the norm for child rearing.

It remains to be seen whether or not we are truly in the midst of a transition or whether the behaviors I have described are part of a passing fad. It is unlikely that all women in industrialized countries will be interested in or able to adopt these customs. Similar behaviors, while part of past hominid environments of adaptedness, are not necessarily compatible with current environments of adaptedness. Technological developments and advances in biomedical research have further increased the behavioral flexibility that is the hallmark of our species. We have an array of choices in our lives that no species or population before us has ever experienced. In preparation for birth, we can choose to deliver at home with midwives, but if anything goes wrong, transport to a hospital is possible, and the result is usually a favorable outcome. Increasingly women in developed nations are asking for some of the care and consideration that is provided by midwives of most other cultures of the world. They want to form a close association with their birth attendant, they want to deliver in more familiar surroundings, and they want to have friends and relatives with them during or soon after delivery. It is a pattern that has existed for more than a million years, and it still haunts the laboring woman who feels something is wrong when she is alone in a strange place, frightened and unsure of what will happen next. More and more we realize that our dramatic and welcomed decrease in infant and maternal mortality has not come without costs. Perhaps it is no longer sufficient justification to explain the despair of childbirth as practiced in many Western nations today. Somehow we lost something along the way, and we now clamor to regain it.

BIRTH AND BONDING IN A WIDER CONTEXT

Far from being an isolated event, birth is just one part of the on-going life cycle of two individuals, and the event has a decided impact on the wider kin network and the society in which it takes place. The way that a woman reacts to parturition and her newborn infant is a reflection of the human evolutionary heritage, her genetic constitution, her own birth and early socialization, attitudes her society has toward childbirth and children, her relationship with the child's father, the role of women in her society, and her own personal dreams and expectations. For the infant, what happens during his or her birth and the early hours that follow may have a profound effect on every phase of his or her development and may affect, in turn, the way he or she reacts to the birth of his or her own children. Although most of this book has focused on a small fraction of the human life cycle, and in some ways treats it as an isolated event, the relationship of birth to the rest of the individual's life, to the culture in which it occurs, and to the evolutionary history of the species must be emphasized.

All animals exhibit a special excitement at the time of parturition. Human beings are no exception, and this excitement serves a purpose. The period of heightened emotions in human mothers soon after birth and events during the first hour after birth play a role in the development of the intense bond between the mother and infant that ensures the maternal care necessary for the survival of the infant. It appears that our evolutionary history has provided human mothers with an optimal (or at least a very good) period for bonding in the first hours after birth of an infant, bonding that takes place via behaviors in the visual, aural, and tactual modes. These behaviors and the subsequent mother–infant relationship are part of the overall human reproductive strategy whose features did not evolve independently but as part of a system designed to ensure survival and enhance fitness. Thus, events in the mother's life affect the quality of her interaction with her infant, and the process continues until that infant becomes a parent in turn. For the human species, it can be described in terms of the model presented in Figure 7.1

On the left side of the model are the immediate antecedents of maternal behavior, events during pregnancy, labor, and delivery that contribute to the birth of a healthy infant and to a strong mother–infant bond. These antecedents include positive emotional support from family, friends, and birth attendants, a relaxed environment for giving birth, unmedicated labor and delivery, and provision for constant contact between mother and newborn. Results of several studies suggest that the four antecedents contribute to survival and to a strong attachment both directly and through intermediary steps by enhancing the amount and quality of interaction during the first hour. These factors are characteristic of the "new ways" of giving birth in Western societies, but I have proposed that their roots can be traced as far back as two million years.

Interactions in the first hour that are believed to contribute to a strong mother–infant bond include encompassing and tactile exploration, looking at the infant *en face,* talking to the infant in a high-pitched voice, early nursing, and holding the infant on the left side. The system can be continued beyond the early hours of life to a strong mother–child bond that reinforces breastfeeding and, thus, results in a healthier child. Breastfeeding, in turn, inhibits ovulation and, thus, increases the birth interval, resulting in a healthier population.

Breastfeeding is the crucial link for extension of the model, and we have seen

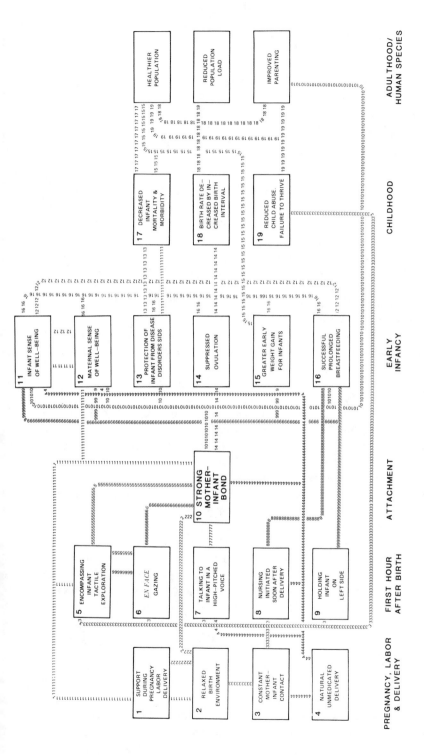

FIGURE 7.1. Birth and bonding in the human life cycle.

that events in the first hour contribute to successful nursing both directly and through the strong mother–infant bond. Our biology indicates that we evolved with the pattern of continuous carrying and feeding. Human milk is low in fat and very low in protein, which is typical of mammals who nurse continuously and are never separated from their infants. Colostrum and the milk itself are replete with antibodies that provide protection to the infant from a myriad of infectious agents in its environment. Prolonged, highly frequent breastfeeding in the absence of any supplemental feeding suppresses ovulation (Konner and Worthman, 1980). This is especially true for women in foraging societies whose nutritional intake is adequate and whose fat reserves are depleted by prolonged lactation. Thus, these women drop below the critical fat level postulated for ovulation (Frisch, 1974) and remain anovulatory for the 2 or 3 years that an infant is nursed. Each child is exposed to the maximal period of attachment and learning without emotional or nutritional competition from siblings. With continuous frequent breastfeeding and no supplementary feeding, the period of postpartum amenorrhea can be extended to 2 or more years in lactating women, regardless of their subsistence level.

The hominid female of the 1980s has inherited from her ancestors difficult parturition, helpless infants, naturally selected behaviors for responding to neonatal needs, emotional and physical dependence on assistance at birth, and the practice of being separated from her infant immediately after birth. At each one of the previously described transitions, maternal and infant mortality were undoubtedly high until adaptation to new challenges took place. This may be true today, as well, as reflected in the high incidence of sudden infant death syndrome of failure of the parent–child bond, and a fertility rate that may soon exceed our ability to adapt.

Our reproductive biology and history indicates that we are "K-strategists," that is, we have relatively few offspring, high parental investment in each offspring, and low infant mortality. Accompanying this strategy, and largely responsible for it, is our long life, slow development, delayed reproduction, and large body size (Pianka, 1970). Most K-strategists, however, have a relatively stable population size, at or near carrying capacity of the environment. It is at this point that humans diverge from the model of K-selection: We now threaten our own survival in that our numbers are beginning to outstrip the resources of the planet that supports us. The system of mother–infant interaction leading to prolonged breastfeeding and increased birth intervals provided the basis for a reproductive strategy compatible with the human environment, but that system has recently broken down.

Our intellectual capabilities may have gotten us to this point in the first place, but it may also be able to help us out of the dilemma. In modern human beings, we have an animal entirely different from those we have been tracing, beginning with the origin of sexual reproduction. Counter to every selective force we have reviewed so far, the human animal can and does refrain from breeding or consciously restricts the offspring produced to very low numbers. Reasons for this are many, and they range from the selfish to the altruistic. Personal rewards are sought in money, material possessions, or careers rather than in parenting. Some are concerned enough about the burgeoning world population that they choose not to have children at all. Others may be concerned enough about a threatening future that they choose not to subject children to a world of resource depletion, crowding, hunger, poverty, terrorism, greed, or nuclear holocaust. The "group-selection" arguments that usually fail to hold up under close scrutiny make sense when we consider the human animal and its ability to think not only of itself but of its fellow human beings. The very fact that we can refrain from breeding "for the good of the species" may be our only solution to overpopulation. It demands a very different reproductive strategy, far removed from the ones that have evolved over the past several million years and that, for our species at least, may have been far too successful.

A

TRANSLATION OF SPANISH DIALOGUES

Birth 2. Hispanic mother

Mother: My child, my child, my child. What is it? Son?

Midwife: I don't know. Look.

Mother: Ay, it's a girl. Ay, my baby. Ya, ya, my child. What a spoiled child. Ya, my child. You are cold. Ya, my child, what's the matter? My poor little child is all crooked.

Midwife: Gloria, nurse your baby.

Mother: She doesn't want it. I can't do it. She's hungry.

Birth 3. Hispanic mother

Mother: What is it?

Midwife: A girl.

Mother: Oh, my love. My love. My little girl. Oh, my little girl. Oh, my love. Ay, my love. My little one, little mother. My love, little one. Ay, my love. Why are your crying, my love, why? My love.

Midwife: Do you have a name for your baby?

Father: Guadalupe.

Midwife: Guadalupe what, nothing else?

Father: Guadalupe. Today is the day of the Virgin of Guadalupe in Mexico.

Birth 4. Hispanic mother

Mother: How pretty is my child, it is mine. What is it? Ay, how beautiful. Ay, how beautiful. Look at how pretty is my child. Ay, how beautiful is my child. Ay, how pretty.

Aunt: It's a boy.

Mother: A boy! Oh, aunt, how happy! Ay, I am saved, my son, my son. No one will take him away from me, no one, no one. My son, my son. How foolish. Ay, how pretty. Is it dark-skinned?

Aunt: No, it's not dark-skinned, it's white.

Mother: White! Ya, ya, ya, my little child. Ya, ya, ya, my little father. Ya, ya, little father. Ya, ya, my little tiny child. Ay, how beautiful. Ay, a boy. Ya, ya, ya little one. Why do you cry? What's the matter? Ya, ya, ya. Ay, how pretty.

Birth 5. Hispanic mother

Mother:	It's a boy, isn't it? My son. It's a boy. Thank you my God. My pretty king. The reason for my life. My little son. My life. Yes, my love. Shshshshshshsh. My pretty thing.
Father:	Look at the big fingernails. Are you tired? It has a very large head. Is it already suckling?

Birth 6. Hispanic mother

Mother:	Thank you, my daughter. Ay, yes. Everything is OK. What is it?
Midwife:	I don't know. Look.
Mother:	Thank you, my God. Thank you, Jesus. In the name of Jesus Christ, your son, I give thanks to these women. Are you going to bathe my daughter or not? What is it? What is it?
Midwife:	Look at your baby.
Mother:	I can't see. What is it?
Midwife:	Look at your baby to see what it is.
Mother:	Female or male?
Midwife:	Look at it.
Mother:	Male. He is hungry.
Midwife:	Give your baby the breast.
Mother:	I don't know how to do it.
Midwife:	But he ought to learn.
Mother:	I don't know how. He is hungry. Meanwhile, give him some water. Meanwhile, give him something, poor little thing.
Midwife:	No.
Mother:	Is it here that you register the name of the children?
Midwife:	The name? Not right now.

BIBLIOGRAPHY

Abegglen, H. and Abegglen, J.J. Field observation of a birth in hamadryas baboons. *Folia Primatologia*, 1976, 26:54–56.

Adachi, M., Saito, R., and Tanioka, Y. Observation of delivery behavior in the rhesus monkey. *Primates,* 1982, 23:583–586.

Adamsons, K. and Towell, M.E. Thermal homeostasis in the fetus and newborn. *Anesthesiology,* 1965, 26:531–548.

Adriani, N. and Kruyt A.C. *The Bare'e-speaking Toradja of Central Celebes,* Vol. I. Amsterdam: Noord-Hollandssche Witgivers Maatschappi (HRAF), 1951.

Ainsworth, M.D.S. *Infancy in Uganda: Infant Care and the Growth of Love.* Baltimore, MD: Johns Hopkins University Press, 1967.

Ainsworth, M.D.S. The development of infant–mother attachment. In B.M. Caldwell and H.M. Ricciuti (Eds.), *Review of Child Development Research,* Vol. 3. Chicago, IL: University of Chicago Press, 1973.

Ainsworth, M.D.S. Attachment theory and its utility in cross-cultural research. In P.H. Leiderman, S.R. Tulkein, and A. Rosenfeld (Eds.), *Culture and Infancy.* NY: Academic Press, 1977.

Alexander, R.D. and Noonan, K.M. Concealment of ovulation, parental care, and human social evolution. In N.A. Chagnon and W. Irons (Eds.), *Evolutionary Biology and Human Social Behavior.* North Scituate, MA: Duxbury Press, 1979.

Alexandre, P. and Binet, J. *Le Groups Dit Pahouin (Fang-Boulou-Beti).* Paris: Presses Universitaires de France (HRAF), 1958.

Altmann, J. *Baboon Mothers and Infants.* Cambridge: Harvard University Press, 1980.

Altmann, S.A. Sociobiology of rhesus monkeys. II: Stochastics of social communications. *Journal of Theoretical Biology,* 1965, 8:490–522.

Anderson, M. Transplantation—Nature's success. *Lancet* (London), 1971, 2:1077–1082.

Anisfeld, E. and Lipper, E. Early contact, social support, and mother–infant bonding. *Pediatrics,* 1983, 72:79–83.

Apgar, V. A proposal for a new method of evaluation of the newborn infant. *Anesthesiology and Analgesia,* 1953, 32:260–267.

Argyle, M. The laws of looking. *Human Nature,* 1978, 1:32–40.

Arms, S. *Immaculate Deception.* Boston, MA: Houghton Mifflin, 1975.

Arney, W.R. Maternal-infant bonding: The politics of falling in love with your child. *Feminist Studies,* 1980, 6:547–570.

Bales, R.F., Strodtbeck, F.L. Mills, T.M., and Roseborough, M.E. Channels of communication in small groups. *American Sociological Review,* 1951, 16:461–468.

Barnett, C.R., Leiderman, P.H., Grobstein, R., and Klaus, M. Neonatal separation: The maternal side of interactional deprivation. *Pediatrics,* 1970, 45:197–205.

Barnett, M.M. and Humenick, S.S. Infant outcome in relation to second stage labor pushing method. *Birth,* 1982, 9(4):221–230.

243

Bartholomew, G.A. Mother-young relations and the maturation of pup behavior in the Alaska fur seal. *Animal Behavior,* 1959, 7:163–171.

Bayley, N. *Bayley Scales of Infant Development.* NY: Psychological Corporation, 1970.

Beaconsfield, P., Birdwood, G., and Beaconsfield, R. The placenta. *Scientific American,* 1980, 243:94–102.

Beck, B.B. The birth of a lowland gorilla in captivity. *Primates,* 1984, 25:378–383.

Beer, A.E. and Billingham, R.E. *The Immunobiology of Mammalian Reproduction.* Englewood Cliffs, NJ: Prentice Hall, 1976.

Bell, R., and Costello, N. Three tests for sex differences in tactile sensitivity in the newborn. *Biologia Neonatorum,* 1964, 7:335–347.

Ben Shaul, D.M. The composition of the milk of wild animals. *International Zoo Yearbook,* 1962, 4:333–342.

Berge, C., Orban-Segebarch, R., and Schmid, P. Obstetrical interpretation of the Australopithecine pelvic cavity. *Journal of Human Evolution,* 1984, 13:573–587.

Bernstein, H., Byerly, H.C., Hopf, F.A., and Michod, R.E. Genetic damage, mutation, and the evolution of sex. *Science,* 1985, 229:1277–1281.

Binford, L.R. Post-Pleistocene adaptations. In L.R. Binford and S.R. Binford (Eds.), *New Perspectives in Archaeology.* Chicago, IL: Aldine, 1968.

Blackburn, D.G. An evolutionary analysis of vertebrate viviparity. *American Zoologist,* 1981, 21:936.

Blackwood, B. *Both Sides of Buka Passage: An Ethnographic Study of Social, Sexual and Economic Questions in the North-Western Solomon Islands.* Oxford: Clarendon Press (HRAF), 1935.

Blakemore, C. and Cooper, G.F. Development of the brain depends on the visual environment. *Nature (London),* 1970, 228:477–478.

Blurton Jones, N.G. Comparative aspects of mother–child contact. In N.G. Blurton Jones (Ed.), *Ethological Studies of Child Behaviour.* Cambridge: Cambridge University Press, 1972.

Bogren, L.Y. Side preference in women and men when holding their newborn child: Psychological background. *Acta Psychiatrica Scandinavia,* 1984, 69:13–23.

Bolinder, G. *Indians on Horseback.* London: Dennis Dobson (HRAF), 1957.

Bolton, R. Child holding patterns. *Current Anthropology,* 1978, 19:134–135.

Boorman, K.E. Deficiency of A births from O mothers. *Annals of Eugenics,* 1950, 15:120.

Boserup, E. *The Conditions of Agricultural Growth.* Chicago, IL: Aldine, 1965.

Bowden, D., Winter, P., and Ploog, D. Pregnancy and delivery behavior in the squirrel monkey *(Saimiri sciureus)* and other primates. *Folia Primatologica,* 1967, 5:1–42.

Bowlby, J. The nature of the child's tie to his mother. *International Journal of Psychoanalysis,* 1958, 39:350–373.

Bowlby, J. *Attachment and Loss. Vol I: Attachment.* London: Hogarth Press, 1969.

Bowlby, J. *Attachment and Loss. Vol. II: Separation.* NY: Basic Books, 1973.

Brackbill, Y., Kane, J., Manniello, R.L., and Abramson, D. Fetus, placenta and newborn: Obstetric premedication and infant outcome. *American Journal of Obstetrics and Gynecology,* 1974, 118:377–383.

Brandt, E. and Mitchell, G. Parturition in primates: behavior related to birth. In L. Rosenblum, (Ed.), *Primate Behavior: Developments in Field and Laboratory Research.* NY: Academic Press, 1971.

Brazelton, T.B. Psychophysiologic reactions in the neonate: Effects of maternal medication on the neonate and his behavior. *Journal of Pediatrics,* 1961, 58:513–518.

Brazelton, T.B. The early mother–infant adjustment. *Pediatrics,* 1963, 32:931–938.

Brazelton, T.B. *Neonatal Behavioral-Neurological Evaluation.* London: National Spastics Society Monographs, Number 5, 1973.

Brazelton, T.B. Implication of infant development among the Mayan indians of Mexico.

In P.H. Leiderman, S.R. Tulkein, and A. Rosenfield (Eds.), *Culture and Infancy*. NY: Academic Press, 1977.

Brazelton, T.B. Behavioral competence of the newborn infant. *Seminars in Perinatology*, 1979, 3:35–44.

Brazelton, T.B., Scholl, M.L., and Robey, J.S. Visual responses in the newborn. *Pediatrics*, 1966, 37:284–290.

Bridges, R.S., Dibiase, R., Loundes, D.D., and Doherty, P.C. Prolactin stimulation of maternal behavior in female rats. *Science*, 1985, 227:782–784.

Brody, S. The concepts of attachment and bonding. *American Psychoanalytic Association Journal*, 1981, 29:815–829.

Brofenbrenner, U. Early deprivation in mammals: A cross-species analysis. In G. Newton and S. Levine (Eds.), *Early Experience and Behavior*. Springfield, IL: Charles Thomas, 1968.

Bronson, G.W. Structure, status, and characteristic of the nervous system at birth. In P. Stratton (Ed.), *Psychobiology of the Human Newborn*. NY: John Wiley and Sons, 1982.

Bruck, K. Temperature regulation in the newborn infant. *Biologica Neonatorum*, 1962, 3:65–119.

Burley, N. The evolution of concealed ovulation. *American Naturalist*, 1979, 114:835–858.

Burns, J.K. Stress hormones and oestriol in relation to human labour. In L. Carenza, P. Pancheri and L. Zichella (Eds.), *Clinical Psychoneuroendocrinology in Reproduction*. London: Academic Press, 1978.

Caine, N. and Mitchell, G. Behavior of primates present during parturition. In J. Erwin, T. Maple, and G. Mitchell (Eds.), *Captivity and Behavior*, Vol. I. NY: Van Nostrand–Rheinhold, 1977.

Caldeyro-Barcia, R. The influence of maternal position on time of spontaneous rupture of the membranes, progress of labor, and fetal head compression. *Birth and the Family Journal*, 1979, 6:7–15.

Chism, J., Rowell, T.E., and Richards, S.M. Daytime births in captive patas monkeys. *Primates*, 1978, 19:765–767.

Chung, C.S. and Morton, N.E. Selection at the ABO locus. *American Journal of Human Genetics*, 1961, 13:9–27.

Clark, M. *Health in the Mexican-American Culture*. Berkeley, CA: The University of California Press, 1970.

Cohen, M.N. Speculations on the evolution of density measurement and population regulation in *Homo sapiens*. In M.N. Cohen, R.S. Malpass, and H.G. Klein (Eds.), *Biosocial Mechanisms of Population Regulation*. New Haven, CT: Yale University Press, 1980.

Coll, C.G., Sepkoski, C., and Lester, B.M. Cultural and biomedical correlates of neonatal behavior. *Developmental Psychobiology*, 1981, 14:147–154.

Collier, G.E. and O'Brien, S.J. A molecular phylogeny of the Felidae: Immunological distance. *Evolution*, 1985, 39:473–487.

Condon, W.S. and Sander, L.W. Neonate movement is synchronized with adult speech: Interactional participation and language acquisition. *Science*, 1974, 183:99–101.

Connolly, A.M., Pancheri, P., Lucchetti, A., Salmaggi, L., Guerrieri, D., Francalancia, M., Bartoleschi, A. and Zichella, L. Labor as a psychosomatic condition: A study on the influence of personality on self-reported anxiety and pain. In L. Carenza, P. Pancheri, and L. Zichella (Eds.), *Clinical Psychoneuroendocrinology in Reproduction*. London: Academic Press, 1978.

Cosminsky, S. Cross-cultural perspectives on midwifery. In S. Tax (Ed.), *Medical Anthropology*, pp. 229–248. The Hague: Mouton, 1977.

Cosminsky, S. Midwifery and medical anthropology. In B. Velimerovic (Ed.), *Modern*

Medicine and Medical Anthropology in the United States-Mexican Border Population. El Paso: Panamerican Health Organization, 1978.

Crelin, E.S. *Functional Anatomy of the Newborn.* New Haven, CT: Yale University Press, 1973.

Crook, C.K. The organization and control of infant sucking. In H. W. Reese and L. P. Lipsitt (Eds.), *Advances in Child Development and Behavior,* Vol. 14. London: Academic Press, 1979.

Cross, H.A. and Harlow, H.F. Observations of infant monkeys by female monkeys. *Perceptual and Motor Skills,* 1963, 16:11–15.

Daly, M. and Wilson, M.I. Whom are newborn babies said to resemble? *Ethology and Sociobiology,* 1982, 3:69–78.

Daly, M. and Wilson, M. *Sex, Evolution, and Behavior.* Boston, MA: Willard Grant Press, 1983.

David, J.H.M. Observations on mating behavior, parturition, suckling, and the mother–young bond in the Bontebok (*Damaliscus dorcas dorcas*). *Journal of Zoology,* 1975, 177:203–223.

De Chateau, P. The influence of early contact on maternal and infant behavior of primiparae. *Birth and the Family Journal,* 1976, 3:149–155.

De Chateau, P. Left-side preference for holding and carrying newborn infants. *Journal of Nervous and Mental Disease,* 1983, 171:241–245.

De Chateau, P. and Wiberg, B. Long-term effect on mother-infant behavior of extra contact during the first hours postpartum. *Acta Paediatrica Scandinavia* 1977, 66:145–151.

De Chateau, P., Holmberg, H., and Winberg, J. Left-side preference in holding and carrying newborn infants. *Acta Paediatrica Scandinavia,* 1978, 67:169–175.

DeCasper, A.J. and Fifer, W.P. Of human bonding: Newborns prefer their mothers voices. *Science,* 1980, 208:1174–1176.

Denenberg, V.H., Grota, L.J. and Zarrow, M.X. Maternal behavior in the rat: Analysis of cross-fostering. *Journal of Reproduction and Fertility,* 1963, 5:133–141.

Desmond, M.M., Rudolph, A.J., and Phitaksphraiwan, P. The clinical behavior of the newly born. *Journal of Pediatrics,* 1963, 62:307–325.

Desmond, M.M., Rudolph, A.J. and Phitaksphraiwan, P. The transitional care nursery: A mechanism of preventive medicine. *Pediatric Clinics of North America,* 1966, 13:651–668.

Detterman, D.K. The effect of heartbeat sound on neonatal crying. *Infant Behavior and Development,* 1978, 1:36–48.

Devitt, N. The transition from home to hospital birth in the United States, 1930–1960. *Birth and the Family Journal,* 1977, 4:47–58.

DeVore, I. Mother–infant relations in free-ranging baboons. In H. Rheingold (Ed.), *Maternal Behavior in Mammals.* NY: John Wiley and Sons, 1963.

Dixson, A.F. and George, L. Prolactin and parental behavior in a male New World primate. *Nature (London),* 1982, 299:551–553.

Doyle, G.A., Pelletier, A. and Bekker, T. Courtship, mating and parturition in the lesser bushbaby (*Galago senegalensis moholi*) under semi-natural conditions. *Folia Primatologica,* 1967, 7:169–197.

Dubois, C. *The People of Alor,* Vol. I. London: Dennis Dobson (HRAF), 1944.

Dubos, R. *Man Adapting.* New Haven, CT: Yale University Press, 1965.

Dunbar, R.I.M. and Dunbar, P. Behavior related to birth in wild gelada baboons (*Theropithecus gelada*). *Behavior,* 1974, 50:185–191.

Dunn, J.F. and Richards, M.P.M. Observations on the developing relationship between mother and baby in the neonatal period. In H.R. Schaffer (Ed.), *Studies in Mother–Infant Interaction.* NY: Academic Press, 1977.

Egeland, B. and Vaughn, B. Failure of "bond formation" as a cause of abuse, neglect, and maltreatment. *American Journal of Orthopsychiatry*, 1981, 51:78–84.

Eibl-Eibesfeldt, I. *Ethology: The Biology of Behavior*. NY: Holt, Rinehart, and Winston, 1975.

Eisenberg, R.B., Griffin, E.J., Coursin, D.B., and Hunter, M.A. Auditory behavior in the human neonate: A preliminary report. *Journal of Speech and Hearing Research*, 1964, 7:245–269.

Elander, G. and Lindberg, T. Short mother–infant separation during first week of life influences the duration of breastfeeding. *Acta Paediatrica Scandinavia*, 1984, 73:237–240.

Elmer, E. and Gregg, G.S. Developmental characteristics of abused children. *Pediatrics*, 1967, 40:596–602.

Emde, R.N., Swedberg, J., and Zuzuki, B. Human wakefulness and biological rhythms after birth. *Archives of General Psychiatry*, 1975, 32:780–783.

Engel, R., Crowell, D., and Nishijima, S. Visual and auditory response latencies in neonates. In B.N.D. Fernando (Ed.), *Felicitation Volume in Honour of C. DeSilva*. Ceylon: Kularatne and Company, Ltd. Cited In A. Korner, The effect of the infant's state, level of arousal, sex, and ontogenetic stage on the caregiver. In M. Lewis and L. Rosenblum (Eds.), *The Effect of the Infant on Its Caregiver*. NY: John Wiley and Sons, 1968.

Epple, G. Parental behavior in *Saguinus fuscicollis* spp. (Callitricidae). *Folia Primatologica*, 1975, 24:221–238.

Estermann, C. *The Ethnography of Southwestern Angola, Volume 1*. NY: Africana Publishing Company, 1976.

Ewer, R.F. *Ethology of Mammals*. NY: Plenum, 1968.

Fanaroff, A.A., Kennell, J.H., and Klaus, M.H. Follow-up of low birth weight infants— the predictive value of maternal visiting patterns. *Pediatrics*, 1972, 49:288–290.

Fantz, R.L. The origin of form perception. *Scientific American*, 1961; 204:288–290.

Fisher, H. *The Loss of Estrous Periodicity in Hominid Evolution*. Ann Arbor, MI: University Microfilms, 1975.

Fisher, H. *The Sex Contract*. NY: William Morrow, 1982.

Fisher, R.A. *The Genetical Theory of Natural Selection*. Oxford: Clarendon Press, 1930.

Flannery, K.V. The origins of agriculture. *Annual Review of Anthropology*, 1973, 2:271–310.

Forbes, T.R. *The Midwife and the Witch*. New Haven, CT: Yale University Press, 1966.

Fraiberg, S. Blind infants and their mothers: An examination of the sign system. In M. Lewis and L.A. Rosenblum (Eds.), *The Effect of the Infant on Its Caregiver*. N.Y.: John Wiley and Sons, 1974.

Fraser, A.F. *Reproductive Behavior in Ungulates*. NY: Academic Press, 1968.

Freedman, D.G. *Human Infancy: An Evolutionary Perspective*. NY: John Wiley and Sons, 1974.

Freedman, D.G. and Freedman, N. Ethnic differences in babies. *Human Nature*, 1979. 2:36–44.

Friedman, E.A. *Labor: Clinical Evaluation and Management*, 2nd Edition. NY: Appleton-Century-Crofts, 1978.

Frisch, R. *Demographic Implications of the Biological Determinants of Female Fecundity*. Cambridge, MA, Center for Population Studies, Harvard University Research Paper Number 6, 1974.

Frodi, A. Aversive crying and child abuse. In B.M. Lester and C.T. Zachariah Boukydis (Eds.), *Infant Crying*. NY: Plenum, 1985.

Fuchs, A-R. and Fuchs, F. Endocrinology of human parturition: A review. *British Journal of Obstetrics and Gynaecology*, 1984, 91:948–967.

Fuchs, A-R., Fuchs, F., Husslein, P., Soloff, M.S., and Fernstrom, M.J. Oxytocin receptors and human parturition: A dual role for oxytocin in the initiation of labor. *Science*, 1982, 215:1396–1398.

Galdikas, B.M.F. Wild orangutan birth at Tanjuing Puting Reserve. *Primates*, 1982, 23:500–510.

Garn, S. Fat, body size, and growth in the newborn. *Human Biology*, 1958, 30:265–280.

Gayton, A.H. *Yokuts of Western Mono*. Berkeley, CA: University of California (HRAF), 1948.

Gill, N.E., White, M.A. and Anderson, G.C. Transitional newborn infant in a hospital nursery—from first oral cue to first sustained cry. *Nursing Research*, 1984, 33:213–217.

Gillman, J. and Gilbert, C. The reproductive cycles of the chacma baboon (*Papio ursinus*) with special reference to the problems of menstrual irregularities as assessed by the behavior of the sex skin. *South African Journal of Medical Sciences*, 1946, 11:1–54.

Ginsburg, H.J., Fling, S., Hope, M.L., Musgrove, D., and Andrews, C. Maternal holding preferences: A consequence of newborn head-turning response. *Child Development*, 1979, 50:280–281.

Goland, R.S., Wardlaw, S.L., Stack, R.I., and Frantz, A.G. Human plasma beta-endorphin during pregnancy, labor, and delivery. *Journal of Clinical Endocrinology and Metabolism*, 1981, 52:74–78.

Goldberg, S. Infant development and mother–infant interaction in urban Zambia. In P.H. Leiderman, S.R. Tulkin, and A. Rosenfeld (Eds.), *Culture and Infancy*. NY: Academic Press, 1977.

Goodall, J. *In the Shadow of Man*. NY: Dell, 1971.

Goodall, J. and Athumani J. An observed birth in a free-living chimpanzee (*Pan troglodytes schweinfurthii*) in Gombe National Park, Tanzania. *Primates*, 1980, 21:545–549.

Goodman, M. On the emergence of intra-specific differences in the protein antigens of human beings. *American Naturalist*, 1960, 94(875):153–166.

Goodman, M. The role of immunochemical differences in the phenetic development of human behavior. *Human Biology*, 1961, 33:131–161.

Goodman, M. Immunochemistry of the primates and primate evolution. *Annals of the New York Academy of Sciences*, 1962, 102:219–234.

Gordon, J.E., Gideon, H., and Wyon, J.B. Childbirth in rural Punjab, India. *American Journal of Medical Science*, 1964, 247:344-357.

Gordon, J.E., Gideon H., and Wyon, J.B. Midwifery practice in rural Punjab, India. *American Journal of Obstetrics and Gynecology*, 1965, 93:734–742.

Goren, C.C., Sarty, M., and Wu, P.Y.K. Visual following and pattern discrimination of face-like stimuli by newborn infants. *Pediatrics*, 1975, 56:544–549.

Gorer, G. *Himalayan Village* (HRAF), 1938.

Goswell, M.J. and Gartlan, J.S. Pregnancy, birth and early infant behaviour in the captive patas monkey (*Erythrocebus patas*). *Folia Primatologica*, 1965, 3:189–200.

Gould, S.J. *Ontogeny and Phylogeny*. Cambridge, MA: Harvard University Press, 1977.

Gouzoules, H.T. Group responses to parturition in *Macaca arctoides*. *Primates*, 1974, 15:287–292.

Graham-Jones, O. and Hill, W.C.O. Pregnancy and parturition in a Bornean orangutan. *Proceedings of the Zoological Society of London*, 1962, 139:503–510.

Granquvist, H.N. *Birth and Childhood Among the Arabs: Studies in a Muhammadan Village in Palestine*. Helsingfors, Finland: Soderstrom and Company (HRAF), 1947.

Greenberg, M. and Morris, N. Engrossment: The newborn's impact upon the father. *American Journal of Orthopsychiatry*, 1974, 44:520–531.

Griffiths, W.G. *The Kol Tribe of Central India*. Calcutta: Royal Asiatic Society of Bengal (HRAF), 1946.

Gubernick, D.J. Maternal "imprinting" or maternal "labelling" in goats? *Animal Behavior,* 1980, 27:314–315.

Gubernick, D.J. Parent and infant attachment in mammals. In D.J. Gubernick and P.H. Klopfer (Eds.), *Parental Care in Mammals.* NY: Plenum, 1981.

Gucwinska, H. and Gucwinska, A. Breeding the Zanzibar galago, *Galago senegalensis zanzibaricus,* at Wroclaw Zoo. *International Zoo Yearbook,* 1968, 8:111–114.

Gutierrez de Pineda, V. *Organizacion Social en la Guajira.* Bogata (HRAF), 1950.

Haith, M.M. *Rules that Babies Look By.* Hillsdale N.J.: Lawrence Erlbaum, 1980.

Hanks, J.R. *Maternity and Its Rituals in Bang Chan.* Ithaca: Cornell University: Department of Asian Studies, Southeast Asia Program Data Paper #51 (HRAF), 1963.

Harlow, H.F. The nature of love. *The American Psychologist,* 1958, 13:673–685.

Harlow, H.F. and Harlow, M.K. The affectional systems. In A.M. Schrier, H.F. Harlow, and F. Stollnitz (Eds.), *Behavior of Nonhuman Primates,* Vol. II. NY: Academic Press, 1965.

Harlow, H.F., Harlow, M.K. and Hansen, E.W. The maternal affectional system of rhesus monkeys. In H.L. Rheingold (Ed.), *Maternal Behavior in Mammals.* NY: John Wiley and Sons, 1963.

Harned, H.S. Respiration and the respiratory system. In U. Stave (Ed.), *Physiology of the Perinatal Period.* NY: Appleton-Century-Crofts, 1970.

Hart, D.V. From pregnancy through birth in a Bisayan Filipino vllage. In D.V. Hart, P.A. Rajadhohn, and R.J. Coughlin, *Southeast Asian Birth Customs.* New Haven, CT: HRAF Press, 1965.

Hart, D.V., Rajadhon, P.A., and Coughlin, R.J. *Southeast Asian Birth Customs.* New Haven, CT: HRAF Press, 1965.

Harvey, P.H. and Clutton-Brock, T.H. Life history variation in primates. *Evolution,* 1985, 39:559–581.

Hazell, L. *Birth Goes Home.* Seattle, WA: Catalyst Press, 1974.

Henneborn, W.J. and Cogan, R. The effect of husband participation on reported pain and probability of medication during labor and birth. *Journal of Psychosomatic Research,* 1975, 19:215–222.

Herbert, M., Sluckin, W., and Sluckin, A. Mother-to-infant "bonding." *Journal of Child Psychology and Psychiatry,* 1982, 23:205–221.

Hersher, L., Richmond, J.B., and Moore, A.U. Maternal behavior in sheep and goats. In H. Rheingold (Ed.), *Maternal Behavior in Mammals.* NY: John Wiley and Sons, 1963.

Hickman, M.A. *Midwifery,* 2nd Edition. Oxford: Blackwell Scientific, 1985.

Hilger, M.I. *Araucanian Child Life and Its Cultural Background.* Washington, D.C.: Government Printing Office (HRAF), 1957.

Hill, S.T. and Shronk, L.K. The effect of early parent–infant contact on newborn body temperature. *Journal of Obstetric and Gynecologic Nursing,* 1979, 8:287–290.

Hill, S.D. and Smith, J.M. Neonatal responsiveness as a function of maternal contact and obstetrical drugs. *Perceptual and Motor Skills,* 1984, 58:859–866.

Hinde, R.A. *Biological Bases of Human Social Behavior.* NY: McGraw-Hill, 1974.

Hogarth, P.J. *Biology of Reproduction.* NY: John Wiley and Sons, 1978.

Holmberg, A.R. *Nomads of the Long Bow: The Siriono of Eastern Bolivia.* Smithsonian Institute: Institute of Social Anthropology Publication #10, (HRAF), 1950.

Hopf, S. Notes on pregnancy, delivery and infant survival in captive squirrel monkeys. *Primates,* 1967, 8:323-332.

Howell, N. The population of the Dobe area !Kung. In R. Lee and I. DeVore (Eds.), *Kalahari Hunter-Gatherers.* Cambridge, MA: Harvard University Press, 1976.

Howell, N. *Demography of the Dobe !Kung.* NY: Academic Press, 1979.

Howell, L.H., Heidrich, A.G., and Apployniaire, S. Labour and parturition in feral olive baboons *Papio anubis.* In D.J. Chivers and J. Herbert (Eds.), *Recent Advances in Primatology. Vol. 1: Behaviour.* NY: Academic Press, 1978.

Hrdy, S.B. *The Langurs of Abu.* Cambridge, MA: Harvard University Press, 1977.

Hrdy, S.B. and Williams, G.C. Behavioral biology and the double standard. In S.K. Wasser (Ed.), *Social Behavior of Female Vertebrates.* NY: Academic Press, 1983.

Huheey, J.E. Concerning the origin of handedness in humans. *Behavior Genetics,* 1977, 7:29–32.

Jacklin, C., and Maccoby, E. Length of labor and sex of offspring. *Journal of Pediatric Psychology,* 1982, 7:355–360.

Jacklin, C., Snow, M., and Maccoby, E. Tactile sensitivity and muscle strength in newborn boys and girls. *Infant Behavioral Development,* 1982, 4:261–268.

Janszen, K. Meat of life. *Science Digest,* 1980, November/December.

Jensen, E. Iban birth. *Folk,* 1967, 8–9:165–178.

Johnson, D.B. Breastfeeding at one hour of age. *American Journal of Maternal and Child Nursing,* 1976, 1:12–14.

Jolly, A. Hour of birth in primates and man. *Folia Primatologica,* 1972, 18:108–121.

Jolly, A. Primate birth hour. *International Zoo Yearbook,* 1973, 13:391–397.

Jolly, A. *Evolution of Primate Behavior.* NY: MacMillan, 1985.

Jordan, B. *Birth in Four Cultures.* Montreal: Eden Press Women's Publications, 1978.

Jordan, B. Biology and culture: Some thoughts on universals in childbirth. Paper presented at the 84th Annual Meeting of the American Anthropology Association, Washington, D.C., 1985.

Kadam, K.M. and Swayamprabha, M.S. Parturition in the slender loris (*Loris tardigradus lydekkerianus*). *Primates,* 1980, 21:567–571.

Kaiser I.H., and Halberg, F. Circadian periodic aspects of birth. *Annals of the New York Academy of Sciences,* 1962, 98:1056–1067.

Kay, M.A. *Anthropology of Human Birth.* Philadelphia, PA: F.A. Davis, 1982.

Kaye, K. Toward the origin of dialogue. In H.R. Schaffer (Ed.), *Studies in Mother–Infant Interaction.* London: Academic Press, 1977.

Kemps, A. and Timmermans, P. Parturition behavior in pluriparous Java macaques (*Macaca fascicularis*). *Primates,* 1982, 23:75–88.

Kennell, J.H., Jerauld, R., Wolfe, H., Chesler, D., Kreger, N.C., McAlpine, W., Steffa, M., and Klaus, M.H. Maternal behavior one year after early and extended post-partum contact. *Developmental Medicine and Child Neurology,* 1974, 16:172–179.

Kimball, C.D. Do endorphin residues of beta lipotropin in hormone reinforce reproductive functions? *American Journal of Obstetrics and Gynecology,* 1979, 134:127–132.

Kimble, G.A. and Garmezy, N. *Principles of General Psychology,* 3rd Edition. NY: Ronald Press, 1968.

King, J.A. Maternal behavior in *Peromyscus.* In H. Rheingold (Ed.), *Maternal Behavior in Mammals.* NY: John Wiley and Sons, 1963.

Klaus, M.H. and Kennell, J.H. Parent-to-infant attachment. In V.C. Vaughan, III, and T.B. Brazelton (Eds.), *The Family—Can it be Saved?* Chicago, IL: Yearbook Medical Publishers, 1975.

Klaus, M.H. and Kennell, J.H. *Mother-Infant Bonding.* St. Louis, MO: Mosby, 1976.

Klaus, M.H. and Kennell, J.H. *Parent-Infant Bonding.* St. Louis, MO: Mosby, 1982.

Klaus, M.H., Kennell, J.H., Plumb, N., and Zuehlke, S. Human maternal behavior at the first contact with her young. *Pediatrics,* 1970, 46:187–192.

Klaus, M.H., Jerauld, R., Kreger, N.C., McAlpine, W., Steffa, M., and Kennell, J.H. Maternal attachment: Importance of the first post-partum days. *New England Journal of Medicine,* 1972, 286:460–463.

Klaus, M.H., Trause, M.A., and Kennell, J.H. Does human maternal behavior after birth show a characteristic pattern? *Parent-Infant Interaction.* Ciba Foundation Symposium 33. Amsterdam: Elsevier, 1975.

Klein, M. and Stern, L. Low birth weight and the battered child syndrome. *Journal of Diseases of Childhood,* 1971, 122:15–18.

Klopfer, P.H. Mother love: What turns it on? *American Scientist,* 1971, 59:404–407.

Konner, M.J. Aspects of the developmental ethology of a foraging people. In N. Blurton Jones (Ed.), *Ethological Studies of Child Behavior.* Cambridge: Cambridge University Press, 1972.

Konner, M.J. Newborn walking: additional data. *Science,* 1973, 179:307.

Konner, M.J. Maternal care, infant development, and behavior among the !Kung. In R. Lee and I. DeVore (Eds.), *Kalahari Hunter-Gatherers.* Cambridge, MA: Harvard University Press, 1976.

Konner, M.J. Biological bases of social development. In M.W. Kent and J.E. Rolf (Eds.), *Social Competence in Children.* Hanover, NH: Univ. Vermont Press, 1979.

Konner, M. and Worthman, C. Nursing frequency, gonadal function, and birth spacing among !Kung hunter-gatherers. *Science,* 1980, 207:788–791.

Kontos, D. A Study of the effects of extended mother-infant contact on maternal behavior at one and three months. *Birth and the Family Journal,* 1978, 5:133–140.

Korner, A.F. Neonatal startles, smiles, erections and reflex sucks as related to state, sex and individuality. *Child Development,* 1969, 40:1039–1053.

Korner, A.F. Sex differences in newborns with special reference to differences in the organization of oral behavior. *Journal of Child Psychology and Psychiatry,* 1973, 14:19–29.

Korner, A.F. The effect of the infant's state, level of arousal, sex, and ontogenetic stage on the caregiver. In M. Lewis and L.A. Rosenblum (Eds.), *The Effect of the Infant on its Caregiver.* NY: John Wiley and Sons, 1974.

Kroeber, A.L. *Handbook of the Indians of California.* Berkeley: California Book Company (HRAF), 1953.

Kron, R.E., Stein, K.E., and Goddard, K.E. Newborn suckling behavior affected by obstetric sedation. *Pediatrics,* 1966, 37:1012.

Kuhn, C.M., Butler, S.R., and Schanberg, S.M. Selective depression of serum growth hormone during maternal deprivation in rat pups. *Science,* 1978, 201:1034–1036.

Kummer, H. *Social Organization of Hamadryas Baboons.* Basel: Karger, 1968.

Kummer, H. *Primate Societies: Group Techniques of Ecological Adaptation.* Chicago, IL: Aldine Atherton, 1971.

Laitman, J.T. The anatomy of human speech. *Natural History,* 1984, 93:20–27.

Lamb, M.E. Early contact and maternal bonding: One decade later. *Pediatrics, 1982,* 70:763–768.

Lamb, M.E. Early mother-neonate contact and the mother-child relationship. *Journal of Child Psychology and Psychiatry,* 1983, 24:487–494.

Lancaster, J.B. *Primate Behavior and the Emergence of Human Culture.* NY: Holt, Rinehart and Winston, 1975.

Lancaster, J.B. and Lancaster, C.S. Parental investment: The hominid adaptation. In D.J. Ortner (Ed.), *How Humans Adapt: A Biocultural Odyssey.* Washington, D.C.: Smithsonian Institution Press, 1983.

Lang, R. *Birth Book.* Palo Alto, CA: Genesis Press, 1972.

LeBoeuf, B.J., Whiting, R.J. and Gantt, R.E. Perinatal behavior of northern elephant seal females and their young. *Behavior,* 1972, 43:121–156.

Le Gros Clark, W.E. *The Antecedents of Man.* Edinburgh: Edinburgh University Press, 1959.

Lee, R.B. and DeVore, I. *Man the Hunter.* Chicago, IL: Aldine, 1968.

Leiderman, P.H., Leifer, A.D., Seashore, M.J., Barnett, C.R., and Grobstein, R. Mother–infant interaction: Effects of early deprivation, prior experience, and sex of infant. *Early Development,* 1973, 51:154–175.

Leutenegger, W. Newborn and pelvic dimensions in *Australopithecus. Nature (London),* 1972, 240:548–569.

Leutenegger, W. Gestation period and birth weight of *Australopithecus. Nature (London),* 1973, 243:548.

Leutenegger, W. Functional aspects of pelvis morphology of simian primates. *Journal of Human Evolution,* 1974, 3:207–222.

Leutenegger, W. Encephalization and obstetrics in primates with particular reference to human evolution. In E. Armstrong and D. Falk (Eds.), *Primate Brain Evolution: Methods and Concepts.* NY: Plenum, 1981.

LeVine, R.A. Child rearing as cultural adaptation. In P.H. Leiderman, S.R. Tulkin, and A. Rosenfeld (Eds.), *Culture and Infancy.* NY: Academic Press, 1977.

Lewin, R. How did humans evolve big brains? *Science,* 1982, 216:840–841.

Lewin, R. Were Lucy's feet made for walking? *Science,* 1983, 220:700–702.

Lewis, M. State as an infant-environment interaction: An analysis of mother–infant behavior as a function of sex. *Merrill-Palmer Quarterly,* 1972, 18:95–121.

Lind, J., Vuorenkoski, V., and Wasz-Hacker, O. 1973. Cited in Klaus, M.H. and J.H. Kennell. *Parent-Infant Bonding.* St. Louis, MO: C.V. Mosby, 1982.

Lindburg, D.G. and Hazell, L.D. Licking of the neonate and duration of labor in great apes and man. *American Anthropologist,* 1972, 74:318–325.

Love, J.A. A note on the birth of a baboon (*Papio anubis*). *Folia Primatologica,* 1978, 29:303–306.

Lovejoy, C.O. Biomechanical perspectives on the lower limb of early hominids. In R.H. Tuttle (Ed.), *Primate Morphology and Evolution.* The Hague: Mouton, 1975.

Lovejoy, C.O. The origin of man. *Science,* 1981, 211:341–350.

Lozoff, B. Birth and bonding in non-industrial societies. *Developmental Medicine and Child Neurology,* 1983, 25:595–600.

Lozoff, B., Brittenham, G.M. Trause, M.A., Kennell, J.H., and Klaus, M.H. Mother-newborn relationship—limits of adaptability. *Journal of Pediatrics,,* 1977, 1:1–13.

Lozoff, B., Wolf, A.W., and Davis, N.S. Cosleeping in urban families with young children in the United States. *Pediatrics,* 1984, 74:171–182.

Luckett, P.W. Reproductive development and evolution of the placenta in primates. *Contributions to Primatology,* 1974, 3:142–234.

Luckett, W.P. Ontogeny of the fetal membranes and placenta. In W.P. Luckett and F.S. Szalay (Eds.), *Phylogeny of the Primates.* NY: Plenum Press, 1975.

Lynch, G., Hechtel, S., and Jacoles, D. Neonate size and evolution of brain size in the anthropoid primates. *Journal of Human Evolution,* 1983, 12:519–522.

McBride, A.F. and Kritzler, H. Observations on pregnancy, parturition, and post-natal behavior in the bottle-nose dolphin. *Journal of Mammology,* 1951, 32:251–266.

McBryde, A. Compulsory rooming-in in the ward and private newborn service at Duke Hospital. *Journal of the American Medical Association,* 1951, 145:625–627.

McDonald, D.L. Paternal behavior at first contact with the newborn in a birth environment without intrusions. *Birth and the Family Journal,* 1978, 5:123–132.

McDonald, J.N. *North American Bison.* Berkeley, CA: Univ. California Press, 1981.

MacFarlane, J.A. *The Psychology of Childbirth.* Cambridge, MA: Harvard University Press, 1977.

McGraw, M.B. *The Neuromuscular Maturation of the Human Infant.* NY: Columbia University Press, 1943.

McKenna, J. Perinatal behavior and parturition of a Colobinae, *Presbytis entellus entellus* (hanuman langur). *Laboratory Primate Newsletter,* 1974, 13(3): 13–15.

Mackey, W.C. The adult male-child bond: An example of convergent evolution. *Journal of Anthropological Research,* 1976, 32:58–73.

Mackey, W.C. The placenta: The celibate sibling. *Journal of Human Evolution,* 1984, 13:449–455.

Manion, J. A study of fathers and infant caretaking. *Birth and the Family Journal,* 1977, 4:174–179.

Marieskind, H.I. *An Evaluation of Caesarean Section in the United States.* Washington, D.C.: Department of Health, Education, and Welfare, 1979.

Martin, R.D. The evolution of reproductive mechanisms in primates. *Journal of Reproduction and Fertility Supplement,* 1969, 6:49–66.

Matsunaga, E. Selection in ABO polymorphism in Japanese populations. *American Journal of Human Genetics,* 1959, 11:405–413.

Maynard Smith, J. The origin and maintenance of sex. In G.C. Williams (Ed.), *Group Selection.* Chicago, IL: Aldine, 1971.

Maynard Smith, J. *On Evolution.* Edinburgh: Edinburgh University Press, 1972.

Mayr, E. Biological classification: Toward a synthesis of opposing methodologies. *Science,* 1981, 214:510–516.

Mead, M. *Growing Up in New Guinea.* NY: William Morrow, 1930.

Mead, M. *New Lives for Old.* NY: William Morrow, 1956.

Mehl, L.E. Statistical outcomes of home births in the United States; Current status. In D. Stewart and L. Stewart (Eds.), *Safe Alternatives in Childbirth.* Chapel Hill, NC: NAPSAC, Inc.

Meier, G.W. Behavior of infant monkeys: differences attributable to mode of birth. *Science,* 1964, 143:968–970.

Miller J.A. Brain already busy while in the womb. *Science News,* 1984, 126:247.

Miranda, S.B. Visual abilities and pattern preferences of premature and full-term neonates. *Journal of Experimental Child Psychology,* 1970, 10:189–205.

Mitchell, G. *Behavioral Sex Differences in Nonhuman Primates.* NY: Van Nostrand Reinhold, 1979.

Mitchell, G. and Brandt, E.M. Behavior of the female rhesus monkey during birth. In G.H. Bourne (Ed.), *The Rhesus Monkey,* Vol. 2. NY: Academic Press, 1975.

Moller, M.S.G. Custom, pregnancy, and child rearing in Tanganyika. *Journal of Tropical Pediatrics,* 1961, 7:66–80.

Moltz, H. and Leon, M. Birth processes and maternal behavior in some familiar laboratory mammals. In J.G. Howells (Ed.), *Modern Perspectives in Psycho-Obstetrics.* NY: Brunner/Mazel, 1972.

Mongeau, G., Smith, H., and Maney, A. The "granny" midwife: Changing role and functions of a folk practitioner. *American Journal of Sociology,* 1960, 66:497–505.

Montagu, A. Neonatal and infant immaturity in man. *Journal of the American Medical Association,* 1961, 178:56–57.

Montagu, A. *Life Before Birth.* NY: The New American Library, 1964.

Montagu, A. *Touching: The Human Significance of the Skin.* NY: Columbia University Press, 1971.

Moss, H.A. Sex, age and state as determinants of mother-infant interaction. *Merrill-Palmer Quarterly,* 1967, 13:19–36.

Moss, I.R., Conner, H., Yee, W.F.H., and Scarpelli, E.M. Human beta-endorphin-like immunoreactivity in the perinatal–neonatal period. *Journal of Pediatrics,* 1982, 101:443–446.

Myles, M. *Textbook for Midwives,* 8th Edition. Edinburgh: Churchill Livingston, 1975.

Nadler, R.D. Periparturitional behavior of a primiparous lowland gorilla. *Primates,* 1974, 15:55–73.

Nash, L.T. Parturition in a feral baboon (*Papio anubis*). *Primates,* 1974, 15:279–285.

Newman, L.F. *Childbirth and Infancy.* Sociological Symposium Number, 1972, 8:51–63.

Newman, L.F. The culture of birth. Paper presented at the 74th Annual meeting of the American Anthropological Association, San Francisco, 1975.

Newton, N. *Maternal Emotions*. NY: P.B. Hoeber, Inc., 1955.

Newton, N. Psychologic differences between breast and bottle feeding. *American Journal of Clinical Nutrition*, 1971, 24:993–1004.

Newton, N. and Modahl, C. Pregnancy: The closest human relationship. *Human Nature*, 1978, 1:40–49.

Newton, N. and Newton, M. Mother's reactions to their newborn babies. *Journal of the American Medical Association*, 1962, 181:206–211.

Nicholson, B. Does kissing aid human bonding by semiochemical addiction? *British Journal of Dermatology*, 1984, 3:623–627.

Nisbett, R. and Gurwitz, S. Weight, sex, and the eating behavior of human newborns. *Journal of Comparative Physiology and Psychology*, 1970, 73:245–253.

Nissen, L.T. and Yerkes, R.M. Reproduction in the chimpanzee: Report on forty-nine births. *Anatomical Record*, 1943, 86:567–578.

Odent, M. *Birth Reborn*. NY: Pantheon Books, 1984.

Oppenheimer, J.R. *Presbytis entellus:* Birth in free-ranging primate troop. *Primates*, 1976, 17:541–542.

Osgood, K., Hochstrasser, and Deuschle, K. Lay midwifery in southern Appalachia. *Archives of Environmental Health*, 1966, 12:759–770.

Oster, H. Facial expressions and affect development. In M. Lewis and L.A. Rosenblum (Eds.), *The Development of Affect*. NY: Plenum, 1978.

Oxorn, H. and Foote, W.R. *Human Labor and Birth*, 3rd Edition. NY: Appleton-Century-Crofts, 1975.

Paige, K.E. and Paige, J.M. *The Politics of Reproductive Ritual*. Berkeley, CA: University of California Press, 1981.

Papousek, H. and Papousek, M. Integration into the social world: Survey of research. In P. Stratton (Ed.), *Psychobiology of the Human Newborn*. NY: John Wiley and Sons, 1982.

Parker, S.T. Piaget's sensorimotor series in an infant macaque: A model for comparing unstereotyped behavior and intelligence in human and nonhuman primates. In S. Chevalier-Skolnikoff and F.E. Poirier (Eds.), *Primate Bio-social Development*. NY: Garland, 1977.

Passingham, R.E. Changes in the size and organization of the brain in man and his ancestors. *Brain, Behavior and Evolution*, 1975, 11:73–90.

Pedersen, C.A. and Prange, A.J., Jr. Induction of maternal behavior in virgin rats after intracerebroventricular administration of oxytocin. *Proceedings of the National Academy of Sciences*, 1979, 76:6661–6665.

Pedersen, C.A., Ascher, J.A., Monroe, Y.L., and Prange, A.J. Oxytocin induces maternal behavior in virgin female rats. *Science*, 1982, 216:648–649.

Peterson, G.H. and Mehl, L.E. Some determinants of maternal attachment. *American Journal of Psychiatry*, 1978, 135:1168–1173.

Phillips, C.R.N. Neonatal heat loss in heated cribs vs mothers' arms. *Child and Family*, 1974, 13:307–314.

Pianka, E.R. On r- and K- selection. *American Naturalist*, 1970, 104:592–597.

Poindron, P., Martin, G.B., and Hooley, R.D. Effects of lambing induction on the sensitive period for the establishment of maternal behavior in sheep. *Physiology and Behavior*, 1979, 23:1081–1087.

Pond, C.M. The significance of lactation in the evolution of mammals. *Evolution*, 1977, 31:177–199.

Porter, R.H., Cernock, J.M., and McLaughlin, F.J. Maternal recognition of neonates through olfactory cues. *Physiology and Behavior*, 1983, 30:151–154.

Prechtl, H.F.R. and O'Brien, J. Behavioral states of the full-term newborn: The emergence of a concept. In P. Stratton (Ed.), *Psychobiology of the Human Newborn.* NY: John Wiley and Sons, 1982.

Prechtl, H.F.R., Theorell, K., and Blair, A.N. Behavioral state cycles in abnormal infants. *Developmental Medicine and Child Neurology,* 1973, 15:606–615.

Raphael, D. *The Tender Gift: Breastfeeding.* NY: Schockin Books, 1973.

Raum, O.F. *Chagga Childhood: A Description of Indigenous Education in an East African Tribe.* London: Oxford University Press (HRAF), 1940.

Rawlins, R.G. Parturient and postpartum behavior of a free-ranging monkey (*Macaca mulatta*). *Journal of Mammalogy,* 1979, 60:432–433.

Rheingold, H. Maternal behavior in the dog. In H. Rheingold (Ed.), *Maternal Behavior in Mammals.* NY: John Wiley and Sons, 1963.

Richard, A.F. Preliminary observations on the birth and development of *Propithecus verreauxi* to the age of six months. *Primates,* 1976, 17:357–366.

Richards, M.P.M. Some effects of experience on maternal behavior in rodents. In B.M. Foss (Ed.), *Determinants of Infant Behavior,* Vol. IV. London: Methuen and Co. Ltd., 1969.

Ringler, N.M., Kennell, J.H., Jarvella, R., Navojosky, B.J., and Klaus, M.H. Mother-to-child speech at 2 years—effect of early postnatal contact. *Journal of Pediatrics,* 1975, 86:141–144.

Ringler, N.M., Trause, M.A., and Klaus, M.H. Mother's speech to her two-year old, its effect on speech and language comprehension at five years. *Pediatric Research,* 1976, 10:307.

Rivinus, H.A. and Katz, S.H. Evolution, newborn behavior and maternal attachment. *Comments on Contemporary Psychiatry,* 1971, 1(3):95–104.

Robinson, J.T. *Early Hominid Posture and Locomotion.* Chicago, IL: University of Chicago Press, 1972.

Robson, K.S. The role of eye-to-eye contact in maternal-infant attachment. *Journal of Child Psychology and Psychiatry,* 1967, 8:13–25.

Rosenberg, K.R. *The Functional Significance of Neanderthal Pubic Morphology.* Ann Arbor, MI: University Microfilms, 1986.

Rosenblatt, J.S. Prepartum and postpartum regulation of maternal behavior in the rat. *Parent-Infant Interaction.* Ciba Foundation Symposium 33. Amsterdam: Elsevier Publishing Company, 1975.

Rosenblatt, J.S. and Lehrman, D.S. Maternal behavior of the laboratory rat. In H.L. Rheingold (Ed.), *Maternal Behavior in Mammals.* NY: John Wiley and Sons, 1963.

Rosenblatt, J.S. and Siegel, H.I. Hysterectomy-induced maternal behavior during pregnancy in the rat. *Journal of Comparative Physiology and Psychology,* 1981, 89:685–700.

Rosenblum, L.A. Sex and age differences in response to infant squirrel monkeys. *Brain, Behavior, and Evolution,* 1972, 5:30–40.

Rossi, A.S. A biosocial perspective on parenting. *Daedelus,* 1977, 106:1–31.

Rothe, H. Further observations on the delivery behavior of the common marmoset (*Callithrix jacchus*). *Zeitschrift Fuer Saeugetierkund,* 1974, 39:135–142.

Rovee-Collier, C.K. and Lipsitt, L.P. Learning, adaptation, and memory in the newborn. In P. Stratton (Ed.), *Psychobiology of the Human Newborn.* NY: John Wiley and Sons, 1982.

Rubin, R. Maternal Touch. *Nursing Outlook,* 1963, 11:328–331.

Russell, C. and Russell, W.M.S. Language and animal signals. In W.L. Anderson and N.C. Stageberg (Eds.), *Introductory Readings on Language.* NY: Holt, Rinehart and Winston, 1975.

Sacher, G.A. and Staffeldt, E.F. Relation of gestation time to brain weight for placental mammals: Implications for the theory of vertebrate growth. *American Naturalist*, 1974, 108(963):593–615.

Sadow, J.I.D. *Human Reproduction: An Integrated View*. Chicago, IL: Yearbook Medical Publishers, 1980.

Saigal, S., Nelson, N.M., Bennett, K.J., and Enkin, M.W. Observations on the behavioral state of newborn infants during the first hour of life. *American Journal of Obstetrics and Gynecology*, 1981, 139:715–719.

Salariya, E.M., Easton, P.M., and Cater, J.E. Duration of breastfeeding after early initiation and frequent feeding. *Lancet*, 1978, p. 1141.

Sale, J.B. Observations on parturition and related phenomena in the hyrax. *Acta Tropica*, 1965, 22:37–54.

Salk, L. The effects of the normal heartbeat sound on the behavior of the newborn infant: Implications for mental health. *World Mental Health*, 1960, 12:168–175.

Salk, L. The critical nature of the postpartum period in the human for the establishment of the mother–infant bond: A controlled study. *Diseases of the Nervous System*, 1970, 31:110–116.

Sameroff, A.J. and Chandler, M.J. Reproductive risk and the continuum of caretaking casuality. In F.D. Horowitz (Ed.), *Review of Child Development*, Vol. 4. Chicago, IL: University of Chicago Press, 1975.

Schaller, G.B. *The Serengeti Lion: A Study of Predator-Prey Relations*. Chicago: University of Chicago Press, 1972.

Schneirla, T.C., Rosenblatt, J.S., and Tobach, E. Maternal behavior in the cat. In H. Rheingold (Ed.), *Maternal Behavior in Mammals*. NY: John Wiley and Sons., 1963.

Schreiber, J.M. On becoming human. *Reviews in Anthropology*, 1977, 4:378–385.

Schreiber, J.M. and Philpott, L. Who is a legitimate health care professional? Changes in the practice of midwifery in the lower Rio Grande Valley. In B. Velimirovic (Ed.), *Modern Medicine and Medical Anthropology in the United States-Mexico Border Population*. El Paso: Panamerican Health Organization, 1978.

Schultz, A.H. Sex differences in the pelves of primates. *American Journal of Physical Anthropology*, 1949, 7:401–424.

Sekulic, R. Birth in free-ranging howler monkeys *Alouatta seniculus*. *Primates*, 1982, 23:580–582.

Short, R.V. The evolution of human reproduction. *Proceedings of the Royal Society of London*, 1976, B 195:3–24.

Shostak, M. *Nisa: The Life and Words of a !Kung Woman*. Cambridge, MA: Harvard University Press, 1981.

Siegel, E. Early and extended maternal-infant contact. *American Journal of Diseases of Childhood*, 1982, 136:251–257.

Sinclair, J.C. Metabolic rate in temperature control. In C.A. Smith and and N.M. Nelson (Eds.), *The Physiology of the Newborn Infant*, 4th Edition. Springfield: Charles C. Thomas, 1978.

Slater, A. and Findlay, J. Binocular fixation in the newborn baby. *Journal of Experimental Child Psychology*, 1975, 20:248–273.

Sousa, P.L., Barros, F.C., Gazalle, R.V., Begeres, R.M., Pinheiro, G.N., Menezes, S.T., and Arruda, L.A. Cited in M.H. Klaus and J.H. Kennell, *Maternal Infant Bonding*. St. Louis, MO: C.V. Mosby, 1976.

Stave, U. *Physiology of the Perinatal Period*. NY: Appleton-Century-Crofts, 1970.

Stern, J.T., Jr. and Susman, R.L. The locomotor anatomy of *Australopithecus afarensis*. *American Journal of Physical Anthropology*, 1983, 60:279–317.

Stevenson, M.F. Birth and perinatal behaviour in family groups of the common marmoset (*Callithrix jacchus jacchus*), compared to other primates. *International Zoo Yearbook*, 1976, 16:110–116.

Stewart, K.J. The birth of a wild mountain gorilla (*Gorilla gorilla beringei*). *Primates,* 1977, 18:965–976.

Stewart, K.J. Parturition in wild gorillas: Behavior of mothers, neonates, and others. *Folia Primatologica,* 1984, 42:62–69.

Stratton, P. Significance of the psychobiology of the human newborn. In P. Stratton (Ed.), *Psychobiology of the Human Newborn.* NY: John Wiley and Sons, 1982. (a)

Stratton, P. Emerging themes of neonatal psychobiology. In P. Stratton, *Psychobiology of the Human Newborn.* NY: John Wiley and Sons, 1982. (b)

Stratton, P. Biological preprogramming of infant behavior. *Journal of Child Psychology and Psychiatry,* 1983, 24:301–309.

Sugiyama, Y. An artificial social change in a hanuman langur troop. *Primates,* 1966, 7:41–72.

Svejda, M.J., Campos, J.J., and Emde, R.N. Mother-infant "bonding": failure to generalize. *Child Development,* 1980, 51:775–779.

Tague, R.G. and Lovejoy, C.O. The Australopithecine obstetric pelvis. Paper presented at the 84th Annual Meeting of the American Anthropological Association, Washington, D.C., 1985.

Takeshita, H. On the delivery behavior of squirrel monkeys (*Saimiri sciurea*) and a mona monkey (*Ceropithecus mona*). *Primates,* 1961–1962, 3(1):59–72.

Tamminen, T., Verronen, P., Saarikoski, S., Goransson, A., and Toumiranta, H. The influence of perinatal factors on breastfeeding. *Acta Paediatrica Scandinavia,* 1983, 72:9–12.

Tanner, J. Variability of growth and maturity in newborn infants. In M. Lewis and L. Rosenblum (Eds.), *The Effect of the Infant on Its Caregiver.* NY: John Wiley and Sons, 1974.

Tanner, N. and Zihlman, A. Women in evolution. Part I: Innovation and selection in human origins. *Signs,* 1976, 1:585–608.

Theorell, K., Prechtl, H.F.R., Blair, A.W., and Lind, J. Behavioral state cycles of normal newborn infants: A comparison of the effect of early and late cord clamping. *Developmental Medicine and Child Neurology,* 1973, 15:597–605.

Thevenin, T. *The Family Bed.* Minneapolis, MN: Thevenin, 1976.

Thoman, E.B., Leiderman, P.H. and Olson, J.P. Neonate–mother interaction during breastfeeding. *Developmental Psychology,* 1972, 6:110–118.

Thoman, E.B., Turner, A.M., Barnett, C.R., and Leiderman, P.H. Neonate–mother interaction: Effects of parity on feeding behavior. *Child Development,* 1971, 42:1471–1483.

Thomas, E.M. *The Harmless People.* NY: Alfred A. Knopf, Inc., 1958.

Thomson, M.E., Hartsoch, T.G., and Larson, C. The importance of immediate postnatal contact: Its effect on breastfeeding. *Canada Family Physican,* 1979, 25:1374–1378.

Thomson, M.E. and Kramer, M.S. Methodologic standards for controlled clinical trials of early contact and maternal-infant behavior. *Pediatrics,* 1984, 73:294–300.

Tindale, N. *Aboriginal Tribes of Australia.* Berkeley, CA: University of California Press, 1974.

Tinklepaugh, O.L. and Hartman, C.G. Behavioral aspects of parturition in the monkey (*Macacas rhesus*). *Comparative Psychology,* 1930, 11:63–98.

Titiev, M. *Araucanian Culture in Transition.* Ann Arbor, MI: University of Michigan Press (HRAF), 1951.

Tonkinson, R. *The Mardujara Aborigines.* NY: Holt, Rinehart, and Winston, 1978.

Townsend, T.W. and Bailey, E.D. Parturitional, early maternal, and neonatal behavior in penned white-tailed deer. *Journal of Mammalogy,* 1975, 56:347–362.

Trevarthen, C. Facial expressions of emotion in mother–infant interaction. *Human Neurobiology,* 1985, 4:21–32.

Trevathan, W.R. *Observations of Mother-Infant Interaction in the First Hour after Birth.* Ann Arbor, MI: University Microfilms, 1980.

Trevathan, W.R. Maternal touch at first contact with the newborn infant. *Developmental Psychobiology,* 1981, 14:549–558.

Trevathan, W.R. Maternal lateral preference at first contact with her newborn infant. *Birth,* 1982, 9:85–90.

Trevathan, W.R. Maternal *en face* orientation during the first hour after birth. *American Journal of Orthopsychiatry,* 1983, 53:92–99.

Trevathan, W.R. Factors influencing the timing of initial breastfeeding. *Medical Anthropology,* 1984, 8:302–307.

Trevathan, W.R. and Udick, L.L. A biocultural approach to human birth practices. Paper presented at the 80th Annual Meeting of the American Anthropology Association, Los Angeles, 1981.

Trezenem, F. *Notes Ethnographiques sur les Tribus Fan du Moven Ogooue (Gabon).* *Societe des Africanistes Journal,* 1936, 6:65–93 (HRAF).

Trinkaus, E. Neandertal pubic morphology and gestation length. *Current Anthropology,* 1984, 25:509–513.

Trivers, R.L. Parent-offspring conflict. *American Zoologist,* 1974, 14:249–264.

Turkewitz, B., Moreau, T., and Birch, H.G. Relation between birth condition and neuro-behavioral organization in the neonate. *Pediatric Research,* 1968, 2:243–249.

Uchendu, V.C. *The Igbo of Southeast Nigeria.* NY: Holt, Rinehart, and Winston, 1965.

Udick, L.L. and McCallum, W.T. A biocultural approach to birth practices. Paper presented at the Western Social Science Association, Denver, 1978.

Van der Erden, M.L. *Maternity Care in a Spanish-American Community of New Mexico.* Berkeley, CA: University of California Press, 1959.

Van Tienhoven, A. *Reproductive Physiology of Vertebrates.* Ithaca, NY: Cornell University Press, 1983.

Vogt, J.L., Carlson, H., and Menzel, E. Social behavior of a marmoset (*Saguinus fuscicollis*). Group I: Parental care and infant development. *Primates,* 1978, 19:715–726.

Vorys, L. The age-old discrimination against midwives. *Mothering,* 1977, 5:50–56.

Walser, E.S. Some aspects of maternal behavior in mammals. *Medical Biology,* 1978, 56:262–271.

Waterhouse, J.A.H. and Hogben, L. Incompatibility of mother and foetus with respect to the isoagglutinogen A and its antibody. *British Journal of Social Medicine,* 1947, 1:1–17.

Waters, E. and Deane, D. Infant–mother attachment: Theories, models, recent data, some tasks for comparative developmental analysis. In L. W. Hoffman, R. Gandelman, and H.R. Schiffman (Eds.), *Parenting: Its Causes and Consequences.* Hillsdale, NJ: Lawrence Erlbaum, 1982.

Weaver, K.F. The search for our ancestors. *National Geographic,* 1985, 168:560–623.

Weiland, I. and Serber, Z. Patterns of mother-infant contact: The significance of lateral preference. *Journal of Genetic Psychology,* 1970, 117:157–165.

Wennberg, R.P., Woodrum, D.E., and Hodson, W.A. The perinate. In D.W. Smith and E.L. Bierman. *The Biologic Ages of Man.* Philadelphia, PA: W.B. Saunders, 1973.

Westbrook, M.T. The reactions to childbearing and early maternal experience of women with differing marital relationships. *British Journal of Medicine and Psychobiology,* 1978, 51:191–199.

Whittlestone, W.G. The physiology of early attachment in mammals: Implications for human obstetric care. *Medical Journal of Australia,* 1978, 1:50–53.

Williams, G.C. *Sex and Evolution.* Princeton, NJ: Princeton University Press, 1975.

Willoughby, D.P. *The Empire of Equus.* NY: A.S. Barnes, 1974.

Wilson, E.O. *Sociobiology: The New Synthesis.* Cambridge, MA: Harvard University Press, 1975.

Winberg, J. and De Chateau, P. Early social development: studies of infant–mother interaction and relationships. In W.W. Hartup (Ed.), *Review of Child Development Research,* Vol. 6. Chicago, IL: University of Chicago Press, 1982.

Wolff, P.H. Observations on newborn infants. *Psychosomatic Medicine,* 1959, 21:110–118.

Wolff, P. Sucking patterns of infant mammals. *Brain, Behavior and Evolution,* 1968, 1:354–367.

Wolpoff, M. *Paleoanthropology.* NY: Alfred A. Knopf, 1980.

Woodson, R.H. Newborn behavior and the transition to extrauterine life. *Infant Behavior and Development,* 1983, 6:139–144.

Wooldridge, F.L. *Colobus guerza:* Birth and infant development in captivity. *Animal Behavior,* 1971, 19:481–486.

Young, J.Z. *The Life of Mammals: Their Anatomy and Physiology.* Oxford: Clarendon Press, 1975.

Yu, V. Effect of body position on gastric emptying in the neonate. *Archives of Diseases of Childhood,* 1975, 50:500–504.

Zarrow, M.X., Gandelman, R., and Denenberg, V.H. Prolactin: Is it an essential hormone for maternal behavior in the mammal? *Hormones and Behavior,* 1971, 2:343–354.

Zelazo, P.R., Zelazo, N.A., and Kolb, S. "Walking" in the newborn. *Science,* 1972, 176:314–315.

INDEX

A

ABO blood group, 11–12, 121
AL–288, 26–27
Aborigine, Australian, 138, 232
Abortion, 11–12, 21, 108, 113
Adaptive radiation, 13
Adoption
  in humans, 109, 186, 203, 205
  in mammals, 195–198
Adrenal corticosteroids, 10
Ainsworth, M. D. S., 36, 39
Albumin, 14–15
Alor, 38
Altmann, J., 83
Altmann, S. A., 152
Altricial young, 16–17, 31–32, 145,
    166, 184, 203
  and bonding, 193–196
  secondarily, 218, 219, 221,
    223–224
Amniotic sac
  in mammals, 73–74, 149
  in primates, 77, 79, 85
  rupture of, 70
Anagenesis, 13–14
Anemia, 11
Anencephalic fetus, 67
Anesthesia, 23, 122, 192
Apgar score, 44, 54, 61, 138, 141,
    164, 168, 180–181
Araucanian, 37
Armadillo, 10–11

A

Asexual reproduction, 2, 33
Asphyxia, 93–94, 122, 229
Asynclitism, 27
Attachment
  behaviors, 53–56, 129–136, 151,
    166, 169, 177, 181, 185, 188
  father–infant, 114–115
  sensitive period for, 201, 203,
    207, 210–213, 230–231, 234,
    236
  theory, 35–36, 39, 191–194, 234,
    236
Australophithecines, 23, 25–29, 136,
    221–222, 227
Australopithecus afarensis, 26
Australopithecus africanus, 23
Aymara, 107

B

Baboon, 12
  anubis, 82–83, 92, 105
  chacma, 83, 89
  gelada, 83, 109, 112
  hamadryas, 83, 109–110, 112
  yellow, 83
Bahaya, 112
Bilirubin, 121, 180
Bipedalism, 136, 218, 219
  and parturition, 17–29, 89, 96,
    108, 144, 221–223, 225
Birds, 3, 67, 178, 199, 206
Birth attendant, 87–88, 103, 108,